The Subfertility Handbook

A Clinician's Guide

Second Edition

The Subfertility Handbook

A Clinician's Guide

Second Edition

Edited by

Gab Kovacs

International Medical Director, Monash IVF, and Professor of Obstetrics and Gynaecology, Monash University, Victoria, Australia

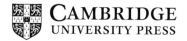

CAMBRIDGE
UNIVERSITY PRESS

CAMBRIDGE UNIVERSITY PRESS
Cambridge, New York, Melbourne, Madrid, Cape Town, Singapore,
São Paulo, Delhi, Dubai, Tokyo, Mexico City

Cambridge University Press
The Edinburgh Building, Cambridge CB2 8RU, UK

Published in the United States of America by Cambridge University Press, New York

www.cambridge.org
Information on this title: www.cambridge.org/9780521147842

First edition published by Cambridge University Press 1997
This edition published by Cambridge University Press 2011

Printed in the United Kingdom at the University Press, Cambridge

A catalogue record for this publication is available from the British Library

Library of Congress Cataloguing in Publication data
The subfertility handbook : a clinician's guide / edited by Gab Kovacs. – 2nd ed.
    p. ; cm.
Includes bibliographical references and index.
ISBN 978-0-521-14784-2 (pbk.)
1. Infertility – Handbooks, manuals, etc.   I. Kovacs, Gabor, MRCOG, FRACOG.
[DNLM: 1. Infertility – diagnosis.   2. Infertility – therapy.   WP 570]
RC889.S83   2011
618.1'78–dc22
                                                                    2010030609

ISBN 978-0-521-14784-2 Paperback

Contents

The color plates will be found between pages 182 and 183.

Foreword

This, the Second Edition of *The Subfertility Handbook – A Clinician's Guide* is published 14 years after the First Edition appeared in print in 1997. Its editor, Gab Kovacs, has assembled a team of expert contributors from Australia, Europe, North America, and Singapore.

A number of conditions impacting on the fertility of subfertile couples are reviewed, including age, lifestyle, immunization status, genetic counseling, history, and other medical conditions. A plan for the couple's first interview including history and physical examination as well as the required investigations, is proposed. In the female patient, investigations involve ovulation, endocrine factors, and tubal patency by conventional or by more modern techniques. Ultrasound can be used to detect abnormalities in the ovary, the uterus, the Fallopian tubes, and the peritoneum. A number of new techniques involving 2D or 3D images have recently been introduced.

In the male partner, a full history and physical examination will be complemented by laboratory tests on semen; furthermore, genetic factors, the post-coital test, sperm function tests, DNA fragmentation, and biopsy of the testis may also need investigation. The diagnostic range spans from normal status to azoospermia and many conditions in between. Therapeutic options for male-factor infertility may, or may not, involve ART (sometimes conventional IVF, but mostly ICSI with ejaculated or non-ejaculated sperm from either epididymis or testis). Since ICSI became available, the use of artificial insemination with donor sperm has substantially decreased and is now used mostly where ICSI has proved unsuccessful.

Several management options for anovulation with Polycystic Ovary Syndrome (PCOS) are reviewed in depth. A first-line treatment option involves Intrauterine Insemination (IUI) with partner semen and the factors influencing success of IUI are discussed. The chapter on conventional IVF discusses in detail: indications, controlled ovarian stimulation and the different clinical techniques used.

The handbook also discusses early pregnancy loss, diagnostic, and therapeutic options for endometriosis as well as the current place of reconstructive surgery in the female. An overview is also provided on the indications, procedures, and outcome of the use of *in vitro* matured oocytes, especially in PCOS.

The chapter on oocyte donation discusses the indications, the results, the screening of oocyte donors, the ethics of using donor oocytes, and the application in Turner patients. Practice and ethics of embryo donation are also discussed.

Without doubt, the inclusion of a detailed chapter on laboratory techniques earns its place in such a handbook. Clinicians should have some insight into what is going on in the laboratory. This description includes the laboratory set-up, the techniques used, the expertise required for IVF, ICSI, blastomere biopsy, *in vitro* culture to different stages of development, and the cryopreservation of oocytes and embryos.

The last chapter discusses vital aspects of subfertility management, i.e., the psychology of infertility, the psycho-social evaluations of different strategies, and the necessary counseling in general, but especially for third-party reproduction.

Each chapter is supported by an up-to-date list of references, and the comprehensive index covers all items used in the handbook.

The book will no doubt prove invaluable for clinicians dealing with couples facing subfertility as well as for Reproductive Endocrinology and Infertility Fellows and Residents, who will find a comprehensive overview for the clinical practices of a fertility clinic.

Professor-Emeritus André Van Steirteghem
Vrije Universiteit Brussels
Editor-in-Chief *Human Reproduction*

Contributors

G. David Adamson
Fertility Physicians of Northern California, San Jose, CA, USA

Majed Al Hudhud
Clinical Research Fellow, IVF, Hammersmith Hospital, London, UK

Baris Ata
Clinical and Research Fellow, Division of Reproductive Endocrinology and Infertility, Department of Obstetrics and Gynecology, McGill University, Montreal, Canada

Pedro N. Barri
Service of Reproductive Medicine, Department of Obstetrics, Gynecology and Reproduction, Institut Universitari Dexeus, Barcelona, Spain

Christopher L. R. Barratt
Assisted Conception Unit, NHS Tayside and Reproductive & Developmental Biology Group, Division of Maternal and Child Health Sciences, Ninewells Hospital, University of Dundee, Dundee, Scotland

Elisabet Clua
Service of Reproductive Medicine, Department of Obstetrics, Gynecology and Reproduction, Institut Universitari Dexeus, Barcelona, Spain

C. Dechanet
Médecine de la Reproduction, Département de Gynécologie-Obstétrique, Pôle Naissances et Pathologies de la Femme, Academic hospital A. de Villeneuve (CHU Montpellier), Faculté de Médecine, Université Montpellier, Montpellier, France

H. Déchaud
Médecine de la Reproduction, Département de Gynécologie-Obstétrique, Pôle Naissances et Pathologies de la Femme, Academic hospital A. de Villeneuve (CHU Montpellier), Faculté de Médecine, Université Montpellier, Montpellier, France

Didier Dewailly
Department of Endocrine Gynaecology and Reproductive Medicine, Hôpital Jeanne de Flandre, and Faculty of Medicine of Lille, Université de Lille II, France

Marion Dewailly
Department of Radiology, Hôpital Jeanne de Flandre, and Faculty of Medicine of Lille, Université de Lille II, France

David K. Gardner
Department of Zoology, The University of Melbourne, Victoria, Australia

Linda Hammer Burns
Associate Professor, University of Minnesota Medical School, Department of Obstetrics, Gynecology, and Women's Health, Reproductive Medicine Center Minneapolis, MN, USA

B. Hédon
Médecine de la Reproduction, Département de Gynécologie-Obstétrique, Pôle Naissances et Pathologies de la Femme, Academic hospital A. de Villeneuve (CHU Montpellier), Faculté de

Médecine, Université Montpellier,
Montpellier, France

Wayland Hsiao
Fellow in Reproductive Medicine,
Weill Cornell Medical College, Department
of Urology and Center for Reproductive
Medicine, New York, NY, USA

Vanessa J. Kay
Consultant in Obstetrics and Gynaecology,
Assisted Conception Unit, NHS Tayside
and Reproductive & Developmental
Biology Group, Ninewells Hospital and
Medical School, Dundee,
Scotland

Gab Kovacs
International Medical Director, Monash
IVF, and Professor of Obstetrics and
Gynaecology, Monash University, Victoria,
Australia

Robert I. McLachlan
Department of Obstetrics and Gynaecology,
Monash University, Prince Henrys Institute
of Medical Research, Andrology Australia,
and Monash IVF, Epworth Hospital,
Richmond, Australia

Vicki Nisenblat
PhD Candidate, the Robinson Institute,
Discipline of Obstetrics and Gynaecology,
School of Paediatrics and Reproductive
Health, The University of Adelaide,
Australia

Robert J. Norman
Director, the Robinson Institute, and
Professor, Discipline of Obstetrics and
Gynaecology, The University of Adelaide,
Australia

W. Ombelet
Genk Institute for Fertility Technology,
Department of Obstetrics and Gynaecology,
Genk, Belgium

Edouard Poncelet
Department of Radiology, Hôpital
Jeanne de Flandre, and Faculty of
Medicine of Lille, Université de Lille II,
France

Shauna Reinblatt
Clinical and Research Fellow, Division
of Reproductive Endocrinology and
Infertility, Department of Obstetrics and
Gynecology, McGill University, Montreal,
Canada

Anthony J. Rutherford
Consultant in Reproductive Medicine
and Surgery, Leeds Centre for
Reproductive Medicine, Seacroft Hospital,
Leeds, UK

Peter N. Schlegel
Urologist in Chief, James Buchanan Brady
Foundation, Weill Cornell Medical College,
Department of Urology and Center for
Reproductive Medicine, New York, NY,
USA

Wendy B. Shelly
Fertility Physicians of Northern California,
San Jose, CA, USA

F. Shenfield
Reproductive Medicine Unit, Elizabeth
Garrett Anderson Obstetric Hospital,
London, UK

Joe Leigh Simpson
Executive Associate Dean for Academic
Affairs, Professor of Human & Molecular
Genetics and Professor of Obstetrics and
Gynecology, Wertheim College of
Medicine, Florida International University,
Miami, Florida, USA

Anna Smirnova
Department of Obstetrics and Gynecology,
Russian Medical Academy of Postgraduate
Education, IVF & Genetics Centre
"FertiMed", Moscow, Russia

Seang Lin Tan
James Edmund Dodds Professor and Chairman, Department of Obstetrics and Gynecology, McGill University, Montreal, Canada

George A. Thouas
Department of Zoology, The University of Melbourne, Victoria, Australia

Geoffrey Trew
Consultant in Reproductive Medicine, Hammersmith Hospital, London, UK

P.C. Wong
Department of Obstetrics and Gynecology, National University of Singapore, Singapore

Cheng Toh Yeong
The Tow Yung Clinic, Singapore

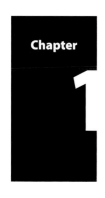

Chapter 1

Subfertility – a logical approach

Gab Kovacs

The introductory point I would like to make is that the term "infertility" is no longer applicable and we should be referring to "subfertility". The Oxford Dictionary defines "infertility" as "not capable of producing offspring; barren". With the advances in treatment over the last three decades, the development of IVF, the use of intracytoplasmic sperm injection (ICSI), application of testicular biopsy, oocyte donation, sperm donation and surrogacy, there is no couple who cannot potentially conceive, so the term "infertility" should no longer be used. Therefore, this book is called the "Subfertility Handbook".

The probability of conception depends on the success rate of the particular treatment, and the number of cycles of treatment that a couple undertake. This has been applied to the "life-table" analysis of repeated treatment cycles by donor insemination [1], ovulation induction [2], and IVF [3]. The "life-table" concept, which takes into consideration what may happen to couples who have not yet had all their treatment cycles, suggests that if a couple keep trying, they should eventually all conceive. The concept of "if at first you don't succeed, try, try, try again" was proven by a report of a woman who successfully conceived after 37 cycles of IVF treatment (fresh and frozen) [4].

The investigation and treatment of a couple who have failed to conceive is like putting a jig-saw together. There are the three main fertility parameters (eggs, sperm, and tubes) (Figure 1.1), and if these are found to be relatively normal and the couple still does not conceive, we have what is termed "unexplained or idiopathic subfertility". If a problem is identified, then that should be corrected. The first factor is "are sufficient number of normal sperm placed in the right place at the right time"? As described in detail in Chapter 3 this requires determining that the timing of intercourse is appropriate and that penetration is adequate. The next step then is to assess sperm quality by semen analysis. If there is a significant male factor, there is only a small chance that an effective treatment to improve semen quality is available (Chapter 7), but fortunately it has been recognized for 25 years now that IVF has an important place in the treatment of male factor subfertility. Using standard IVF can be described as "taking the mountain to Mohammed", where many men have sufficient sperm to fertilize their partner's oocyte in vitro whereas they cannot do so naturally [5]. With the development of ICSI [6] men with very few sperm and even men with azoospermia can have a handful of sperm extracted and can now fertilize oocytes. The only men who cannot produce embryos are those with a total lack of sperm. Even this may be overcome in the future with haploidization of human cells [7] or the cloning of sperm cells.

The Subfertility Handbook: A Clinician's Guide, Second Edition ed. Gab Kovacs. Published by Cambridge University Press. © Cambridge University Press 2011.

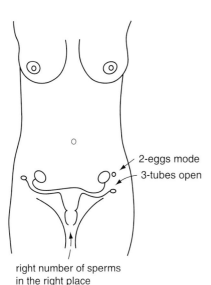

Figure 1.1 The three basic fertility parameters.

2-eggs mode

3-tubes open

right number of sperms
in the right place
at the right time

In the presence of potentially fertile semen, the next step to confirm is that ovulation is occurring, with regular ovulatory cycles of 25 to 32 days. Longer cycles or cycles with inadequate luteal phase should all be treated with the aim of producing regular cycles close to 28 days. Even in the presence of sub-normal semen it is worthwhile optimizing ovulation, which then may achieve a pregnancy. Many women who present with subfertility have polycystic ovarian syndrome (PCOS) with irregular or infrequent ovulation. There seems to be a tendency amongst some IVF specialists to treat these couples with IVF as a first line of treatment. In my opinion, this is over-treatment, and if there is a clear explanation for the inability to conceive, that is infrequent/inadequate ovulation, then initial treatment should be directed at the cause, and a course of ovulation induction should first be tried. If there is another recognized problem such as male factor or tubal disease then of course IVF is indicated as a first choice. Some of these couples will still fail to conceive after several ovulations, and then moving on to IVF is certainly indicated. How many cycles would depend on the woman's age, and the availability and affordability of treatment.

The third part of the jig-saw is that the "tubes should be patent and normal". At what stage this should be undertaken and by which method is discussed fully in Chapter 4. What defines "tubal infertility" is harder to define. Bilateral tubal obstruction is clearly a barrier to conception, but does unilateral patency, peritubal adhesions, endometriosis, or abnormal "tortuous tubes" mean that there is a tubal factor? The treatment of these factors is described in Chapters 16 and 17. If after appropriate treatment and sufficient time a pregnancy has not been achieved, IVF is the fall-back treatment, and whether it is defined as "tubal" or "unexplained" subfertility is irrelevant.

If the three basic fertility parameters "sperm", "eggs" and "tubes" are adequate, and a pregnancy has still not been achieved, the subfertility is defined as "unexplained".

Explaining "unexplained" subfertility requires us to work through the potential steps required for a pregnancy to be conceived. Apart from three basic fertility factors, sperm, eggs and tubes, there is the fourth "transport" factor, where sperm, oocytes and the subsequent embryo need to be transported. Once the sperm and oocytes are together, the fifth factor is that "fertilization" has to take place. IVF clearly has a role in overcoming transport problems, and also diagnoses whether the fertilization rate is within normal (>50%). In cases where fertilization appears to be the problem, subsequent cycles can be undertaken using ICSI, which usually overcomes the problem. Thus the most effective option to proceed to next if unexplained subfertility is diagnosed is IVF. Whether controlled ovarian hyperstimulation (COH) with intrauterine insemination (IUI) should be performed first, again depends on local facilities. This is described in Chapter 9. Whilst this does not totally overcome transport problems and gives no information on fertilization, it does sometimes result in pregnancies. The final sixth factor is "implantation". With IVF the embryo enters from a different perspective trans-cervically, but implantation is still a problem, with only one out of three transfers being successful.

In order to improve the investigation and treatment of subfertile couples in a busy gynecology clinic, a protocol using a flow chart was first developed in 1977 [8]. At that stage, many of the pathways ended in a question mark. With the development of IVF, the last option along any branch of the flow chart in 2010 is IVF, highlighting that IVF is the last option for whichever cause of subfertility the couple is experiencing.

Such a flow-chart, outlining a logical approach to managing subfertility, is shown in Figure 1.2.

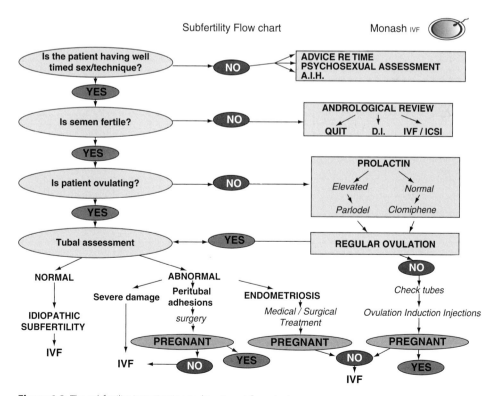

Figure 1.2 The subfertility investigation and treatment flow chart.

This book provides a comprehensive approach to each of the possible factors that act as a barrier to conception.

References

1. Kovacs G, Baker G, Burger H, *et al.* AID with cryopreserved semen: a decade of experience. *Brit J Obstet Gynaecol* 1988; **95**: 354–60.

2. Kovacs GT, Phillips SE, Healy DL, Burger H G. Induction of ovulation with gonadotrophin releasing hormone (GnRH) – life table analysis of 50 courses of treatment. *Med J Aust* 1989; **151**: 21–6.

3. Kovacs GT. The likelihood of pregnancy with in vitro fertilization and GIFT in Australia and New Zealand. *Med J Aust* 1993; **158**: 805–7.

4. Kovacs GT, Howlett D. If at first you don't succeed, try, try, try again – A successful birth after 37 cycles of ART over 11 years. *Aust NZ J Obstet Gynaecol* 2004; **44**: 580–2.

5. de Kretser DM, Yates C, Kovacs GT. The use of in vitro fertilization in the management of male infertility. *Clinics in Obstet Gynecol* 1986; **12**: 767–73.

6. Palermo G, Joris H, Devroey P, Van Steirteghem A C. Pregnancies after intracytoplasmic injection of a single spermatozoon into an oocyte. *Lancet* 1992; **340**: 17–18.

7. Palermo GD. Haploidisation of somatic cells. *Gynecol Obstet Biol Reprod (Paris)* 2005; **34** (1 Pt 2): 1S50–4.

8. Kovacs GT. Infertility: a flow chart approach. *Aust NZ J Obstet Gynaecol* 1979; **4**: 220–4.

Chapter

2

Pre-pregnancy counseling and treatment

Vicki Nisenblat and Robert J. Norman

Preconception care is an essential component of preventive health care that seeks to promote the health of a woman and her partner before pregnancy. Preconception care is defined as "interventions that aim to identify and modify biomedical, behavioral and social risks to a woman's health or pregnancy outcome through prevention and management" [1]. Its main goals are to optimize fertility and to maximize health outcomes for parents and their future children.

Lifestyle behaviors and environmental influences have significant impact on fertility at least in one partner. According to a Center for Disease Control and Prevention report, more than a third of pregnancies are complicated by maternal health issues, 11% of women smoke and 10% drink alcohol during the pregnancy, 69% do not take folate supplements, 31% are obese, 3% take medications that are known teratogens [1]. There is clear evidence that preconception interventions for women with chronic diseases, poor reproductive history and adverse lifestyle behaviors may lead to improved fertility and pregnancy outcomes [1–4].

Preconception counseling should be provided early. Given that most women do not recognize that they are pregnant until well after their "missed period", they are unaware of their pregnancy during the most vulnerable period for the fetus and many issues related to maternal and fetal health are addressed too late. Infertility clinics serve an excellent modality for providing a preconception evaluation, in particular because the pregnancy is planned and timing of conception can be delayed in order to improve the woman's health and to create a more favorable environment for future fetuses.

Medical, genetic and reproductive health conditions should be addressed. Preconception assessment includes risk variables pertaining to age, nutritional status, lifestyle, psychosocial factors, medical, reproductive and family history in both partners. Strategies to improve peri-conceptional health include healthy weight achievement, cessation of smoking, alcohol and illicit drug use, folate supplementation, immunizations, optimizing chronic disease control, genetic counseling, dental care and psychological support. Review of coital practices and education for optimizing of natural fertility may be beneficial before further extensive evaluations and treatments are undertaken.

Age

Relative fertility is decreased by half in women in their late 30s compared with women in their early 20s. Several large observational studies reported longer periods taken to conceive following increase in maternal age, with significant decline in natural pregnancy rate after 35

The Subfertility Handbook: A Clinician's Guide, Second Edition ed. Gab Kovacs. Published by Cambridge University Press. © Cambridge University Press 2011.

years [5]. The success of infertility treatments accordingly reduces with age. IVF cannot reverse the effect of age on fertility, and live birth following IVF diminishes by 2% for each year of female age. The live birth rate is about 26–40% per IVF cycle in women less than 35 years old and declines to about 6% per cycle in women over age 40 [6,7]. Cumulative live birth after 2–3 IVF cycles approaches 50–60% for women under 35 years old with gradual decrease to about 30% after age of 40. The incidence of spontaneous miscarriages and genetic abnormalities substantially increases with maternal age both in spontaneous and treatment-associated pregnancies. The risk of chromosomal abnormalities for women delivering at age 20 is 1:526, but for women delivering at 45 is 1:21. Pregnancies of women aged 35 and older are more often complicated by preeclampsia, gestational diabetes, placental abruption, fetal malposition, intrauterine growth restriction and stillbirth. This can be partially attributed to underlying health problems increasing with age; however, maternal age itself is a strong independent factor for increase in pregnancy risks. Advanced paternal age is associated with an appreciable decline in male fertility, increased risk of genetic mutations and possibly autism-related disorders, mainly after the age of 45–50 [5].

- An increased risk for experiencing infertility later in life should be an important part of routine preconception counseling in women and men. Theoretic benefits of conception sooner rather than later should be discussed. Evaluations and treatments for infertility, usually postponed for after the first year of natural attempts, are justified after 6 months in women over 35 years old. Evaluations for medical comorbidities and discussion of genetic antepartum screening have to be addressed in the advanced age group. No specific guidelines recommend an otherwise different management approach based solely on age-related risks.

Lifestyle

Weight

More than half of the general population in developed countries is overweight and more than a third is obese [8]. Obesity (BMI $\geq 30\,\text{kg/m}^2$) is associated with increased risk of diabetes mellitus, hypertension, heart disease, osteoarthritis, respiratory impairment, sleep apnea and certain types of cancer. Being underweight (BMI $\leq 18\,\text{kg/m}^2$) is prevalent among women with eating disorders or who undertake strenuous exercise, and poses significant health risks related to nutrient deficiencies, cardiac arrhythmias, low bone mass and excess death. Both obesity and being underweight are associated with a decline in natural fertility, mainly through chronic anovulation. A lower fecundity is also present even in ovulating obese women and may be partly attributed to hyperinsulinemia [2]. In the Nurses' Health Study, a cohort of 116 678 women, an increase in BMI resulted in a higher risk of infertility with relative risk of 3.7 [95% CI 2.0–3.7] for BMI ≥ 30 [9]. The rate of infertility in obese women increases by 4% per each kg/m^2 BMI [10]. Obesity significantly reduces the success of fertility treatments, associated with half the chance of pregnancy rate after IVF treatment compared with normal-weight individuals. The combination of reduced responsiveness to stimulation protocols, higher cycle cancellation rate, reduced embryo quality and impaired implantation are responsible for poorer outcomes in obese patients. This is particularly prominent in abdominal adiposity; pregnancy rate decreases by 30% per cycle for each 0.1 increase in waist/hip ratio. Obesity has been also linked to increased rates of early pregnancy loss, gestational diabetes, hypertensive disease in pregnancy, large for gestational age infants and higher rate of operative deliveries. Low pre-pregnancy weight increases risks for preterm birth and low birth weight both associated with significant neonatal morbidity. An increase in birth defects has been reported in association with abnormal maternal weight, including gastroschisis in underweight and neural tube or cardiac malformations in obese women [3].

In men obesity relates to impaired sexual function, abnormalities in sperm count and higher DNA fragmentation index, particularly for BMI $\geq 35\,kg/m^2$. The pathogenetic mechanisms may include increased testicular temperature due to fat deposition and a decrease in circulating testosterone due to sleep apnea, hyperinsulinemia and dysregulation of the hypothalamo-pituitary axis by increased estrogen.

Achievement of healthy weight reduces metabolic risks, increases chances for conception and improves pregnancy outcomes. Guidelines for obesity management recommend an initial weight loss of at least 5–10% and maintaining a reduction in weight of 10–20% with waist circumference of less than 88 cm [8,10]. Even mild weight loss results in favorable reproductive results; however, severely obese women should reduce their BMI at least to $35\,kg/m^2$ before conception to minimize associated risks. Weight loss in men results in normalizing of hormonal profile, but there are limited data on the extent that weight loss in infertile men effectively restores fertility. The primary managing strategies for weight reduction and maintenance include lifestyle modifications through either diet or exercise or both. Overall lowering caloric intake is more important for weight reduction than the actual composition of diet. Dietary treatment is better tolerated if designed for gradual weight loss and tailored on an individual basis considering personal eating habits. Pharmacological treatment with weight-reduction drugs and bariatric surgery are reserved for patients who fail to achieve the established weight loss goals with lifestyle changes or whose BMI exceeds $40\,kg/m^2$. In BMI exceeding $50\,kg/m^2$, bariatric surgery is recommended as a first-line option. Stress reduction and elevation of self esteem have been found to contribute to the success of weight-loss programs. Several studies on multifactorial lifestyle interventions, which incorporated diet, exercise and behavioral therapy and were provided by a multidisciplinary team, showed beneficial metabolic and reproductive effect [2].

- All women should be counseled about risks to their health and future pregnancies, including infertility in regard to their BMI. The worldwide standard of care in obese women of reproductive age is advice on weight loss prior to conception. Obese women should be advised that it will take longer to conceive and weight loss is likely to increase their chances for conception. Women with BMI $\geq 25\,kg/m^2$ should be offered life-modifying strategies based on decrease in caloric intake and increase in physical activity, preferably within structured weight-loss programs. Women with BMI $\leq 19\,kg/m^2$ should be assessed for eating disorders and referred to a specialist in the field and/or to a nutrition specialist.

Nutritional composition

There is little evidence that dietary variations, including vitamin-enriched, herbal remedies, vegetarian or low-fat diets, improve fertility [3]. The safety of many of the dietary supplements in pregnancy has not been established, while most data available are gained from case reports, retrospective or animal studies. A balanced diet usually addresses most of daily nutritional requirements.

Supplementation of folic acid for women of reproductive age has been associated with clear success in reducing neural tube defects (NTD) in offspring by up to 70% [11].

Iron deficiency anemia increases risk for preterm birth, growth restriction in the fetus as well as poor maternal well-being. Inadequate maternal iodine levels can affect neurological development in the fetus. Despite iodine food fortification programs, iodine intake in women of reproductive age is insufficient in many areas worldwide. Maternal vitamin D deficiency is associated with rickets and convulsions in neonates and is common in individuals with dark skin or limited exposure to sun. Vegans and individuals with poor intestinal absorption or heavy alcohol consumption are more prone to other vitamin deficiencies.

Certain food products should be avoided due to potential harmful effects on the fetus [12]. Elevated blood mercury levels associated with heavy sea-food consumption have been linked to infertility and neurological impairment in offspring. Consumption of raw meat and fish carries a risk of toxoplasmosis. Unpasteurized milk product intake can be associated with the risk of *Listeria* infection.

- All women should be assessed for nutritional and caloric adequacy. Women should be asked about use of vitamins, minerals, herbs and other remedies and advised in light of evidence available. Intake of supplements in excess of recommended daily allowances or of unproven safety should be discouraged. All women of reproductive age should be advised to ingest 0.4 mg of folic acid or a folic-acid-containing multivitamin supplement and to consume a balanced healthy diet of folate-rich food. Women who have previously had a child with a NTD or take anti-epileptic drugs should take 4 mg folic acid a day. All women should be screened for iron-deficiency anemia. Screening for vitamin deficiencies should be provided to individuals at risk. Maintenance of adequate iodine intake prior to conception and in pregnancy should be encouraged (200–250 μg a day). Calcium supplements should be recommended if dietary sources are inadequate. Women considering conception should avoid fish high in methylmercury and soft cheeses, and eliminate contact with raw fish, poultry and meat.

Exercise

Regular physical activity modifies cardio-metabolic risk factors, improves body composition, and helps to reduce and control weight. Exercise also has a favorable impact on eating behaviors, bone health and general well-being. Although direct benefits of physical activity before conception on reproductive health are unclear, weight control and mood stability have clear indirect plausible beneficial effects. The combination of exercise with diet on weight reduction in obese adults is more beneficial than either diet or exercise as sole intervention. In obese anovulatory women an exercise training program for 20–24 weeks leads to significant improvement in free androgen index, restoration of menstrual cycles with increase in ovulation and pregnancy rates either as a single intervention or in combination with diet [2,3]. Physical activity and leanness in men have been associated with reduced risk for erectile dysfunction.

Current guidelines vary between a minimum of 30 min exercise at least three times a week to 30–90 min activity daily with strong agreement on continuity and adherence to a physical activity combined with healthy eating habits [3,10].

- Moderate-intensity physical activity, such as 30 minutes brisk walking on most days, or at least three times a week, should be recommended to all adults during the preconception period and beyond.

Smoking

Smoking leads to a significant risk of death from neoplastic, ischemic heart and cerebrovascular diseases. Deleterious effects on fertility are observed in active and passive smokers either through decreased ovarian function or adverse effect on sperm. According to the results of a large meta-analysis comparing 10 928 smoking with 19 128 non-smoking women, infertility was more common in smoking populations with odds ratio of 1.60 [95% CI 1.34–1.91] [13]. Smoking has been associated with significant delayed conception with odds ratio of 1.54 [95% CI 1.19–2.01] in active smokers and 1.14 [95% CI 0.92–1.45] in passive smokers compared to non-smokers [14]. Smokers have a higher risk of menstrual abnormalities, increased baseline FSH levels, lower pregnancy rates and earlier menopause. There is compelling evidence of a negative effect of smoking on IVF outcomes with decreased response to stimulation, significant decline in pregnancy and live birth rate and an increase in number of treatment cycles. It takes two times longer for smokers to achieve pregnancy with IVF; the risk of treatment failure increases with each year of smoking. Smoking in men has been associated with deterioration in all semen parameters and a higher rate of DNA damage in addition to exposure of their female partner to passive smoking. Smoking-related risks in pregnancy include preterm births, miscarriages, stillbirths, growth restriction, placental abruption and placenta previa [15].

- All couples should be counseled to avoid smoking and to eliminate exposure to passive smoking. Those who smoke should be offered smoking-cessation interventions based on behavioral and pharmacotherapy.

Alcohol

The maximum recommended alcohol consumption is no more than one standard drink per day for adult women and no more than two standard drinks per day for adult men [15]. In women alcohol has been associated with anovulation and impaired implantation. Reduced libido, impotence and abnormal sperm parameters have been linked with alcohol intake in men. However, the literature is controversial; dose–effect associations vary within reports and some studies failed to support an alcohol–infertility relationship. Alcohol intake in pregnancy is linked to risks of miscarriage, growth restriction and fetal alcohol syndrome. There is no established safe level of alcohol in pregnancy. Due to the deleterious effects on fetal development alcohol consumption in pregnancy should be discouraged. The Australian National Health and Medical Research Council recommend zero alcohol intake in pregnancy.

- All women should be assessed for alcohol use and advised of the risks to fertility and to the fetus. Women should be informed that there is no safe level of alcohol exposure in pregnancy. Interventions to reduce alcohol use should be delivered to the women who exceed recommended alcohol limits prior to conception.

Caffeine

The literature on the effects of caffeine on fertility and pregnancy remains confusing, mainly due to the lack of well-designed randomized controlled trials, individual differences in caffeine metabolism and difficulties in estimating caffeine consumption. Although caffeine has been associated with a decline in fertility, spontaneous abortions, growth restriction and stillbirth, after adjustment for various confounders there is little evidence to support an adverse effect of mild to moderate caffeine consumption. Overall, caffeine consumption of 200–400 mg a day is not associated with negative impact on general or reproductive health. The safe level of caffeine intake in pregnancy remains unclear. It is prudent to recommend to women who are trying to conceive or who are pregnant that they reduce their caffeine intake to 100–200 mg per day, which is equivalent to less than two cups of coffee or 3–4 cups of tea per day [16].

- Caffeine consumption in the peri-conception period and pregnancy should be reduced to 100–200 mg a day.

Illicit drugs

Recreational drugs have been associated with reduced fertility and negative effect on pregnancy rate [15]. Marijuana leads to lower fertility and intellectual impairment in offspring. Abnormal sperm counts and sexual dysfunction have been demonstrated in heroin-addicted males. Cocaine use in pregnancy increases risk of prematurity, growth restriction, stillbirth and placental abruption. Anabolic steroids lead to suppression of hypothalamo-gonadal axis, erectile dysfunction and decreased sperm quality that last up to one year after the use is discontinued.

- Couples should be counseled on the risk of illicit drug use before and during the pregnancy. Pregnancy should be delayed until individuals are drug free.

Environmental pollutants

Exposure to pesticides, household glues, glycol ethers, heavy metals and solvents used in dry-cleaning or the printing industry has been associated with reduced fertility in both men and women [2,3].

- Those planning pregnancy should be questioned and counseled about reducing their peri-conceptional exposure to pollutants at home, in their community and at work.

Psychosocial stress

Growing evidence suggests that chronic psychosocial stress may disturb ability to conceive and successfully maintain pregnancy. Indirect effects of stress include depression, violence, higher risks of substance abuse, transient sexual dysfunction, lower compliance with pre-conception care and maternal suicide. Stress may directly suppress reproductive function via endocrine, immune and autonomic nervous systems. Higher stress levels in the preconception period have been linked to lower pregnancy and live birth rates and higher risk of miscarriage. The effects on pregnancy may include preterm birth, lower birth weight, lower Apgar scores and poor neurological performance in infants. In IVF patients, higher stress levels have been related to lower number of retrieved oocytes and lower implantation and pregnancy rates. Severe depression or significant acute stress in men may lead to decreased testosterone levels and impaired spermatogenesis [17]. Stress reduction and elevation of self esteem contribute to the success of lifestyle modifications, such as weight loss and stopping smoking. However, others have found no relationship between stress and stress-relieving interventions and reproductive outcomes.

- Screening for socioeconomic and psychosocial risks helps to identify women with depression, domestic violence or social instability. Exposure to stress should be limited before conception. Referral to appropriate resources can help to decrease stress and improve social support.

Immunizations

Proper immunization status in women of reproductive age offers protection from potentially serious illnesses, grants fetal resistance to intrauterine infection and confers passive immunity to the newborn via maternal immunoglobulins. The assessment of the woman's vaccination history is strongly recommended before beginning the treatment of infertility [18]. Protection should be universally provided for the following diseases: measles, mumps, rubella, tetanus, diphtheria and pertussis. Vaccination for varicella, recommended to all women who might be pregnant during the varicella season (autumn/winter), should be reviewed annually and updated as needed. For all women ≤ 26 years human papillomavirus vaccination is recommended. Other vaccinations should be considered based on individual risk assessment, which includes health, lifestyle, traveling and occupational risks. Immunization should be completed before conception as some vaccines should not be administered during pregnancy. However, there is no convincing evidence linking vaccination in pregnancy with congenital malformations or intrauterine infection. An unintentional administration of any listed vaccine is not an indication for pregnancy termination.

- All women of reproductive age should be assessed for immunization status and offered vaccines recommended for adults.

Genetic counseling

History provides a non-invasive screening for assessment of risk for genetic disorders and birth defects. Identified risk factors that require referral to genetic counseling include developmental delay, congenital anomalies or any genetic family disorders, chromosomal anomalies or known genetic conditions in at least one member of a couple. An additional set of tests address an assessment for carrier status based on increased carrier frequency among certain ethnic groups. The majority of these disorders are autosomal recessive; carriers themselves are asymptomatic and show no signs of family history. The list of common ethnicity-based tests is presented in Table 2.1. Individuals of mixed ancestry can be offered relevant testing. Testing for cystic fibrosis should be offered to patients of all races. Avoidance of pregnancy, use of donor gametes, preimplantation genetic diagnosis and oriented antenatal diagnosis can be discussed in a relevant context.

Table 2.1 Genetic counseling by ethnicity [26]

Ethnicity	Recommended testing
All ethnicities	Cystic fibrosis
Ashkenazi Jewish	Cannavan disease, familial dysautonomia, Tay-Sachs disease, Gaucher's disease, Newman-Pick disease type A, Bloom syndrome, Fanconi anemia group C
African	Sickle cell disease, Thalassemia
Mediterranean, Asian, Indian	Thalassemia
French-Canadian, Cajun	Tay-Sachs disease

- All couples should be aware of the availability of genetic screening for cystic fibrosis and ethnicity-based conditions. If genetic risk factors present, a referral to genetic counseling should be offered.

Reproductive history

Previous reproductive experience is important in identifying factors related to previous poor outcomes that may be amenable to intervention prior to future conceptions [3]. Women with a previous preterm pregnancy have an increased risk of subsequent preterm birth. Interventions to improve subsequent pregnancy outcomes include stabilizing of underlying chronic conditions or diagnosis and treatment of cervical incompetence. Previous growth-restricted infants suggest evaluation for risk factors with subsequent improvement in nutrition and health status. Women with a history of delivering a baby with congenital malformations should be counseled regarding recurrence and preventive options in subsequent pregnancies. Appropriate work-up is mandatory to identify the potential cause of previous stillbirth or recurrent pregnancy losses. Even if there is inability to identify or to eliminate potential risks, psychological support and a close monitoring plan in the next pregnancy can be provided.

- Women with adverse outcomes in previous pregnancies should be counseled regarding recurrence of another event and preventive strategies. Repeat miscarriages, stillbirth or preterm delivery necessitate work-up to identify the cause; prior congenital anomalies may require genetic counseling.

Chronic medical conditions

Women with chronic medical conditions are of particular concern due to increased risk for pregnancy-related morbidity and adverse outcomes. Multidisciplinary links in the context of specific disease are often necessary to review the woman's health and provide high-quality information to the couple. Maternal fetal medicine specialists or physicians with expertise in the care of complicated pregnancies can be involved at preconception stages. For the majority of chronic diseases, optimal control prior to conception is associated with favorable maternal and neonatal outcomes [19]. Others, such as pulmonary hypertension, Eisenmenger's syndrome, Marfan's syndrome with aortic involvement or severe renal insufficiency possess high risk of significant morbidity and mortality in pregnancy. Women with inherited disorders, such as cystic fibrosis, hemoglobinopathy or Huntington disease, should be offered pre-implantation or antenatal diagnosis and referred to a genetic counselor.

Effective treatment of the underlying condition should be weighed against any possible effect on pregnancy outcome. Clear teratogenic effects have been found in about 30 medications and they should be withdrawn prior to conception. Although many medicines can be given when indicated, effects on the human fetus are unclear in most, which creates difficulties in assessing all potential levels of risk. Self-discontinuation of medications can lead to exacerbation of disease with increasing risk for mother or fetus and should be discouraged. The list of most common medical conditions, their effects on pregnancy and key-points in preconception care are presented in Table 2.2.

Table 2.2 Preconception care for women with chronic medical conditions

Medical condition	Effect on reproduction/pregnancy	Preconception considerations
Chronic hypertension	Worsening in blood pressure (BP), renal deterioration, cardiac decompensation, preeclampsia/eclampsia, cerebral hemorrhage, preterm birth, growth restriction, placental abruption, stillbirth	Assess baseline renal function, retinopathy, ventricular hypertrophy Goal BP < 150/100 Stop ACE inhibitors, angiotensin receptor blockers
Diabetes mellitus	Pregnancy-induced hypertension, pregnancy loss, fetal malformations, growth restriction, preterm birth, macrosomia, operative deliveries	Baseline assessment for nephropathy, neuropathy, retinopathy, vascular disease Good glycemic control 1 month before conception (HbgA1C < 6–7%) Proper weight maintenance, diet, physical activity
Epilepsy	Increase in frequency of seizures (mainly due to discontinuation of treatment), congenital malformations, pregnancy loss, growth restriction, neonatal hemorrhagic disorders, developmental disabilities in offspring, perinatal death	Seizure control Lowest-dose monotherapy preferable If medication withdrawal – commence 6 months before conception Avoid carbamazepine/valproic acid if possible Avoid self-discontinuation of treatment Folic acid 4 mg daily 1 month before conception
Thyroid disorders	Anovulation, preeclampsia, heart failure, thyroid crisis, placental abruption, preterm birth, low birth weight, stillbirth, impaired cognition in the offspring, neonatal hypo-/hyperthyroidism	Euthyroid before conception Thyroid stimulating/ antithyroid antibodies PTU preferred over methimazole Avoid radioactive iodine ablation 6 months before conception
Phenylketonuria	Microcephaly, congenital heart disease, intrauterine growth restriction, mental and developmental delay in offspring	Strict metabolic control with low-phenylalanine diet Phenylalanine levels < 6 mg/dl before and throughout pregnancy
Rheumatoid arthritis	Subfertility in men and women mainly due to antirheumatic drugs, 80% of remission in pregnancy, growth restriction (mainly in corticosteroid treatment), 90% flare postpartum	Advise on the natural history of disease in pregnancy Stop methotrexate, cyclophosphamide, leflunomide before conception Avoid cyclosporine and azathioprine if possible
Systemic lupus erythematosus (SLE)	Exacerbation of disease in > 50%, pregnancy loss, stillbirth, intrauterine growth restriction, preterm birth, neonatal lupus.	Remission 6 months before conception Baseline renal and cardiovascular function Hydroxychloroquine is preferable to cytotoxic agents Low-dose aspirin to prevent adverse fetal consequences
Chronic renal disease	Worsening of renal function, chronic hypertension, preeclampsia, anemia, pregnancy loss, stillbirth, growth restriction, preterm delivery	Normal blood pressure before conception Assess baseline renal and cardiovascular functions Stop ACE inhibitors, angiotensin receptor blockers

Table 2.2 (cont.)

Medical condition	Effect on reproduction/pregnancy	Preconception considerations
Cardiovascular disease	Cardiac decompensation, thromboembolism, pregnancy loss, stillbirth. NYHA[a] > 2, ejection fraction < 40%, left heart obstruction, prior cardiac event – increased risk of adverse maternal/fetal outcome. Fetal heart anomalies if parents with congenital heart disease	Baseline cardiac function Correction of structural lesions prior to conception Optimum control before conception Substitute warfarin for heparin or low molecular weight heparin prior to conception and in early pregnancy Genetic counseling in congenital conditions
Thrombophilia	Venous and arterial thrombosis, preeclampsia, recurrent pregnancy loss, placental abruption, placental infarcts, intrauterine growth restriction, fetal stroke, stillbirth	Assess need for prophylaxis in pregnancy/ postpartum/during infertility treatments Substitute warfarin prior to conception and in early pregnancy Genetic counseling in hereditable disorders
Asthma	Increase severity of the disease (30%), preeclampsia, hypertension, hyperemesis gravidarum, preterm birth, growth restriction, stillbirth, neonatal hypoxia In well-controlled disease – outcomes similar to general population	Baseline pulmonary functions Aggressive treatment of active disease in preconception/pregnancy Inhaled corticosteroids are prophylaxis of choice in persistent disease in pregnancy
Psychiatric disorders	Exacerbation in pregnancy (mainly due to self-discontinuation of treatment), postpartum depression	Avoid paroxitine, other SSRI preferred Avoid carbamazepine/valproic acid if possible

[a] NYHA, New York Heart Association functional classification.

- All women with chronic medical conditions should be counseled about the effect of their disease on pregnancy and the effect of pregnancy on the disease. Optimal disease control should be achieved prior to conception. Medications should be limited to minimal effective dose, teratogenic medicines should be avoided and self-discontinuation of treatment should be discouraged.

Infectious diseases

Screening for infections in the preconception period can identify certain risks for women's reproductive health and future pregnancies [20]. A summary of screening policies in the preconception period is presented in Table 2.3.

- All women should be assessed for the risk of infectious diseases. Risk assessment of STD should be based on the sexual history of both partners. Strategies include patient education for primary prevention, immunization, indicated testing and treatment.

Coital practices

Whereas short abstinence periods of several days do not appear to affect sperm morphology or counts, longer periods of above 5–10 days may have an adverse effect. Daily or alternate day

Table 2.3 Screening for infectious diseases in preconception period

Disease	Population to be tested
HIV, HBV, Syphilis	Universal routine screening
Chlamydia	≤ 25 years old or risk for STD[a]
Gonorrhea	High risk for STD
HSV	Genital herpes in partner
HCV	Drug users, blood product recipients, healthcare workers, hemodialysis, born to infected mothers, infected partner, multiple partners, migrants from endemic areas
Tuberculosis	Personal contact with someone having active disease, migrants from endemic areas, drug users, healthcare workers, immune-compromised individuals
Toxoplasma	Universal screening not advised Counseling for prevention: avoid exposure to raw meat and excretions of cats, wash fruits/vegetables
CMV	Universal screening not advised Counseling for prevention: avoid close contact with urine and saliva of young children, hand hygiene
Asymptomatic bacteriuria	All pregnant women No evidence on efficacy of pre-pregnancy screening
Bacterial vaginosis	All symptomatic women No evidence regarding screening/treatment in asymptomatic women Weak evidence in risk group for preterm birth
Periodontal disease	All women; however, sparse evidence of effect of treatment on pregnancy outcome
GBS	Pregnant women (universally 35–37 weeks or high-risk group) No evidence on efficacy of pre-pregnancy screening

[a] STD, sexually transmitted disease.

intercourse results in the highest cycle pregnancy rates, 37% and 33%, respectively, with a decline to 15% with weekly frequency [3]. However, frequent intercourse may be associated with elevated stress levels; the optimal frequency should be estimated considering couple preferences. Common misperceptions that remaining supine after coitus or particular positions at the time of intercourse improve fertility have not been proved. Sperm appears in the cervical canal seconds after ejaculation, regardless of position. Female orgasm can promote sperm transport; however, there is no relationship between orgasm and fertility or between coital practices and offspring gender. Certain vaginal lubricants reduce sperm motility, such as saliva and water-based products (KY Jelly, Touch, Astroglide). This effect has not been observed with mineral oil, canola oil or hydroxyethylcellulose-based lubricants [3]. Pregnancy is more likely to be achieved when intercourse occurs within the "fertile window" spanning 6 days and ending on the day of ovulation, particularly 2–3 days within ovulation. The monitoring of ovulation may be difficult and associated with additional unnecessary stress and costs. Clinical signs, such as changes in mood, libido, pain or changes in cervical mucus, help to establish ovulation in more than 50% of women. Commercial kits for ovulation detection estimate the mid-cycle luteinizing hormone (LH) peak and are mainly based on monitoring urinary LH. The false-positive rates of these kits average 7% of cycles and may result in the necessity for multiple checks [3].

- In order to maximize the probability of conception couples should be advised on regular intercourse commencing after cessation of menses for a period of 7–10 days in women with "regular periods" or more in elongated cycles, preferably every 1–2 days. Estimation of ovulation time with LH kits should be reserved for couples having infrequent intercourse.

Preconception care for men

Men are active partners in family planning. Men should be targeted because their lifestyle and general health affect semen quality and the health of their offspring and influence women's compliance with recommendations. There is no consensus on delivery of such care to men and recommendations for men are sparse [21].

- Each male planning pregnancy with their partner should undergo medical evaluation and preconceptional education in order to detect and modify high-risk behaviors and poorly controlled diseases.

Other considerations

Leiomyoma

Uterine leiomyomas may be associated with impaired fertility and reduced success of IVF cycles [22]. During pregnancy, myomas are associated with increased risk of malpresentation, cesarean section, preterm delivery, placental abruption, spontaneous miscarriages or pain related to myoma degeneration. Treatment prior to pregnancy can be considered in symptomatic women, in recurrent pregnancy loss after exclusion of other potential causes or in large intramural myomas distorting the uterine cavity. Myomectomy, the most common treatment in women wanting to preserve fertility, achieves symptom relief in up to 80% of women, with a recurrence rate of 30% within 10 years. The majority of women conceive within one year after myomectomy with a reported pregnancy rate of 40–50%. There is no convincing evidence that myomectomy reduces the incidence of adverse obstetrical outcomes or the miscarriage rate. Non-invasive treatments, including uterine artery embolization, Doppler-guided mechanical compression of uterine arteries and myolysis with MRI-guided focused ultrasound, provide symptom relief and an effective decrease in myoma size. However, the data regarding fertility and pregnancy after these procedures are still limited and none of them is currently recommended in women planning to conceive [22].

Hydrosalpinx

Hydrosalpinx has been related to infertility and reduced success of IVF treatments; the mechanism is still unclear; however, flushing and the embryotoxic effect of tubal fluid may be important. Salpingectomy has been shown to improve the pregnancy rate and can be considered in patients with repeat failures to conceive [23].

Uterine anomalies

Uterine anomalies occur in 7–8% of the general population and in 25% of women with pregnancy losses. Uterine anomalies are also associated with preterm birth, malpresentation, growth restriction, dystocia, uterine rupture, postpartum hemorrhage and higher rate of cesarean deliveries. Some evidence suggests lower pregnancy rates in the IVF cycle for women with uterine anomalies. Surgical correction may be advised in some cases; however, strong evidence regarding significantly plausible effects of treatment on reproductive performance exists only for patients with uterine septum greater than 1 cm [24]. If infertility treatments are planned in such patients, special considerations should be undertaken to avoid the chance of multiple gestations.

Polycystic ovary syndrome (PCOS)

PCOS is a common endocrine disorder associated with anovulation, androgen excess and insulin resistance. More than half of women with PCOS are obese. Women diagnosed with PCOS and their first-degree relatives have a higher incidence of adverse metabolic profiles. Lifestyle modifications are the treatment of first choice; even small weight losses restore ovulation and improve androgen levels, lipid profile, insulin sensitivity and hirsutism. Metformin may have an additional beneficial effect and can be considered in conjunction with lifestyle improvements. Screening for metabolic derangements should be performed in all women with PCOS and considered in daughters of mothers diagnosed with the disorder [25].

Summary

Preconception counseling is far beyond providing information about pregnancy to women prior to conception. It is an ultimate period for risk assessment, health promotion and medical/psychosocial interventions.

References

1. Center for Disease Control and Prevention. Recommendations for improving preconception health and healthcare: United States: a report of the CC/ATSDR Preconception Care workgroup and the Select Panel on Preconception Care. *MMWR Morb Mortal Weekly Rep* 2006; **55**: 1–23.

2. Homan GF, Davies M, Norman RJ. The impact of lifestyle factors on reproductive performance in the general population and those undergoing fertility treatment: a review. *Hum Reprod Update* 2007; **13**: 209–23.

3. Practice Committee of the American Society for Reproductive Medicine in collaboration with the Society for Reproductive Endocrinology and Infertility. Optimizing natural fertility. *Fertil Steril* 2008; **90**: S1–S6.

4. Health Council of the Netherlands. *Preconception Care: A Good Beginning*. The Hague: Health Council of the Netherlands, 2007; publication no. 2007/19E.

5. Heffner LJ. Advanced maternal age – How old is too old? *N Engl J Med* 2004; **351**: 1927–9.

6. Wright FC, Schieve LA, Reynolds MA, *et al.* Assisted reproductive technology survelliance – United States 2002. *MMWR Surveill Summ* 2005; **54**: 1–24.

7. Bryant J, Sullivan E, Dean J. *Assisted Reproductive Technology in Australia and New Zealand 2002*. Assisted Reproductive Technology Series Number 8. Sydney: Australian Institute of Health and Welfare, National Perinatal Statistics Unit, 2004.

8. World Health Organization. *Obesity: Preventing and Managing the Global Epidemic*. Report of a WHO consultation. Technical report series no. 894. Geneva: World Health Organization, 2000.

9. Rich-Edwards JW, Goldman MB, Willett WC. Adolescent body mass index and infertility caused by ovulatory disorder. *Am J Obstet Gynecol* 1994; **171**: 171–7.

10. National Institute for Clinical Excellence. *Obesity: Guidance on the Prevention,*

Identification, Assessment, and Management of Overweight and Obesity in Adults and Children. NICE Clinical Guideline 43. London: NICE, 2006.

11. Lumley J, Watson L, Watson M, Bower C. Periconceptional supplementation with folate and/or multivitamins for preventing neural tube defects. *Cochrane Database Syst Rev* 2001; **3**: CD001056.

12. Gardiner PM, Nelson L, Shellhaas CS, *et al.* The clinical content of preconception care: nutrition and dietary supplements. *Am J Obstet Gynecol* 2008; **199**(6 Suppl 2): S345–56.

13. Augood C, Duckitt K, Templeton AA. Smoking and female infertility: a systematic review and meta-analysis. *Hum Reprod* 1998; **13**: 1532–9.

14. Hull MG, North K, Taylor H, *et al.* Delayed conception and active and passive smoking. The Avon Longitudinal Study of Pregnancy and Childhood Study Team. *Fertil Steril* 2000; **74**: 725–33.

15. Floyd RL, Jack BW, Cefalo R, *et al.* The clinical content of preconception care: alcohol, tobacco, and illicit drug exposures. *Am J Obstet Gynecol* 2008; **199**(6 Suppl 2): S333–9.

16. Nisenblat V, Norman RJ. The effects of caffeine on fertility and pregnancy outcomes. *UpToDate*, 2009.

17. Klerman LV, Jack BW, Coonrod DV, *et al.* The clinical content of preconception care: care of psychosocial stressors. *Am J Obstet Gynecol* 2008; **199**(6 Suppl 2): S362–6.

18. Practice Committee of the American Society for Reproductive Medicine.

Vaccination guidelines for female infertility patients. *Fertil Steril* 2008; **90**: S169–71

19. Dunlop AL, Jack BW, Bottalico JN, *et al.* The clinical concept of preconception care: women with chronic medical conditions. *Am J Obstet Gynecol* 2008; **199**(6 Suppl 2): S310–27.

20. Coonrod DV, Jack BW, Stubblefield PG, *et al.* The clinical content of preconception care: infectious diseases in preconception care. *Am J Obstet Gynecol* 2008; **199** (6 Suppl 2): S296–309.

21. Frey KA, Navarro SM, Kotelchuck M, *et al.* The clinical content of preconception care: preconception care for men. *Am J Obstet Gynecol* 2008; **199**(6 Suppl 2): S389–95.

22. The Practice Committee of the American Society for Reproductive Medicine in collaboration with the Society of Reproductive Surgeons. Myomas and reproductive function. *Fertil Steril* 2008; **90**: S125–30.

23. Strandell A, Lindhard A, Waldenstrom U, *et al.* Hydrosalpinx and IVF outcome: cumulative results after salpingectomy in a randomized controlled trial. *Hum Reprod* 2001; **16**: 2403–10.

24. Stubblefield PG, Coonrod DV, Reddy UM, *et al.* The clinical concepts of preconception care: reproductive history. *Am J Obstet Gynecol* 2008; **199**(6 Suppl 2): S373–83.

25. Norman RJ, Dewailly D, Legro RS, *et al.* Polycystic ovary syndrome. *Lancet* 2007; **370**: 685–97.

26. Solomon BD, Jack BW, Feero GF. The clinical content of preconception care: genetics and genomics. *Am J Obstet Gynecol* 2008; **199**(6 Suppl 2): S340–4.

The first interview with a new couple

Majed Al Hudhud and Geoffrey Trew

The first interview with a specialist for any patient is important – it allows a bond of trust to be established and the patient to gain confidence in the advice and strategies that the specialist recommends. This bond is even more important with infertility patients. The whole area of infertility is deeply personal and can have profound effects on the couple. The first interview therefore has to be handled in an even more sensitive fashion than most other clinical situations. Several areas around the first appointment have to be thought about.

Fertility management includes decisions for investigations and treatment which concern both partners. For that reason it is advisable to see couples seeking fertility treatment together if at all possible.

It is also advisable to see the couple in a dedicated unit for fertility management rather than a general gynecological clinic. This can not only improve the efficiency and effectiveness of treatment but also be reassuring to the couple. It should allow a multidisciplinary approach with specialists present who can see and investigate both the male and female partners. The infertility clinic should not share a waiting room with users of antenatal clinics or classes for obvious reasons.

Bearing in mind the stress and anxiety associated with fertility problems support in this regard is essential. This support should be offered at any stage. The treatment itself is stressful, with the waiting time before starting it or awaiting its results sometimes adding more stress especially if the treatment has been unsuccessful [1].

Adequate provision of clear information about the investigations planned and treatment steps involving both partners in the management plan are essential to minimize the emotional burdens of anxiety and stress of the couple. It may be helpful as well to offer the couple contact details of a fertility support group.

Furthermore, counseling services should form an integral part of the fertility management team. Counselors should have professional counseling qualifications and should not be directly involved in the management of the couple's fertility problems. It is important to offer the counseling option at an early stage of the course of the management. This will give the patients the opportunity to access it before, during or after the investigation or the treatment phases irrespective of the outcome of these procedures.

Different kinds of counseling are available. In addition to support counseling there is implication counseling, which aims to enable the couple to understand the implications of proposed treatments and consequent actions for themselves, their families and for any children born as a result and anyone else affected by the donation or the treatment.

The Subfertility Handbook: A Clinician's Guide, Second Edition ed. Gab Kovacs. Published by Cambridge University Press. © Cambridge University Press 2011.

Table 3.1 Consider early investigation in a couple with any of the following

Female
  Age over 35 years
  Amenorrhea/oligomenorrhea
  Previous abdominal /pelvic surgery
  Previous STI, PID
  Abnormal pelvic exam
  Presence of substantial fibroid

Male
  Previous genital pathology
  Previous urogenital surgery
  Previous STI
  Varicocele
  Significant systemic disease
  Abnormal genital exam

If there is a need for genetic counseling an appropriate referral should be made to a qualified genetic counselor [2].

According to the World Health Organization (WHO) infertility (clinical definition) is a disease of the reproductive system defined by the failure to achieve a clinical pregnancy after 12 months or more of regular unprotected sexual intercourse [3]. However, diagnosis of infertility based on this definition can exaggerate the risk of infertility, since about 50% of women who do not conceive in the first year are likely to do so in the second year.

On the other hand, if there is any obvious factor affecting the chances of spontaneous pregnancy it may warrant investigation of the problem earlier (e.g. women over 35 years, history of tubal damage, oligomenorrhea, previous pelvic surgery, history of testicular maldescent or orchidopexy, history of sexually transmitted infection, etc.) (Table 3.1).

A common definition of sub- and infertility is very important for the appropriate management of infertility. Subfertility generally describes any form of reduced fertility with prolonged time of trying to conceive. Infertility may be used synonymously with sterility with only sporadically occurring spontaneous pregnancies. Three major factors affect the spontaneous probability of conception: the duration of subfertility, age of the female partner and the cause of subfertility [4].

One of the important points during the first consultation is to provide a friendly environment to the couple. This will break the ice, release the tension and encourage them to answer some sensitive questions. They may find some of the questions embarrassing and it is important to keep them aware of the nature of the questions beforehand, asking them in a constructive manner and seeking the best way of helping them.

History-taking

A good starting point in history-taking is to enquire about the couple's occupations. This is an area about which they both know more than the doctor and therefore can discuss it confidently. Moving on from here, one should ask about the biographical data of the couple. Religious, ethnic or cultural background may determine the way they are evaluated and could exclude certain treatment options. It is also important to ask the couple about the duration of the fertility problem and any previous history of conception.

The next step should be taking the female partner's history including her age, the age of menarche, menstrual history (regularity, amount and duration of the period and the presence of any kind of dysmenorrhea). Regular, painful cycles, especially if associated with premenstrual symptoms, usually suggest ovulatory cycles. Secondary dysmenorrhea is suggestive of endometriosis.

Other relevant points in the female's history include any previous pregnancy, miscarriage or termination, and any method of contraception used before trying to get pregnant. Cervical smear history (dates and results) is important and the patient should be up to date with cervical screening before commencing any fertility treatment. Her past medical history should be ascertained, especially with any history of sexually transmitted infection, appendicitis or any pelvic surgery. Any medication or allergy as well as the family history are also relevant. Some medications can inhibit ovulation (e.g. nonsteroidal anti-inflammatory drugs); others may be contraindicated during the peri-conception period. Chemotherapy can induce ovarian failure.

Personal and lifestyle details, the extent of stress in the patient's life, exercise regime (type, regularity and duration of exercise), caffeine consumption, smoking status, alcohol intake, any recreational drugs (marijuana and cocaine can adversely affect ovulatory and tubal function), current and recent occupation should all be noted.

The woman's current weight and any change (10% or more within the last 12 months) should be noted. The body mass index (weight in kilograms divided by height in meters squared) should be calculated. Ideal BMI is between19 and 25. Low BMI is a recognized cause of hypoestrogenic amenorrhea. Weight loss of over 15% of ideal body weight is associated with menstrual dysfunction. Women who are underweight are at increased risk of preterm delivery and small for gestational age babies.

On the other side, BMI over 30 has a negative impact on spontaneous conception, miscarriage, pregnancy and the long-term outlook of both mother and child due to both an increased rate of congenital anomalies and the possibility of metabolic disease later in life [2].

Metabolic-wise, the distribution of body fat is more important than the actual body weight. Visceral fat is more metabolically active and an increase in waist circumference (waist : hip ratio) (WHR) correlates better than BMI with both metabolic risk and long-term disease.

To measure the WHR ratio the waist measurement is taken 2.5 cm above the umbilicus in centimeters. Next, the hip measurement is taken at the top of the iliac bone in centimeters on the right front of the body. The level will be slightly lower than the umbilicus. Unfortunately, WHR is difficult to measure in obese patients due to increased possibility of error, while BMI is more consistent.

With respect to the male partner the history is less complicated. Again, occupation needs to be explored, with the possibility of any noxious influences. Stress may affect the couple's relationship, libido and the frequency of sexual intercourse.

Some occupations involve exposure to hazards (heat, X-ray, chemicals, etc.) that can affect fertility.

Any history of systemic medical disease (e.g. diabetes, upper respiratory tract disease), any surgery on the testes or scrotum (indication and outcome), childhood illnesses and development history need to be explored. Additionally, any history of sexually transmitted infection, trauma, medication, chemotherapy as well as alcohol, smoking or other drug intake all need to be identified. Questions also should be asked about the family history, physical activity and social habits.

BMI should be obtained for the male partner as there is evidence that men with a BMI more than 29 are likely to have reduced fertility. Obesity may have a deleterious effect on erectile function in men with existing vascular risk factors such as heart disease and diabetes.

Finally, the couple's coital habit needs to be explored. It may be best to leave it to the end of the history-taking, by which time they have got to know the clinician a bit better. Frequency of intercourse and its timing in relation to the ovulation period should be documented. Enquiry should be made about any erectile dysfunction, premature ejaculation, difficult penetration or pain during intercourse. Any superficial or deep dysparunia, the use of any lubricants (which may be spermicidal) and the adequacy of ejaculation should be explored. Keeping in mind the environment in which investigation of fertility problems takes place should enable people to discuss sensitive issues such as sexual abuse.

The best sperm motility has been found in semen emission every three to four days on average. Coitus every two to three days is likely to maximize the overall chance of natural conception, as spermatozoa survive in the female reproductive tract for up to seven days after insemination.

This is also a good time to dispel some of the old myths the patients may have been erroneously told about; that the female doesn't have to stay lying down for 30 minutes after intercourse, that pillows under the bottom after sex don't help, that sexual position doesn't have a detrimental or beneficial impact on fertility and finally that losing some fluid after sex is normal and it's not the "good" sperm that is being lost but rather the seminal fluid. This also gives the couple the opportunity to ask about other concerns regarding the sex itself that might worry them.

The next step should be directed towards the result of any previous fertility investigation, starting from less to more invasive ones such as blood tests and their timing in relation to the menstrual cycle, then any pelvic ultrasound scan or hysterosalpingogram and their results. Additionally, one should ask about any previous surgical investigations/operations and their findings (diagnostic laparoscopy, dye test, ovarian drilling or management of endometriosis). A similar approach should be followed regarding the male partner's history of any investigations, starting with semen analysis, blood tests or ultrasound, and moving on to any surgical intervention such as testicular biopsy, varicocele ligation or orchidopexy, etc.

Physical examination

After completing the history-taking one should proceed with a physical examination. An explanation of the nature and the purpose of the examination should be made clear to the couple to obtain their consent for it and to put them at ease during the course of the examination.

For the female, a general examination should include vital signs, assessment of the development of secondary sexual characteristics and any sign of endocrine disorders (e.g. acne, hirsutism, balding, acanthosis nigricans, virilization, goiter or other signs of thyroid disease). A Ferriman and Gallway Hirsute Score (Table 3.2) is useful in assessment of hirsutism. All sites of excessive hair growth should be inspected. In white Caucasian women a score greater than 6 indicates abnormal hair distribution and may be associated with hyperandrogenism. Hyperandrogenic hirsutism may have an adrenal origin (congenital adrenal hyperpiasia, Cushing's syndrome or adrenal tumor) or an ovarian origin (polycystic ovarian syndrome, hyperthecosis, functional ovarian tumor, intersex with ovotestis).

Table 3.2 Ferriman–Gallway Hirsute Score

Site	Grade	Definition
Upper lip	1	A few hairs at outer margin
	2	A small moustache at outer margin
	3	A mustache extending halfway from outer margin
	4	A mustache extending to mid line
Chin	1	A few scattered hairs
	2	Scattered hairs with small concentrations
	3 and 4	Complete cover, light and heavy
Chest	1	Circumareolar hairs
	2	With mid-line hair in addition
	3	Fusion of these areas, with three-quarter cover
	4	Complete cover
Upper back	1	A few scattered hairs
	2	Rather more, still scattered
	3 and 4	Complete cover, light and heavy
Lower back	1	A sacral tuft of hair
	2	With some lateral extension
	3	Three-quarters cover
	4	Complete cover
Upper abdomen	1	A few mid-line hairs
	2	Rather more, still midline
	3 and 4	Half and full cover
Lower abdomen	1	A few mid-line hairs
	2	A mid-line streak of hair
	3	A mid-line band of hair
	4	An inverted V-shaped growth
Arm	1	Sparse growth affecting less than a quarter of the limb surface
	2	More than this: cover still incomplete
	3 and 4	Complete cover, light and heavy
Thigh	1–4	As for arm

Grade 0 at all sites indicates absence of terminal hair.

Hirsutism is common in patients with hypothyroidism, acromegaly or porphyria and in women who are taking drugs such as phenytoin, diazoxide and glucocorticoids.

Chest examination should include assessment of breast development, the presence of peri-areolar hirsutism or galactorrhea and to rule out lumps. Tanner staging of breast development should be noted (Table 3.3).

An abdominal examination should be carried out to note any scars, hirsutism, striae or masses.

Pelvic examination should be followed by inspection of the vulva and vagina to rule out any congenital abnormalities. Speculum examination should be done to obtain a high vaginal swab (HVS) and an endocervical swab to detect the presence of *Chlamydia trachomatis* as the evidence suggests that screening for and treating cervical chlamydial infection can reduce the incidence of pelvic inflammatory disease in women at increased risk of *Chlamydia* [2]. A cervical smear can also be taken if the patient is due for one.

Table 3.3 The Tanner staging of breast and pubic hair development

Stage	Breast changes	Pubic hair changes
1	Papillary elevation	Lanugo hairs
2	Elevation of breast bud and papilla	Dark terminal hair on labia majora
3	Further enlargement of breast tissue and papilla	Terminal hair covering the labia majora and spreading to the mons pubis
4	Elevation of papilla and areolar unit over the breast: papilla is at or above the equator of the breast	Terminal hair covering the labia majora and the mons pubis fully
5	Areola is recessed into the breast and/or papilla is below the equator of the breast	Terminal hair covering the labia majora, mons pubis, and inner thigh

Bimanual examination then should be carried out to assess the uterine size, position and mobility and note any abnormality, masses or tenderness. Any nodules in the pouch of Douglas or a fixed retroverted uterus would suggest endometriosis. The examination of the female partner is further discussed in Chapter 4.

When fertility evaluation is directed by a gynecologist, physical examination of the male partner may be deferred pending the results of the first semen analysis when there is no element of abnormal reproductive history. If indicated, examination may be conducted by a gynecologist with proper training and experience, but is most often performed by a urologist or other specialist in men's reproduction.

Physical examination of the male should begin with assessing the secondary sexual characteristics, including body habitus, hair distribution and breast development.

Genital examination should start with assessing the penis, locating the urethral meatus, then palpation of the testes and measurement of their size (usually firm and measure 15–25 ml in volume). The next step is to check the presence and consistency of both the vas deferens and epididymides and to check for the presence of any varicocele. Finally, if appropriate, digital rectal examination determines the size and symmetry of the prostate and may reveal the presence of midline cysts or dilated seminal vesicles suggesting ejaculatory duct obstruction.

This is discussed in detail in Chapter 5.

Investigations

By the end of the physical examination, a provisional plan of the investigations and treatment options should be discussed. It would be helpful to draw a diagram to show the female pelvic anatomy and to explain the ovulation and fertilization physiology. This will help the couple to understand the process very well.

The parameters that need to be assessed on the female side are the ovulation and the ovarian reserve, tubal patency, uterine cavity and the abdominal cavity.

Ovarian reserve will be considered here, whilst investigation of pelvic normality is considered in detail in Chapter 4.

Assessment of ovarian reserve is essential before embarking on any fertility treatment. It aims to assess the female fecundability, which is related to the total number of primordial follicles remaining within the ovaries (referred to as ovarian reserve). The number of primordial follicles declines with age. Increasing age is associated significantly with reduced implantation and pregnancy rates.

Women aged 40 years or older have the poorest pregnancy outcomes when compared with those aged under 40 [5].

One of the indirect measurements to estimate the ovarian reserve is day 2–3 basal serum FSH. It has been reported that pregnancy rates decline significantly as basal FSH rises in women aged over 35 years. The clomiphene citrate challenge test is another test that has been used historically to demonstrate a correlation with the probability of conception in these populations [6], but is less used today as it has been surpassed by the other more practical tests below.

In addition to basal FSH, an ultrasound scan should be carried out to assess the ovarian volume (normal volume 5–10 ml) and antral follicle count (AFC) (normally 5–10 antral follicles). Diminished ovarian volume and/or antral follicle count are associated with poor ovarian reserve. The advantage of pelvic ultrasound is that additional information can be obtained regarding any pelvic pathology and the position and accessibility of both ovaries.

Recently, more evidence has emerged in favor of measuring the anti-Müllerian hormone (AMH) serum level to assess the ovarian reserve especially in patients with expected poor ovarian response. Additional studies are to be awaited to learn whether the test's capacity may prove to be superior to current tests such as basal FSH and the AFC. One of the advantages of AMH measurement is that the test can be done on any day of the menstrual cycle.

One of the other tests available is serum inhibin B. The value of assessing serum inhibin B is uncertain and therefore it is not recommended [2,6].

Other investigations

Rubella and varicella immunity status needs to be checked during the course of the investigations and non-immune patients should be advised to have the vaccination against rubella and/or varicella and if so it is recommended not to get pregnant for at least one month after the rubella vaccine [2] and one month after each dose of varicella vaccine [7].

The male partner should be asked to produce a semen sample for analysis following two to three days of abstinence in a masturbated specimen delivered promptly to the laboratory.

New World Health Organization reference values for human semen characteristics have been published recently [8]. See Table 3.4.

Table 3.4 WHO reference values for semen analysis, 2010

Semen volume	1.5 ml or more
Total sperm number	39 million per ejaculate or more
Sperm concentration	15 million per ml or more
Vitality	58% or more live
Progressive motility	32% or more
Total (progressive + non-progressive) motility	40% or more
Morphologically normal forms	4%

An abnormal semen analysis test should be repeated. This is because of its low specificity and high false positivity. Ideally, the second sample should be at least three months after the first analysis, which is the duration of the spermatozoa formation cycle. However, this delay may cause anxiety and the timing of the second sample should take into consideration the preferences of the man. If azoospermia or severe oligozoospermia is reported in the initial semen analysis, a repeat test should be undertaken within two to four weeks [9]. Investigation of the male partner is discussed in detail in Chapter 5.

The value of post-coital testing for cervical mucus for the presence of motile sperm is controversial and is subject to debate. It is not recommended to perform it routinely because it has no predictive value for the pregnancy rate [10].

Tubal assessment

The result of semen analysis and assessment of ovulation should be known before testing for tubal patency is performed.

Towards the end of the assessment, the doctor should be able to assess the couple regarding the "welfare of the unborn child", which is a very crucial issue, before embarking on any assisted fertility treatment.

Now, according to the history and physical examination certain problems may become apparent for each individual couple. These issues need to be explained to the couple and they need to be guided through the best available evidence on how to deal with it. Such problems not only reduce the chances of achieving pregnancy but may also affect the long-term health of the couple and of the fetus during the pregnancy and during childhood.

The first general advice should be about encouraging the couple to have a healthy diet and to exercise. (This is discussed in detail in Chapter 2.) There is a large body of evidence relating to the impact of lifestyle on reproductive performance. However, motivating patients to modify their lifestyle can be difficult and challenging. Changing lifestyle behaviors requires time, considerable effort and motivation. A patient-centered approach to counseling and advice has been shown to produce the best outcomes [11].

The couple should be informed that there is some evidence that consumption of caffeine is associated with reduced fecundity in the general population. Although the mechanism is unclear, caffeine may affect female reproduction by targeting ovulation and corpus luteal function and higher early follicular estrogen levels [11].

Discussing the effect of smoking is another important point. Smoking (including passive smoking) is associated with reduced fertility among females and reduced sperm quality in men [11]. There is also significant association between maternal cigarette smoking in pregnancy and increased risks of small for gestational age infants, still birth and infant mortality. In fact, it is strongly recommended to offer the couple referral to a smoking-cessation program to support their efforts in stopping smoking.

Women should be informed that drinking no more than one or two units of alcohol once or twice per week, avoiding episodes of intoxication, reduces the risk of harming the fetus [2].

Men should also be advised that excessive alcohol intake is detrimental to semen quality. It is recommended to limit alcohol intake to 3 to 4 units per day to eliminate harmful effects [2].

The use of recreational drugs (e.g. marijuana and cocaine) can adversely affect ovulatory and tubal function. Anabolic steroids and cocaine can adversely affect semen quality [2].

Special advice in this regard should be made and relevant referral should be offered.

There is a link between increased scrotal temperature and reduced semen quality in the healthy population. A sedentary work position and occupational heat exposure may affect the scrotal temperature. There is also some evidence that wearing tight-fitting underwear, in a fertile population, can impair semen quality. Advice about these issues should be given to the male partner.

It is recommended to advise the female partner to take 0.4 mg of folic acid daily. This dose should be increased to 5 mg per day if there is any current use of antiepileptic medication or the patient has had a child with a neural tube defect.

It is proved that preconception folic acid supplementation up to 12 weeks gestation reduces the risk of having a baby with neural tube defects.

Couples where either of them is known to have chronic viral infection such as hepatitis B , hepatitis C or HIV should be referred to centers that have appropriate expertise and facilities to provide safe risk-reduction investigation and treatments. Counseling provided by a qualified person in such cases is very important regarding the implications of the treatment for the couple and the unborn child.

Many aspects of fertility-related issues are complex and take time to understand and lots of questions arise immediately following the consultation. Thus, verbal discussion needs to be supported by written information to help the patients to cope well and find answers to their concerns. This will also give them the opportunity to make informed decisions regarding their care and treatment via access to evidence-based information. These choices should be recognized as an integral part of the decision-making process.

This sort of management plan usually aids the couple with their subfertility problem. They may have further questions and should be encouraged to write these down and bring them back to the next appointment. The result of the investigations would be discussed at the next interview and, depending on the findings, a management plan decided upon.

Further reading

Adam Balen. *Infertility in Practice*, 3rd edn. Informa Healthcare, 2008.

References

1. Hammerli K, Znoj H, Barth J. The efficacy of psychological interventions for infertile patients: a meta-analysis examining mental health and pregnancy rate. *Hum Reprod Update* 2009; 15(3): 279–95.

2. National Collaborating Centre for Women's and Children's Health. *Fertility: Assessment and Treatment for People with Fertility Problems*, Commissioned by the National Institute for Clinical Excellence. RCOG Press, 2004.

3. Zegers-Hochschild F, Adamson GD, Mouzon J de, *et al.* On behalf of ICMART and WHO. The International Committee for Monitoring Assisted Reproductive Technology (ICMART) and the World Health Organization (WHO) Revised Glossary on ART Terminology, 2009. *Hum Reprod* 2009; 24(11): 2683–7.

4. Gnoth C, Godehardt E, Frank-Herrmann P, *et al.* Definition and prevalence of subfertility and infertility. *Hum Reprod* 2005; 20(5): 1144–7.

5. Baird DT, Collins J, Egozcue J, *et al.*, ESHRE Capri Workshop Group. Fertility and ageing. *Hum Reprod Update* 2005; 11(3): 261–76.

6. Broekmans FJ, Kwee J, Hendriks DJ, Mol BW, Lambalk CB. A systematic review of

tests predicting ovarian reserve and IVF outcome. *Hum Reprod Update* 2006; **12**(6): 685–718.

7. Marin M, Güris D, Chaves S, Schmid S, Seward J. Prevention of Varicella. Recommendations of the Advisory Committee on Immunization Practices (ACIP). *MMWR* 2007; **56**(RR04): 1–40.

8. Cooper TG, Noonan E, von Eckardstein S, *et al.* World Health Organization reference values for human semen characteristics. *Hum Reprod Update* 2010; **16**(3): 231–45.

9. Dohle GR, Jungwirth A, Colpi G, *et al. Guidelines on Male Infertility.* European Association of Urology, 2007.

10. Oei SG, Helmerhorst FM, Bloemenkamp KW, *et al.* Effectiveness of the postcoital test: randomised controlled trial. *BMJ* 1998; **317**: 502.

11. Homan GF, Davies M, Norman R. The impact of lifestyle factors on reproductive performance in the general population and those undergoing infertility treatment: a review. *Hum Reprod Update* 2007; **13**(3): 209–23.

Female Fertility Assessment:

Medical record number:	

Surname   Given name(s)

D.O.B   Age   Religion   Marital Status

Height   Weight   **BMI**

m   kg   kg/m²

Subfertility: Primary ☐   Secondary ☐   Duration [   ] months

Previous fertility: Current relation ☐   Previous relations [   ]

Past Obstetric History: _____

Gynecology & Menstrual History:

Menarche [   ]   Cycles [/]   Regularity [   ]

Menstrual bleeding [   ]   Dysmenorrhea [   ]   Premenstrual symptoms [   ]

Cervical screening: date of last smear [   ]   Result [   ]

Contraceptive History: [   ]

Tubal Factors: IUD [   ]   STI [   ]   PID [   ]

Abdominopelvic surgery [   ]

Coital History: Frequency [   ]   Dysparunia [   ]   Fertile period [   ]

Past Medical History:

	Yes	No	Details
Diabetes			
Malignancy			
Other			

Medications	
Allergy	
Family history	
Occupation	

Healthy diet ☐   Exercise ☐   Mental health ☐

Smoking [/day]   Alcohol [Unit/week]   Recreational drugs ☐

Examination Findings:

General Examination _____

Secondary sexual characteristics: Breast development ☐   Hair distribution ☐

Pelvic examination: _____

Investigations:

Chlamydia screening	☐	Rubella	☐	Progesterone	☐
FSH	☐	LH	☐	Estradiol	☐
AMH	☐	Testosterone	☐	SHBG	☐
Free Androgen Index	☐	Prolactin	☐	TFT	☐

Ovulatory status [   ]

Ovarian ultrasound assessment

	R	L		R	L
Volume			Morphology		
AFC			Accessibility		
Pathology					

Comment: _____

Tubal Assessment: HSG ☐   HyCoSy ☐   Fertiloscopy ☐   Falloposcopy ☐
Laparoscopy & dye ☐

Uterine cavity ☐   Patent R tube ☐   L tube ☐
Intra-abdominal adhesions ☐   Endometriosis ☐   stage ☐

Comment: _____

Male Factor: Yes ☐   No ☐   Unexplained subfertility [Yes | No]

Management Plan: _____
_____
_____

Male Fertility Assessment

Medical record number: [   ]

Surname	Given Name(s)	D.O.B
[ ]	[ ]	[ ]

Partner's Surname	Given Name(s)	D.O.B
[ ]	[ ]	[ ]

Marital status [   ]   Duration [   ]

Subfertility   Primary [ ]   Secondary [ ]   Duration [Months]

Previous fertility: Current relation [   ]   Previous relations [   ]

Past Medical History:

	Yes	No	Details
Diabetes			
Malignancy			
Recent Pyrexia			
Other			

Infectious Disease:

STI [   ]   UTI [   ]   Epididymitis [   ]   Orchitis [   ]

Past Surgical History:

	Yes	No	Rt	Lt	Date	Comment
Maldescence of testes						
Varicocele ligation						
Vasectomy						Reversal
Genital injury/surgery						
General surgery						

Medications	
Allergy	
Family history	

Coital History:

Libido [   ]   Frequency [   ]   Erection [   ]

Ejaculation [   ]   Timing of intercourse: Random [   ]   Fertile phase [   ]

Occupation [   ]

Exercise [ ]   Smoking [ ] /day   Alcohol [ ] Unit/wk   Recreational drugs [   ]

Physical Examination:

General: _____

Weight	Height	BMI
kg	m	kg/m²

Androgen status [   ]   Gynaecomastia [   ]

Genital Examination:

Penis [   ]   Urethral meatus [   ]   Scrotum [   ]

	Rt	Lt	Comment
Testes			
Epididymis			
Vas deferens			
Varicocele			

Investigations:

Semen Analysis:

Semen volume	ml	Progressive motility	%
Total sperm number	million	Total motility	%
Sperm concentration	million/ml	Normal forms	%
Vitality	%		

Blood tests:

Testosterone [   ]   FSH [   ]   Cystic fibrosis screening [   ]

Prolactin [   ]   LH [   ]   Karyotyping [   ]

Ultrasound scan: _____

Testicular Biopsy: _____

Other: _____

Diagnosis: Normal [   ]   Abnormal [   ]

Principal: 1-

Secondary: 1-

2-

3-

Management Plan: _____

_____

_____

Investigation of the female patient

Anna Smirnova and Gab Kovacs

Usually investigation for infertility is carried out by gynecologists, because if a couple failed to conceive it has been traditionally expected that the woman has a problem and should visit a doctor. As described in Chapter 3 it is preferable to interview both partners together, but in some cases women prefer to answer questions about previous pregnancies, history of sexually transmitted infections and previous contraception in the absence of their partners.

The first subject for investigation is "is the couple really infertile" and the second subject is "what is the cause of infertility".

The duration of infertility is counted in months as the total number of consecutive months with unprotected intercourse. Months where contraception has been used as well as periods of abstinence and separation are subtracted. We expect that women under 35 years should become pregnant within 12 months of regular unprotected coitus. Women after 35 should be referred for investigation for infertility earlier – after 6 months of regular unprotected coitus without pregnancy. Patients with amenorrhea or sexual dysfunction should be investigated immediately.

Fertility declines with the increasing age of both partners, especially in women after 35 years and men after 50 years. Among women younger than 25, 75% had achieved pregnancy within six menstrual cycles, whereas only 25% of women older than 35 had achieved pregnancy in the same period of time.

A woman is considered to have primary infertility if she has never been pregnant. Secondary infertility is considered in a woman who previously has been pregnant in the same or in a previous relationship, independent of the pregnancy outcome.

The key points of investigation (as described in Chapter 1) are history, examination and investigations – ovulation assessment, assessment of tubal patency, tuboperitoneal lesions and intrauterine pathology which may affect implantation, and semen analysis. A clear schedule of examination should be planned at the first visit in order to make a diagnosis in a short period of time and avoid unnecessary and repetitive investigations.

According to data from a WHO study, 8.9% of couples achieved pregnancy during the period of investigation [1].

History

The general information about personal and medical history can be obtained from a questionnaire completed by the patient before consultation. The history that needs to be taken at the first interview is described in detail in Chapter 3.

The Subfertility Handbook: A Clinician's Guide, Second Edition ed. Gab Kovacs. Published by Cambridge University Press. © Cambridge University Press 2011.

Examination

The general examination starts when the patient comes into the consulting room from observations of body habitus, skin, hair excess, gait and posture. This has again been covered in Chapter 3.

The gynecological examination should be performed on all patients. External and internal genitalia are examined.

The vulva is inspected for evidence of normal anatomy, with particular reference to cliteromegaly (glans greater than 1 cm or clitor greater than 2 cm), labial fusion, and presence of inflammation or papillomas. Very rarely patients achieve reproductive age without a diagnosis of imperforate hymen or vaginal agenesis. Intact hymen is another rare finding in patients with infertility and usually indicates sexual difficulties with absence of vaginal intercourse. An assessment of hair and pigment distribution should be made with reference to the Tanner staging of pubic hair development (see Chapter 3). Vaginismus may be found in some women, which makes it impossible to examine the genitalia adequately.

Inspection of the vagina for the presence of any discharges is performed. A vaginal swab should be sent for microbiological examination if there is any sign of inflammation or infection. Tests for *Chlamidia trachomatis*, *N. gonorrhea* and *Mycoplasma genitalium* are necessary for diagnostic classification.

Lack of secretion and atrophy of vaginal mucus are common in estrogen-deficient women. Occasionally a vaginal septum may be found as a congenital abnormality.

The cervix is inspected for the shape, size and evidence of laceration, state of ectocervical and endocervical epithelium and evidence of normal cervical secretions for that stage of the menstrual cycle. A Pap-smear test is recommended to reveal any atypical cells or cervical dysplasia. Purulent discharges should be investigated by appropriate bacteriological microscopy and culture.

Bimanual palpation of the uterus and adnexa is carried out to assess the size, shape and consistency of the uterus as well as its mobility. A uterus may appear to be enlarged due to pregnancy, fibroids, adenomyosis, or multiparity. Obesity and retroversion make assessment difficult. The adnexa are examined for evidence of thickening of the utero-sacral ligaments which may be caused by endometriosis. Enlargement of an ovary or both ovaries may be found and their mobility and tenderness should be noted. In the case of pelvic tenderness questions about persistence of pain on physical examination in the past or pain with intercourse or on defecation or urination should be asked.

Ultrasonography is a more accurate method compared with bimanual examination so more precise data about ovaries and uterus may be obtained with a transvaginal ultrasound probe than with palpation.

Investigations

Ovulation assessment

The assessment of ovulation involves history, examination and investigation. Of couples who present with infertility up to 30% have disorders of ovulation.

A patient with a menstrual cycle of between 21 and 35 days, with bleeding lasting from 2 to 7 days, who experiences midcycle stretchy mucus and premenstrual breast tenderness is likely to be ovulatory.

Symptoms of ovulation

Premenstrual syndrome (mastalgia, swelling, pelvic pain, etc.) is caused by progesterone effects and suggests normal ovulatory menstrual cycles.

Regular midcycle pain (mittleschmerz) also suggests ovulation. It may be caused by bleeding from the ovulating follicle and irritation of peritoneal surfaces.

Cervical mucus consistency and viscosity change during follicular and luteal phases. The transparent, liquid and stretchy mucus can usually be noted before ovulation, indicating maximum fertility. After ovulation the thick, scant, viscous mucus is due to progesterone secretion [2].

The cervical score, which is correlated with the degree of follicle maturity and estrogen level, was described by V. Insler [3]. Each of the following factors is gauged by scoring from 0 to 3: the cervix should be open and the volume of mucus should be good (although every woman will be different in both these parameters, they will be consistent in one woman from ovulation to ovulation); the mucus should be clear, watery and stretchy; and the mucus should produce a complete "ferning" pattern when it is allowed to dry on a microscope slide. The first two criteria vary at ovulation in different women (so anything above a score of 9 or 10 can be normal), but the same woman should achieve a similar score from one ovulation to the next.

Investigations of ovulation

These include the measurement of basal body temperature (BBT), ultrasound monitoring, progesterone assay and luteinizing hormone (LH) assay, ultrasound follicular tracking and endometrial biopsy.

Basal body temperature

The average basal body temperature is elevated by 0.3 to 0.5 degrees during the luteal phase when compared with the follicular phase. This is a result of the progestogenic effect on the hypothalamus and it starts two days after the LH peak. It is important to measure the temperature immediately after awakening from uninterrupted sleep of at least 6 hours. Unfortunately this technique determines ovulation only retrospectively and has poor prognostic value, but it does help the timing of intercourse, or at least when intercourse need not be continued after the ovulatory rise.

Hormonal assays

Serum progesterone level must be estimated in every patient. Elevated serum progesterone (levels depending on local assays) is a presumptive sign of ovulation, but it doesn't allow an estimation of whether the follicle was ruptured or not. Luteinization of unruptured follicle (LUF syndrome) is characterized by all hormonal signs of ovulation but associated with infertility because the oocyte has not been released from the ovary.

Usually the progesterone is measured in the middle of the luteal phase (day 21 of a 28-day cycle) when the peak of progesterone secretion occurs. In patients with an irregular cycle serial weekly progesterone assays may be necessary. In women with a long regular cycle the progesterone level should be measured approximately seven days before the next menstrual period. If other parameters suggest ovulation but the progesterone level is lower than the ovulatory level, the test should be repeated in a subsequent cycle. A low progesterone level may be due to luteal phase deficiency.

Serum or urinary LH assay allows the determination of the LH "peak" which occurs 24–36 hours before ovulation. Urinary reagent strips are now available which enable patients to test their own urine with convenience, on a regular basis, with greater than 85% accuracy. The test should be carried out at the same time every day, starting three days before expected ovulation. Appearance of the intensely coloured second strip predicts ovulation in 12 to 36 hours. This technique is particularly useful for timing intercourse or artificial insemination.

Endometrial biopsy

Endometrial biopsy is another method of obtaining evidence of probable ovulation. A sample of endometrium aspirated from the uterine cavity in the luteal phase of the cycle should show adequate secretory transformation as a result of progesterone secretion by the corpus luteum. The microscopic picture of the endometrium correlates with the estrogen and progesterone levels, which enables dating of the endometrium with reference to the expected onset of the next menstrual period. For better interpretation of results the endometrial biopsy should be taken on the same day as the serum progesterone.

Luteal phase deficiency may lead to implantation failure or early pregnancy loss. The duration of a normal luteal phase is not less than 10 days. Delay of endometrial maturity assessed by microscopy by three or more days could be considered abnormal. The diagnosis of luteal phase deficiency should be based on abnormal findings in at least two cycles [4].

Current thought is that endometrial biopsy to evaluate the luteal phase should not be offered as there is no evidence that medical treatment of luteal phase defect improves pregnancy rates [5].

Ultrasound to assess ovulation

Repeated transvaginal ultrasound scans performed on different days of the same menstrual cycle allow detection of ovulation, and especially verification of the rupture of the follicle. This is the only method which enables the exclusion of the luteinization of unruptured follicle syndrome.

The preovulatory follicle is seen as a cystic echo-free structure within the ovary. It grows at a linear rate of 2–3 mm per day during 4–5 days and achieves a diameter of 17–25 mm at the time of ovulation. There is a linear correlation between the estrogen level, the size of the dominant follicle and the endometrium thickness. Ultrasound monitoring usually starts two or three days before expected ovulation and is repeated every other day until ovulation criteria are obtained.

Ultrasound features of ovulation are:

- collapse of the follicle with a decrease in the size
- complete disappearance of the follicle
- presence of fluid in the cul-de-sac
- multiple small echo-positive structures in the follicle (blood clots).

After ovulation features of the development of a corpus luteum are present. It appears sonographically as a hyperechogenic structure at the site of the former follicle. No fluid can be found in the cul-de-sac in the case of luteinization of unruptured follicle.

A difference exists between the endometrium in the follicular and luteal phases. In the early proliferative phase it is isoechogenic. Starting 5–6 days before ovulation there is a change from one to three echogenic lines together with an increasing hypoechogenic texture between the lines. At ovulation the endometrium has a thickness of 10–16 mm. Following ovulation the three endometrial lines become indistinguishable owing to increased hyper-echogenecity. Endometrial thickness at the time of ovulation of less than 6 mm is associated with a reduced pregnancy rate.

Endocrine profile

Hormonal assay might be necessary in patients with clinical features of ovarian, thyroid or adrenal dysfunction. The normal values and ranges for all the relevant hormones are different in each laboratory.

The prolactin level should be estimated in every infertile woman. The blood must not be taken early in the morning, after intercourse or breast or pelvic examination. If the level is higher than normal, the blood test for prolactin should be repeated once or twice within one month and the lowest value is taken into account. Repeated significant elevation (more than four times normal) requires imaging of the hypothalamo-pituitary region by X-ray, computer tomography (CT) or MRI to detect or exclude a pituitary or rarely hypothalamic tumor, especially if associated with amenorrhea.

Hyperprolactinemia may lead to galactorrhea. About one-quarter of patients with galactorrhea have hyperprolactinemia but galactorrhea may also occur in a woman with normal prolactin levels. Neuroleptic drugs, antidepressants, hypotensive drugs (reserpine, methyldopa) and drugs for treating gastrointestinal symptoms (cimetidine, metoclopramide, domperidone) may cause hyperprolactinemia. The elevated prolactin level may be associated with low FSH, LH and low/high TSH levels.

Thyroid dysfunction is strongly associated with infertility. The TSH and free thyroxin levels should be measured in women with amenorrhea, oligomenorrhea, polymenorrhea or hyperprolactinemia.

Serum FSH and LH levels should be measured in all patients with amenorrhea. In patients with primary amenorrhea and an elevated FSH level, karyotype examination should be undertaken and may reveal a chromosomal abnormality. In women with secondary amenorrhea an FSH level more than 30 IU/l indicates premature ovarian failure. Low FSH and estrogen levels are common in patients with hypogonadotropic hypogonadism.

The progestogen withdrawal test is useful in patients with secondary amenorrhea. Absence of vaginal withdrawal bleeding after a progestogen administered for 5–7 days orally or intramuscularly indicates a low endogenous estrogen level or intrauterine synechia (Asherman's syndrome).

Elevated serum androgen (testosterone, dehydroepiandrosterone, androstendione, etc.) levels may be found in women with ovarian dysfunction and hirsutism. Hyperandrogenemia may be of adrenal origin (congenital adrenal hyperplasia, Cushing's syndrome or adrenal tumor) or ovarian origin (polycystic ovarian syndrome, hyperthecosis, functional ovarian tumor, intersex with ovotestis).

Assessment of internal genitalia and tubal patency

Ultrasound examination of the pelvis is a first-step procedure in investigation of any case of infertility. A hysterosalpingogram is preferred to investigate tubal patency in women with no history of comorbidity. Alternatively, hysterosalpingo-contrast sonography should be offered where appropriate expertise is available. Both investigations can be done as an outpatient procedure.

A laparoscopy and dye test is more invasive but has higher diagnostic value and is the "gold standard", and should be offered to the woman at high risk of tubal and peritoneal adhesions. Fertiloscopy (transvaginal hydrolaparoscopy) with dye test is another technique to assess tubal patency. It can be done under local anesthetic as an outpatient procedure. Falloposcopy is a transvaginal endoscopy to assess the fallopian tube lumen.

Women without a history of pelvic inflammatory diseases, or sexually transmitted infections should be investigated by minimally invasive outpatient-based methods such as minihysteroscopy and transvaginal hydrolaparoscopy.

Women over 35 with suspected tubal or tuboperitoneal factor of infertility and long duration of infertility should be recommended to be treated directly by IVF.

The only true test of tubal function is pregnancy.

Hysterosalpingography (HSG)

The hysterosalpingography (HSG) may be used to assess uterine and tubal status in women under 35 years with normal ovulation whose partners have normospermia, who have been infertile for less than two years and have no past history of pelvic inflammatory disease or pelvic surgery.

At HSG radio-opaque dye is injected through the small canula via the cervix into the uterine cavity under X-ray screening. The uterine cavity is outlined and if the tubes are patent, the dye is seen to disperse into the peritoneal cavity. The HSG diagnoses the congenital uterine cavity abnormalities and acquired deformities such as polyps, submucous fibroids and intra-uterine adhesions. However, it doesn't make it possible to visualize the fimbriae, ovaries, extratubal adhesions and endometriosis.

Selective salpingography is available at HSG via a catheter placed in the uterine cornua or the first 1 cm of tube. It is a good diagnostic test for proximal tubal occlusion [6]. Tubal recanalization can be performed after selective salpingography under X-ray control.

An HSG should be performed only in the follicular phase of the menstrual cycle after cessation of menstrual bleeding till ovulation (days 6–12 of the menstrual cycle) to avoid X-ray radiation during undiagnosed early pregnancy.

An HSG can be painful in the case of partial or complete tubal obstruction because high pressure is necessary to minimize the risk of a false-positive result. An effective nonsteroidal anti-inflammatory drug (ibuprofen, naproxen, or diclofenac) should be given orally at least one hour before the procedure to decrease discomfort.

Contraindications include a history of pelvic inflammatory diseases, allergy to iodine, bleeding, acute infection, and pregnancy. The HSG should not be carried out during bleeding because of the risk of vascular embolism by oil contrast and the risk of endometrial cell dissemination into the peritoneal cavity. Blood clots in the uterine cavity may imitate polyps or fibroids.

If HSG shows an abnormal finding then laparoscopy or hysteroscopy should be performed. In women with normal HSG who are suspected of having unexplained infertility the laparoscopy should be omitted and cycles of ovarian stimulation and/or intrauterine insemination should be considered (see Chapter 9) before reverting to ART [7].

Ultrasound to assess pelvic normality

Ultrasound examination of ovaries, uterus and tubes is recommended for all infertile women. It is a non-invasive procedure that provides good anatomical information [8]. The investigation should be carried out in the early follicular phase between days 5 and 12 of a 28-day menstrual cycle. The use of a vaginal transducer is mandatory. It allows us to assess ovarian reserve and to reveal most of the pathological conditions associated with infertility such as:

1. ovarian origin: ovarian functional cysts, endometriomas, tumors, polycystic ovaries, premature ovarian failure
2. tubal origin: hydrosalpinx or sactosalpinx
3. uterine origin: congenital abnormalities, fibroids, endometrial polyps, uterine septum, intrauterine adhesions, adenomyosis.

Hysterosalpingo-contrast sonography (HyCoSy) is an alternative procedure for evaluation of uterine cavity pathology and tubal patency. Sterile saline can be used as an echo-negative contrast medium for the assessment of the uterine cavity. For the examination of fallopian tubes the echo-positive contrast agent containing micro-air bubbles is more efficient. Contraindications to HyCoSy include concurrent genital infection, heavy bleeding, and pregnancy.

The concordance between HyCoSy and HSG for the presence of endometrial cavity pathology is up to 90%, but for tubal patency the concordance is lower. HyCoSy classed more examinations of tubal patency as uncertain and HSG more frequently classified tubes as occluded [7]. Both methods had similar sensitivity, specificity, and diagnostic accuracy, but more women reported the pain associated with HyCoSy as mild to moderate. The HyCoSy procedure is well tolerated and can be used as a primary tool for the evaluation of tubal patency in infertile women [9].

Hysteroscopy

Diagnostic hysteroscopy is usually carried out by a 2–5 mm rigid or flexible hysteroscope which enables the direct visualization of the uterine cavity and cervical canal. Office hysteroscopy or mini-hysteroscopy with 2–2.5 mm hysteroscope is a very effective diagnostic procedure that may be performed without cervical dilatation and anesthesia on an outpatient basis. It is well tolerated, less painful and may be recommended for routine use in infertility work-up [10].

Saline solution given under controlled pressure is necessary for the distension of the uterine cavity. Visualization of the uterine cavity allows one to find endometrial abnormalities such as endometrial polyps, submucous fibroids, congenital septum, intrauterine synechia, and local areas of hyperplasia or malignancy. In patients with infertility, diagnostic hysteroscopy is usually combined with laparoscopy.

Contraindications include heavy bleeding, acute pelvic infection, carcinoma of the cervix or endometrium, and cervical stenosis. Complications are rare and include cervical trauma and uterine perforation. Carbon dioxide, which was previously popular, should no longer be used because of the risk of CO_2 embolism.

Laparoscopy

Laparoscopy and chromopertubation are the gold standard for the assessment of tubal patency and pelvic status. They enable direct visualization of the peritoneal cavity and internal genitalia through a 5–10 mm telescope inserted at the umbilicus.

During diagnostic laparoscopy the uterus is inspected for congenital or acquired lesions. The shape of the uterus, the presence, location and size of fibroids, and the presence of scars from previous surgery are recorded. Any adhesions should be noted, with assessment of density (filmy and translucent or dense and thick) and position.

Each tube should be investigated separately and if it is abnormal, the details are specified. The presence and position of constriction, fibrosis, nodularity, dilatation, endometriosis, and adhesions are described before injection of the dye. The fimbriae should be freely mobile, with full access to the whole ovarian surface and no agglutination of the folds or fimbriae themselves. Adhesions reduce fertility by impairing the movement of the fimbriae over the ovarian surface and by inhibiting the normal muscle segmentation that assists gamete and embryo transport.

The testing of tubal patency is performed by passing dye (methylene blue) via a cervical cannula into the uterine cavity and laparoscopically observing how it is flowing down the tube and out through the fimbria. If there is no spill of dye, the site of blockage is assessed. When no dye enters the tube a corneal or intramural block is suspected; when dye passes into the tube but there is no intraperitoneal spill, the site of block and/or dilatation is noted. Sometimes a tube with partial obstruction may be recorded as patent; however, it may have internal lesions that impair its function.

The assessment of ovaries includes their size and mobility, the thickness of the capsula, and the presence of corpus luteum, endometriosis, functional cysts or tumors.

Mild forms of endometriosis can only be diagnosed by direct inspection of pelvic organs by laparoscopy. The site, size, and extension of the endometriotic lesions are scored to determine the degree of endometriosis. All visualized endometriosis should be treated at the initial laparoscopic surgery by coagulation with the laser or diathermy or by surgical excision (see Chapter 16).

As with any surgery, diagnostic laparoscopy has a risk associated with general anesthesia, bleeding, infection, injury of internal organs, phlebitis and venous thromboses. CO_2 insufflation may cause gas embolism and soft tissue emphysema.

Transvaginal hydrolaparoscopy

Transvaginal hydrolaparoscopy (THL) or fertiloscopy is a new procedure to easily and rapidly explore the pelvis [11]. This technique is based on vaginal access to the pouch of Douglas using a needle puncture technique and saline media for distension. It was derived from the culdoscopy method, which was abandoned when laparoscopy showed its superiority in the 1970s. The employment of small-diameter laparoscopes has allowed re-evaluation of transvaginal access for infertility investigation.

Fertiloscopy improves the visualization of the tubo-ovarian structures because the access from the caudal pole with hydroflotation allows inspection of the organs in their normal position without manipulation. THL could be performed on an outpatient basis under local anesthesia. This may reduce the procedure's cost and the incidence of complications associated with general anesthesia. However, laparoscopy remains the gold standard to explore tuboperitoneal infertility or infertility associated with endometriosis.

The success rate of accessing the pouch of Douglas for THL is 90–95%, and the complication rate about 2–5%. The THL diagnosis correlates with that of laparoscopy in 92% of cases. Retroverted uterus should be considered as a relative contraindication to THL [12].

Falloposcopy

Falloposcopy [13] allows the direct visualization of the internal part of the tube using a flexible telescope passed through the cervix, across the uterine cavity and through the tubal ostia into the tube. Falloposcopy provides a unique possibility to visualize endotubal disease and may be used therapeutically for removal of debris and for cutting down filmy intratubal adhesions [14]. However, certain technical problems limit the usefulness of this method in routine clinical practice since it provides images of sufficient quality only in 10–60% of patients [15]. The requirement for considerable expertise and general anesthesia limits its usefulness as a screening test. It is generally concluded that it has not lived up to its expectations.

Genetic testing

Karyotypic analysis and genetic counseling are necessary in couples with recurrent pregnancy loss, stillbirth and in the case of any inherited disease in the family of either partner.

X-chromosome abnormalities may affect fertility in women with Turner syndrome, especially in mosaic form. All patients with primary amenorrhea and elevated FSH level should be recommended for leukocyte karyotype analysis.

Chromosomal translocations in the woman or in her partner significantly decrease the probability of live birth. If a couple with chromosomal translocation has infertility, in vitro fertilization with preimplantation diagnosis of all obtained embryos might be helpful. (This is discussed in detail in Chapter 11.)

Cervical factor testing

The post-coital test (PCT)

Interest in cervical mucus–sperm interaction goes back to the days of J. Marion Sims [16] in 1866, when he first described the inspection of post-coital cervical mucus for the presence of moving sperm. He concluded nearly 150 years ago that if moving sperm were present, then three conclusions could be drawn:

1. there were sperm present and the male was "not barren"
2. the cervix was in the right position to catch the sperm
3. the cervical secretions were not inimical to the spermatozoa.

His work was repeated by Max Huhner, an American urologist, in 1913 [17] and the test has been known ever since as the "Sims-Huhner Test". There have been two schools of thought about the value of the PCT. The proponents of the test maintain that "as the first requirement for pregnancy is that a number of motile sperm should reach the cervix" the PCT is one of the first tests to be undertaken. The critics say that at the time of the PCT, the sperm that is going to fertilize the oocyte should be well on its way to the Fallopian tube and one is looking at the "also rans". Whilst there has been debate about the value of the PCT as a diagnostic test, a study reported by us in 1978 showed that many fertile couples would fail if the criteria of "at least 10 motile sperm per high power field" were applied [18].

A more elegant method for testing sperm–mucus interaction was the in vitro sperm penetration test of Kremer [19], which can be modified to compare the partner's sperm penetration of pre-ovulatory mucus against donor sperm and donor mucus. Whilst the results are more scientific, except for believers of "cervical hostility", who believe in bypassing the cervix by using artificial insemination, the results have little clinical significance. This is discussed in more detail in Chapter 9.

As the treatment of unexplained subfertility, whether that is due to cervical factor (if it does exist) or some other transport mechanism, is usually IVF, tests for cervical factor are now rarely carried out, as they do not change the management.

References

1. Rowe PJ, Comhaire FH, Hargreave TB, Mellows HJ. *WHO Manual for the Standardized Investigation and Diagnosis of the Infertile Couple.* Cambridge University Press, 1993.

2. Billings EL, Brown JB, Billings JJ, Burger HG. Symptoms and hormonal changes accompanying ovulation. *Lancet* 1972; **1**: 282–4.

3. Insler V, Melmed H, Eichenbenner I, Serr D, Lunenfeld B. The cervical score. A semiquantitative method for monitoring the menstrual cycle. *Int J Gynaecol Obstet* 1972; **10**: 223–8.

4. Jones GS. The luteal phase defect. *Fertil Steril* 1976; **27**: 351–6.

5. Coutifaris C, Myers ER, Guzick DS, *et al.* Histological dating of timed endometrial biopsy tissue is not related to fertility status. *Fertil Steril* 2004; **82**: 1264–72.

6. Woolcott R, Fisher S, Thomas J, Kable W. A randomized, prospective, controlled study of laparoscopic dye studies and selective salpingography as diagnostic tests of fallopian tube patency. *Fertil Steril* 1999; **72**: 879–84.

7. Fatum M, Laufer N, Simon A. Investigation of the infertile couple: should diagnostic laparoscopy be performed after normal hysterosalpingography in treating infertility suspected to be of unknown origin? *Hum Reprod* 2002; **17**: 1–3.

8. Ekerhovd E, Fried G, Granberg S. An ultrasound-based approach to the assessment of infertility, including the evaluation of tubal patency. *Best Pract Res Clin Obstet Gynaecol* 2004; **18**: 13–28.

9. Strandell A, Bourne T, Bergh C, *et al.* The assessment of endometrial pathology and tubal patency: a comparison between the use of ultrasonography and X-ray hysterosalpingography for the investigation of infertility patients. *Ultrasound Obstet Gynecol* 1999; **14**: 200–4.

10. Hamed HO, Shahin AY, Elsamman AM. Hysterosalpingo-contrast sonography versus radiographic hysterosalpingography in the evaluation of tubal patency *Int J Gynaecol Obstet* 2009; **105**: 215–7.

11. Gordts S, Campo R, Rombauts L, Brosens I. Transvaginal hydrolaparoscopy as an outpatient procedure for infertility investigation. *Hum Reprod* 1998; **13**: 99–103.

12. Darai E, Dessolle L, Lecuru F, *et al.* Transvaginal hydrolaparoscopy compared with laparoscopy for the evaluation of infertile women: a prospective comparative blind study. *Hum Reprod* 2000; **15**: 2379–82.

13. Kerin JF. Falloposcopy: antegrade imaging in the management of oviductal disease. *J Am Assoc Gynecol Laparosc* 1996; **3** (Supplement): S21.

14. Kovacs GT, Kerin J, Scudamore I, Wood C. Falloposcopy – a non invasive method of salpingostomy case report. *Gynaec Endosc* 1992; **1**: 159–60.

15. Lundberg S, Rasmussen C, Berg AA, Lindblom B. Falloposcopy in conjunction with laparoscopy: possibilities and limitations. *Hum Reprod* 1998; **13**: 1490–2.

16. Sims JM. *Clinical Notes on Uterine Surgery with Special Reference to the Management of the Sterile Condition.* London: Robert Harwicke, 1866.

17. Huhner M. *Sterility in the Male and Female and Its Treatment.* New York: Rebman, 1913.

18. Kovacs GT, Newman GB, Henson GL. The post-coital test: what is normal? *Brit Med J* 1978; **1**: 803.

19. Kremer J, Jager S. The sperm-cervical mucus contact test: a preliminary report. *Fertil Steril* 1976; **27**: 335–40.

Assessment of the male partner

Wayland Hsiao and Peter N. Schlegel

Introduction

Infertility affects up to 15% of couples, with a male factor being the primary or contributing cause in 40–60% of infertility cases. It is important that the male partner should be evaluated concurrently with the female partner. In addition to detecting treatable abnormalities from a fertility standpoint, evaluation of the infertile man is critical to uncover life-threatening problems associated with the symptoms of infertility as well as genetic conditions associated with male infertility that can be transmitted to offspring with the use of assisted reproduction.

This is an exciting time in male infertility; advances in diagnostic testing and refinements in surgical technique have allowed us to treat an increasing number of men once deemed subfertile or ever sterile. With the advent of intracytoplasmic sperm injection (ICSI), men who previously had almost no hope for reproductive success can now be successfully treated with extracted testicular sperm. It is imperative that the modern infertility practitioner has a thorough understanding of the advantages and limitations of various laboratory tests as well as the indications, costs, and success rates of all treatment options.

History and physical examination

A complete history and physical exam is the cornerstone of the evaluation of the infertile male. A complete medical history including any systemic diseases along with current or previous medical and surgical treatments should be noted. Diabetes, thyroid dysfunction, and renal insufficiency are a few of the systemic medical diseases that may impact fertility potential. It takes nearly three months for a stem cell within the testis to proceed through two meiotic divisions, morphologically mature, and travel through the reproductive tract. Therefore, special attention should be paid to systemic illness and high fevers over the last three months, which may cause transient but substantial declines in sperm quality and quantity.

A complete and thorough sexual history is also essential. It should start with a developmental history regarding the onset and progression of puberty since abnormalities may suggest an endocrine cause of infertility. A history of sexually transmitted diseases should be elicited in addition to a history of orchitis or mumps orchitis after puberty. Also, any urological history or history of urologic procedures and surgeries is relevant and should be obtained. Most importantly, a detailed reproductive history including the duration of the problem, previous pregnancies (with current or previous partners), partners' previous pregnancies, frequency and timing of intercourse, erectile function, ejaculatory function, prior methods of birth control, use of vaginal lubricants, and the results of any previous

The Subfertility Handbook: A Clinician's Guide, Second Edition ed. Gab Kovacs. Published by Cambridge University Press. © Cambridge University Press 2011.

fertility evaluation for the patient and his partner are all necessary information to be gathered by the practitioner. Particularly, the use of lubricants should be actively questioned. Some commercially available lubricants such as K-Y Jelly have been shown to inhibit sperm motility, whereas egg whites and vegetable and mineral oils do not appear to have this detrimental effect. There are also commercially available lubricants that do not inhibit sperm motility [1]. Finally, an evaluation of erectile dysfunction and Peyronie's disease may be helpful as these may interfere with sexual activity.

All surgical procedures are relevant to the evaluation of the infertile male, but special attention should be paid to inguinal, scrotal, or urethral surgeries. One of the most common surgeries seen in this setting is orchidopexy performed for cryptorchidism (undescended testis) during childhood. In these patients, low sperm density has been reported in 30% of adults with a history of unilateral cryptorchidism and 50% with bilateral cryptorchidism [2]. The subsequent low fertility potential of these testes may arise from inherently poor testicular quality, iatrogenic obstruction, or testicular ischemia after surgery. Interestingly, it seems that any abnormality or trauma affecting the testis on one side can have deleterious effects on the contralateral "normal" testis as well. For example, torsion, testis cancer or varicocele can all cause abnormal results on semen analysis despite an apparent unilateral abnormality, most likely due to an immunological mechanism [3].

Any operative procedure performed in the inguinal or scrotal region should raise suspicion for vasal injury or testicular artery injury resulting in testicular atrophy. Inguinal hernia repair, performed at any point in life, is a common cause of iatrogenic obstruction and testicular atrophy. Even minor procedures such as testis biopsies or sperm extraction procedures may cause testicular atrophy. Another important point of history to elicit is a history of retroperitoneal surgery. The sympathetic nerves responsible for ejaculation travel down the retroperitoneum before entering the pelvis and innervating the reproductive organs. Therefore, any surgery of the retroperitoneum or pelvis may adversely affect emission or ejaculation. Surgical procedures performed on the prostate or bladder neck can also cause problems with emission and ejaculation.

Finally, exposure to potential gonadotoxins should be identified. Alcohol, tobacco, caffeine, radiation, chemotherapy (especially alkylating agents), marijuana, and anabolic steroids may all adversely affect spermatogenesis. Medications, including cimetidine, sulfa drugs, nitrofurantoin, cholesterol-lowering agents, serotonin reuptake inhibitors and calcium channel blockers, have also been thought to impair semen quality. Environmental exposures including excessive scrotal exposure to heat by routine use of saunas or hot tubs should be discouraged. Undergarment type does not seem to significantly affect sperm production.

Physical examination

A complete physical examination includes an examination of the head, neck, heart, lungs, abdomen, extremities, and nervous system. The full body should be examined with special attention paid to body habitus, limb length, and degree of virulization. Any surgical scars are noted, with special attention paid to the inguinal regions. Sometimes, surgical scars are found from infant or childhood surgeries that the patient forgot to mention or did not know about.

The genital exam should start with an evaluation of the penile skin for any indication of sexually transmitted diseases. Additionally, visualization of white patches may indicate balanitis xerotica obliterans, which can cause severe urethral stricturing. The position and patency of the urethral meatus should be noted since hypospadias may impair the man's ability to deposit an ejaculate deep in the vaginal vault near the cervix. The shaft of the penis is palpated for Peyronie's disease plaques or fibrotic thickening. The testes are examined for size, tenderness as well as consistency. A normal testis is over 4 cm in the long axis and has a volume greater than 16 ml. The seminiferous tubules contain the spermatogenic region of the testis and occupy 80% of its volume. Abnormally soft testis may indicate impairment of spermatogenesis.

The epididymis is palpated next. Any unusual fullness, induration, or tenderness may indicate previous or current infection which can result in epididymal obstruction. The vas is a firm usually easily palpable structure in the cord and should be palpated along its course to evaluate for any areas of discontinuity. Absence of the vas may be due to congenital absence or subsequent atresia. These patients may have a higher incidence of seminal vesicle or renal anomaly.

Varicoceles can also be found on exam of the cord and have been found in up to 40% of men presenting with subfertility. Examination of varicoceles should be performed with the patient standing as well as in the supine position. The patient should be examined in a warm room and it may be helpful to place a heating pad on the scrotum prior to examination to relax the cremasteric muscles. The severity of varicoceles is graded on the following scale: Grade I is palpable only during Valsalva maneuver; Grade II is palpable in the standing position; and Grade III is visible through the scrotal skin. Benign varicoceles should decompress with the patient in the supine position. If a patient has an isolated right varicocele or bilateral varicocele which does not decompress when supine, one should consider imaging of the retroperitoneum to evaluate for retroperitoneal pathology.

The exact mechanism of varicocele-induced infertility remains unknown. Varicoceles may cause testicular dysregulation due to elevated intratesticular temperature, relative hypoxia due to poor venous drainage, dilution of intratesticular testosterone, reflux of adrenal and renal metabolites down the spermatic cord, or increased oxidative stress. However, spermatogenesis in the testes and maturation in the epididymis are highly sensitive to even minor elevations in temperature, and the effect of varicoceles on scrotal temperature has garnered the most support.

The final portion of the exam consists of a digital rectal exam to examine the prostate. Particular attention should be paid to the size and consistency of the prostate gland. A tender or indurated prostate may indicate prostatitis. The seminal vesicles can also be palpated past the base of the prostate and it should be noted whether they are dilated. A markedly dilated seminal vesicle may require further radiological evaluation including a transrectal ultrasound.

Though rare, there are several syndromes relevant to the work-up of the infertile man. Kartagener's syndrome is clinically characterized by situs inversus, frequent respiratory infection and immotile sperm. It is caused by a defective microtubule arrangement in the axoneme of cilia and sperm tails. Without the use of ICSI, reproduction is only rarely reported. Kallmann's syndrome is associated with anosmia, lack of secondary sexual characteristics, and disproportionately long arms and results in hypogonadotropic hypogonadism. It is caused by a failure of gonadotropin releasing hormone (GnRH) secreting neurons to migrate to the hypothalamus during development, which impairs GnRH secretion by the hypothalamus. Treatment in the fertility-seeking patient consists of hormone replacement with human chorionic gonadotropin (hCG) and FSH. It is notable that these patients may be severely osteoporotic given their long history of hypogonadism so it would be prudent to obtain a bone density scan regularly on these patients. Finally, Klinefelter's syndrome is the most common sex chromosome abnormality seen. It is caused by meiotic non-disjunction in developing oocytes or sperm with a resulting 47,XXY karyotype. It is characterized by undervirilization, small firm testes, gynecomastia, and taller than average stature. Of note, these patients develop spermatogenesis at puberty, but the tubules then undergo progressive degeneration, eventually resulting in non-obstructive azoospermia. We have recently reported a 68% sperm retrieval rate in Klinefelter's syndrome patients with non-obstructive azoospermia utilizing microdissection testicular sperm extraction [4].

Laboratory studies

Semen analysis

The semen analysis is critical in the initial evaluation of the infertile man and to a large extent guides further work-up. Substantial fluctuations in seminal quality can occur even in properly collected samples. Therefore, we prefer to see at least two or three separate specimens collected over several months, each with a consistent 48 to 72 hour abstinence period. The entire sample is collected in a cup by masturbation and transported at body temperature (in the patient's pocket) to the lab in less than one hour. Alternatively, collection can take place in the office/clinic so that transport time is minimized.

The physical appearance of the specimen is evaluated including the color, volume, viscosity, pH and liquefaction. Freshly ejaculated semen coagulates and then gradually liquefies over 20 minutes. The seminal vesicles are responsible for 50–80% of the volume of the ejaculate. Its secretions are basic and contain high levels of fructose produced through an androgen-dependent process and are responsible for coagulation of semen. Prostatic secretions are rich in zinc, prostate specific antigen, acid phosphatases and slightly acidic. They are responsible for liquefaction of semen. Patients with seminal vesicle obstruction or absence will have a fructose-negative, low-volume, low-pH ejaculate that does not coagulate. However, the most common cause of low-volume ejaculate is incomplete collection.

Microscopic evaluation of the semen sample is necessary to determine sperm concentration, motility, and morphology. However, when evaluating semen parameters, one must keep in mind that the average semen parameters for normal fertile men far exceed the threshold necessary for conception. Therefore, when discussing semen parameters, one usually refers to "limits of adequacy" rather than "normal values" (Table 5.1). This highlights

Table 5.1 Semen analysis; minimal standards

Volume	1.5–5 ml
Density	> 20 million sperm/ml
Motility	> 50%
Forward progression	> 2 (scale 0–4) or > 30% motile
Morphology	> 30 % World Health Organization criteria > 15% Kruger criteria
Leukocytes	< 1 million
Absence of: significant agglutination, hyperviscosity	

an important difference between subfertility and sterility. As semen quality declines below the limits of adequacy, the chances of pregnancy statistically decrease, but never reach zero, theoretically, until a total absence of motile sperm is demonstrated, at which point the patient is considered sterile without assisted reproduction.

If no sperm are found on routine analysis, the specimen is centrifuged at $3000 \times g$ for 15 minutes and the pellet is resuspended in 10–200 μl volume for further inspection. Absence of sperm in the pellet makes a definitive diagnosis of azoospermia. An extended sperm preparation, allowing detailed microscopic analysis of all portions of this centrifuged semen pellet, may allow detection of rare sperm in men with severely impaired sperm production. At this point, it is important to make the distinction between aspermia (lack of ejaculation or emission) and azoospermia (lack of sperm in an ejaculated sample). Aspermia represents a failure of emission or ejaculation. Spinal cord injury, diabetes mellitus, and multiple sclerosis can cause aspermia as well as retroperitoneal surgery or an inability to reach orgasm. Azoospermia represents either reproductive tract obstruction or a defect in sperm production.

After the sperm count is assessed, the next step involves assessment of motility and morphology. Sperm morphology is usually assessed with either the Kruger criteria or the World Health Organization criteria. Abnormal morphology is referred to as teratospermia. Motility is the amount of flagellar motion and forward motion that a sperm makes. It is best assessed within 1–2 hours of ejaculation. The most commonly used system grades motility on a scale of 0–4. Zero indicates no motility; one denotes sluggish motion with no forward progression; two denotes slow forward progression; three indicates sperm moving in a straight line at a moderate speed; four is moving in a straight line at great speed. If motility is low ($< 30\%$) a viability stain should be performed. Determination of the proportion of viable sperm is important since intracytoplasmic sperm injection (ICSI) is often successful using immotile sperm so long as they are viable. There are two general approaches to viability testing, traditional staining versus the hypo-osmotic swell test. In traditional viability staining, washed sperm are exposed to dyes which penetrate dead sperm but are not taken up in viable sperm. The viability is expressed as a percentage of viable sperm. Unfortunately, stained spermatozoa are destroyed by traditional staining processes and cannot be used for ICSI, thus our estimate of viability is used to estimate the subsequent success of ICSI using unstained sperm. In the second approach, sperm are exposed to a hypo-osmotic solution which causes cellular swelling and a characteristic bulging of the sperm membranes. In fertile males, about 80% of sperm should swell in a hypo-osmotic swell test [5]. The advantage of this approach is that the sperm remain viable and can be used for ICSI. Correlation of this test with SPA and IVF results has been inconsistent [6].

A complete microscopic examination should include an analysis of "round cells", which represent either immature germ cells or leukocytes. While a Pap smear is routinely used during semen analysis, this stain does not distinguish between white blood cells and immature germ cells. A peroxidase stain is a better test for detecting leukocytes, but it has the disadvantage of only identifying granulocytes, not lymphocytes or macrophages. Immunohistochemical techniques are now available which make use of monoclonal antibodies directed against WBC surface antigens [7]. This allows more consistent and accurate evaluation of round cells. It is clinically relevant to make the distinction between leukocytes and immature germ cells because abnormally high levels of leukocytes are suggestive of infection which should be treated with systemic antibiotics. Pyospermia (10^6 leukocytes/ml) should be evaluated further with bacterial cultures including analysis for *Mycoplasma*

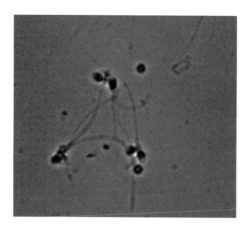

Figure 5.1 Sperm agglutination.

hominis, *Ureaplasma urealyticum* and *Chlamydia trachomatis*. Empirical use of antibiotics for pyospermia has not been shown to have any better chance of decreasing the number of white cells than placebo therapy.

Finally, the semen specimen can be evaluated for sperm agglutination (Figure 5.1). This finding is not uncommon and frequently represents an artifact of specimen collection or processing. For example, when sperm are present at high concentrations, they may appear to agglutinate. Dilution of the semen specimen will allow accurate evaluation of the presence or absence of agglutination. However, persistent agglutination may suggest the presence of antisperm antibodies, which can be performed with further testing for antisperm antibodies.

Urine studies

A urine analysis should be obtained in any patient with symptoms of urinary frequency or urgency, prior infections or suspected anatomic abnormalities. The presence of > 50 WBC/HPF on microscopic exam is suggestive of urinary tract infection and should be followed by a urine culture. Clinically, if infection of the prostate is suspected, a pre- and post-prostatic massage urine can be sent separately for culture. Sterile urine on the pre-massage urine and bacterial growth in the post-massage urine strongly suggest prostatic infection if there is a high enough clinical index of suspicion for prostatitis. If both cultures show growth, then a bladder or kidney source should be considered. Persistent microscopic hematuria (> 3 RBC per HPF on two of three properly collected specimens) or gross hematuria will require urological examination to evaluate for malignancy. Finally, and most importantly for fertility, a postejaculatory urine specimen should be microscopically examined for the presence of spermatozoa in men with low volume, azoospermic semen specimens unless a cause of azoospermia has already been identified. The presence of sperm (> 10/HPF or 20% antegrade ejaculated sperm) in the urine is suggestive of retrograde ejaculation in an oligospermic male. The presence of any sperm at all in the urine of an azoospermic male provides a diagnosis of retrograde ejaculation.

Hormonal studies

Normal spermatogenesis, maturation, and transport require a functioning hypothalamic-pituitary testicular hormonal axis. The first step in this cascade is the pulsatile release of

GnRH by the hypothalamus, which stimulates the release of luteinizing hormone (LH) and follicle stimulating hormone (FSH) from the anterior pituitary. LH stimulates testosterone production in the Leydig cells. FSH acts on the Sertoli cells to maintain spermatogenesis. Conversely, Sertoli cells release inhibin, which modulates FSH release in a negative feedback loop. Also, estradiol and testosterone inhibit LH in a negative feedback loop. Estradiol is formed from testosterone by the enzyme aromatase, which is present in a number of cell types.

Serum FSH reflects the number of Sertoli and germ cells, thereby reflecting the completeness of spermatogenesis in the seminiferous tubules [8]. So a man with normal spermatogenesis in a solitary testis may have a marginally elevated FSH. However, a man with non-obstructive azoospermia associated with diffuse maturation arrest and normal-volume testes will typically have a normal serum FSH level but may have no sperm present whatsoever within the testes. In addition, a man with diffuse Sertoli cell only pattern but isolated pockets of spermatogenesis will typically have an elevated FSH but have an excellent chance of sperm retrieval with testicular sperm extraction (TESE), whereas with maturation arrest (despite a frequently normal FSH), no mature sperm are often found despite intensive efforts at TESE.

Although only 3% of male infertility cases are due to a primary hormonal problem in most clinical series [9], at a minimum, an FSH level and testosterone level should be measured in the work-up of an infertile male. If the FSH level is more than 2–3 times normal values, the patient has some degree of testicular failure and the chance of finding obstruction is very low. High FSH, however, is not a contraindication for microdissection TESE and we have found that FSH level is not related to sperm retrieval in our experience with microdissection testicular sperm extraction [10].

Patients with primary testicular failure (hypergonadotropic hypogonadism) may have low testosterone coupled with significantly elevated gonadotropins, especially FSH, due to the absence of negative feedback. Conversely, if both testosterone and FSH are low, it is most likely due to hypothalamic or pituitary dysfunction. LH and prolactin levels should then be obtained. Prolactin is a pituitary hormone which can decrease LH release and impairs libido if present in excess. Elevated prolactin levels can be idiopathic or due to macroadenomas of the pituitary. If prolactin levels are normal, then low levels of LH, FSH, and testosterone confirm the diagnosis of hypogonadotropic hypogonadism, which suggests pituitary dysfunction caused by pituitary tumor, pituitary adenoma, or Kallman's syndrome. Symptoms such as severe headaches or impaired visual fields should raise clinical suspicion of a macroadenoma and warrant further work-up including an MRI of the brain.

Genetic tests

Karyotype analysis and microdeletion analysis of the Y chromosome are indicated for men with severe oligospermia or azoospermia ($< 10 \times 10^6$ sperm/ml) because of the common detection of genetic anomalies in men with low sperm production [11]. Of men with non-obstructive azoospermia, 15–27% will have definable genetic abnormalities using a screen for Y chromosome microdeletions and standard karyotype analysis. Both are analyzed from peripheral blood leukocytes. Karyotype abnormalities include Klinefelters's syndrome, other sex chromosome anomalies (e.g. XXY), and autosomal translocations. The Y chromosome microdeletion assay is a PCR-based assay. Common defects include deletions of the AZFb, AZFc or AZFa regions of the Y chromosome. For men who have AZFc deletions, sperm are commonly found in the ejaculate or with TESE. So, a detailed search of the ejaculated, centrifuged semen specimen is critical before performing a potentially unnecessary surgical attempt to retrieve sperm from the testes. In contrast, men with AZFa or AZFb deletions are highly unlikely to have sperm found even with extensive TESE procedures [12] and these men should be referred to adoption or the use of donor sperm.

Another genetic test available is for the cystic fibrosis (CF) gene. Men with congenital bilateral absence of the vas deferens (CBAVD) are usually carriers of cystic fibrosis gene mutations, and testing of the female partner is mandatory before proceeding to sperm retrieval with assisted reproduction. CBAVD is also associated with a 10–15% rate of detection of renal anomalies (agenesis or malascent.) Men with idiopathic epididymal obstruction are also frequently carriers of CF gene mutations. If the female partner is a carrier as well, then the chance of having a CF child may approach 50%. If a genetic anomaly is detected, genetic counseling is mandatory before processing to treatment with assisted reproduction. In some cases, preimplantation genetic diagnosis can be used to analyze each embryo during IVF to avoid transfer of genetically abnormal embryos. This process can minimize the risks of transmission of genetic anomalies.

Computer-assisted semen analysis

Computer-assisted semen analysis (CASA) has been developed to overcome the highly subjective nature of conventional analysis of sperm morphology and quality [13]. Advanced time exposure photomicrography, multiple exposure photomicrography, and videomicrography coupled with computer-based analysis have made automated analysis of sperm possible. Like conventional analysis, CASA evaluates sperm count, motility, and morphology. Sperm density can also be measured but superiority over conventional sperm analysis has not been demonstrated. In fact, CASA is far inferior to visual evaluation of sperm concentration for severely oligospermic men. Azoospermic men may be incorrectly classified as having sperm in the ejaculate by CASA. In terms of motility, curvilinear velocity, straight-line velocity, and amplitude of lateral head displacement are commonly reported. CASA also allows the quantification of sperm motility and identification of "hyperactivated" motility, which may also yield insight into the fertilizing capacity of sperm. CASA provides a great deal of detailed information but the value of this tool outside the research laboratory remains to be convincingly demonstrated.

Post-coital test

For natural conception, sperm must travel through cervical mucus to fertilize the ova. The post-coital test evaluates the interaction between sperm and the cervical mucus environment in the woman. Cervical mucus is obtained just prior to ovulation but several hours after sexual intercourse. Cervical mucus is clear and thin just prior to ovulation. The specimen is considered normal if microscopic findings show more than 10 sperm per HPF and 50% or more have progressive motility. Indications for this test include hyperviscous semen, unexplained infertility, extremes of ejaculate volume with good sperm density, and abnormal penile anatomy. Patients with poor-quality semen analysis do not require a post-coital test since results are invariably poor.

By corroborating the results of the post-coital test with the standard semen analysis, one can localize the abnormality to cervical mucus function or male deposition of semen. Variations in this test include cross mucus hostility testing. In this variation, the wife's mucus is placed in contact with both her husband's sperm and normal donor sperm for in vitro comparison. If the interaction is normal with the donor sperm and abnormal with the male partner's sperm, then there is a specific factor hindering that man's sperm. Another variation of this test involves the use of bovine cervical mucus, thereby removing the female factor entirely. The motility of sperm in human and bovine mucus is similar. If post-coital testing shows cervical or male deposition factors, then these couples will most likely benefit from further testing of antisperm antibodies. However, it is also possible to go to IVF or IUI depending on the sperm density.

Antisperm antibody testing

In light of an abnormal post-coital test or in cases of idiopathic infertility, antisperm antibody testing may be obtained. A blood–testis and blood–epididymal barrier exists which prevents exposure of sperm to the immune system. Any insult to the testicle, epididymis, or spermatic cord structures can lead to antibody formation. When these barriers are breached, the sperm may be detected by the man's immune system as "foreign" and antisperm antibody production occurs. An association between antisperm antibodies and infertility has been apparent for many years. Conditions associated with antibody formation include vasectomy, infection, reproductive tract obstruction, testicular cancer, testis biopsy, testicular torsion, cryptorchidism, and varicoceles. Indications for antibody testing include the presence of abnormal sperm agglutination, impaired motility, an abnormal post-coital test or unexplained infertility.

Higher rates of antisperm antibodies occur in infertile men and pregnancy rates are significantly lower for couples with high titers of antisperm antibodies [14]. Various studies have shown that the antibodies of greatest importance are bound to the sperm surface. Antibodies to internal sperm antigens and those found only in serum are of questionable clinical significance.

A number of techniques are available to detect antisperm antibodies. The most widely used and most accurate method is the direct immunobead assay (e.g. Sperm Check Biorad Laboratories, Hercules, CA, USA). Direct tests of antisperm antibodies involve the addition of rabbit anti-human Ig-coated microbeads one μm in size (of either polyacrylamide or latex). Washed sperm are mixed with these beads and binding is evaluated with a phase-contrast or bright field microscopy. An indirect assay can be performed in either a man or a woman and involves mixing donor sperm with the subject's serum. This is then subsequently exposed to anti-human Ig-coated microbeads and again analysis is done with microscopy. The mixed agglutination reaction (SpermMar test, Ortho Diagnostic Systems, Beerse, Belgium) is performed by mixing unwashed patient sperm with red blood cells coated with human antibodies. If antibodies are present, agglutination of RBCs occurs when anti-human antiserum is added. Enzyme-linked immunosorbent assays (ELISA) are also available and easy to use but false-positive results have been problematic.

Sperm function tests

Although sperm may be present in adequate numbers, with normal motility and morphology, there is no guarantee that the sperm are functionally competent to fertilize an ovum. Therefore, several tests of sperm function have been developed. Each has shortcomings but may be useful in certain clinical or experimental situations. In clinical practice, these tests are rarely used or indicated, since the application of ICSI has become so readily available and successful.

Species-specific fertilization is regulated by the zona pellucida, an acellular glycoprotein layer that surrounds the ovum. This layer can be removed, allowing for evaluation of sperm–oocyte interaction using a sperm penetration assay (SPA). The SPA is the most commonly performed sperm function test. In this test, human sperm are combined with hamster oocytes in vitro. A positive (normal) SPA requires that a sperm be capable of capacitation, the acrosome reaction, fusion with the oolemma, and incorporation into the ooplasm. The total number of ova penetrated and the number of penetrations per ova are determined. Normal results vary by laboratory but, in general, 10% of eggs penetrated and greater than five penetrations per egg are considered desirable. The SPA is a nonstandardized bioassay and results have been variable.

The variability in results has led to substantial controversy surrounding indications for SPA and interpretation of results. SPA results correlate with semen analysis, especially motility in most studies and with in vitro fertilization rates [15]. Patients with a positive SPA have a 95% chance of fertilizing human ova in vitro, while patients with a negative SPA have a 50% chance [16]. Other studies have suggested a correlation between SPA results and natural pregnancy as well [17]. However, we rarely apply the SPA in evaluation of infertile men at Weill Cornell since it is uncommon to have this test provide novel information that is not available from standard semen analyses. In addition, SPA is an expensive test that rarely changes clinical management of couples with male infertility. Occasional situations when the SPA may be indicated include cases of unexplained infertility and for couples considering assisted reproduction with IVF where there are borderline indications for intracytoplasmic sperm injection (ICSI). SPA testing is, however, unnecessary when there are clear indications present to proceed with ICSI.

Another less commonly performed test of sperm function is the hemizona assay, which measures the ability of sperm to interact with the zona pellucida, a prerequisite for fertilization. The human zona pellucida is micromanipulated and microscopically divided in half. Each half is then mixed with either the patient's sperm or the sperm of a fertile donor. An index is obtained by counting the total number of sperm bound divided by the number of donor sperm bound to the zona pellucida. A hemizona index less than 60% correlates with decreased chance of successful IVF [18]. The need for human ova is a significant limitation to the usefulness of this procedure. More importantly, the hemizona assay provides limited information that will affect clinical treatment, and this test is not performed often with the advent of ICSI.

Capacitation and the acrosome reaction are other necessary steps for normal fertilization. It is possible to use light microscopy or transmission electron microscopy to identify sperm that undergo the acrosome reaction [19,20]. This information could be used to identify the subgroup of patients whose infertility is secondary to abnormalities in the acrosome reaction. Many of these men are typically treated with ICSI. Of note, many of these men may have already been identified as candidates for ICSI based on severely abnormal morphology.

Sperm DNA fragmentation testing

Largely, sperm can be thought of as highly specialized cells whose purpose is to carry the genetic code intact to the oocyte. During sperm maturation, histones (DNA binding proteins) are replaced with protamine and DNA is tightly packaged to resist DNA damage during conception. Obviously, the use of sperm in IVF or ICSI with grossly abnormal DNA is of concern. Though, in many cases, sperm from semen samples with poor DNA integrity often have abnormal motility, low concentration and abnormal morphology, DNA fragmentation has come to be recognized as the single male factor identified to date that provides predictive information on the chance of successful IVF and ICSI.

Several tests allow assessment of the integrity of DNA within spermatozoa. The TUNEL assay detects the number of DNA breaks within the spermatozoa. The nicked ends of DNA in sperm undergoing apoptosis are identified by terminal deoxynucleotidyl transferase that incorporates dUTP that is conjugated to a fluorescent marker. Results are normally reported as a percentage of sperm with uptake of the tracer. Normal men will typically have DFI (DNA fragmentation index) values less than 10%, but the 30% cut-point has generally been used as a predictive factor for the chance of successful pregnancy with natural intercourse, IUI or IVF/ICSI. In the Comet assay, sperm are placed on an agarose gel, lysed and an electric field is applied, resulting in a "tail" of DNA migrating in the gel. Increased DNA damage results in increased tail length and fluorescence. Unfortunately, this test is not as repeatable as other DNA fragmentation assays.

The sperm chromatin structural assay (SCSA) is an indirect test of DNA fragmentation. It is based on the assumption that damaged DNA chromatin will denature more easily than normal DNA when exposed to acid. The marker acridine orange binds to DNA and is red when it binds to single-stranded DNA and green when it binds to normal double-stranded DNA. Cells are then counted and sorted in a flow cytometer. Results of this test have been correlated with fertilization and pregnancy rates using assisted reproduction.

Meta-analysis of data from published series has suggested that abnormal sperm DNA fragmentation (> 30%) predicts a higher chance of IVF or ICSI failure, even if female age is not controlled. There is also some evidence that high DFI may affect embryo development and miscarriage rates [21,22]. However, no level of abnormal DNA integrity has been identified that precludes any chance of success with IVF or ICSI. The effect of high DFI values (by TUNEL or SCSA) on IVF and ICSI outcomes remains controversial. For fertile men, DNA integrity testing is rarely below a threshold of 30% DFI, whereas men with normal semen parameters and infertility have abnormal DFI in 8% of cases.

Testicular biopsy

An understanding of testicular histology is mandatory for any practitioner of male reproductive medicine. A testicular biopsy is indicated for the evaluation of azoospermic men with palpable vasa and normal FSH levels (< 7.6 IU/L) to differentiate ductal obstruction from abnormal spermatogenesis. It can be accomplished under general or local anesthesia through a small window scrotal incision. Needle biopsy has been performed, but a percutaneous needle biopsy provides so few tubules for analysis that the clinical usefulness of this approach remains debatable. Bilateral biopsy is indicated whenever two testes are present. Testicular biopsy is not indicated in cases of oligospermia since the results will rarely alter therapy.

Microscopic evaluation of biopsy specimens should initially be quantified by evaluating the average number of elongating spermatids per round seminiferous tubule. If more than 15–20 mature spermatids per tubule are present in an azoospermic patient, then a diagnosis of obstruction can be made. Of note, seminiferous tubules are frequently present in a mosaic of different spermatogenic patterns in a single testis.

Histologically, tubules may be generally classified into the following categories: normal, hypospermatogenesis, maturation arrest, Sertoli cell only, and sclerosis. Testicular biopsy findings are rarely pathognomonic and do not, by themselves, provide a clinical diagnosis of the cause of impairment of testicular function. Oftentimes, biopsy simply confirms what is already strongly suspected clinically. Of note, we don't require biopsy prior to microdissection TESE, unless the prognostic value of the biopsy would change a couple's decision to undergo TESE.

Normal

Seminiferous tubules are separated by a thin interstitium containing acidophilic Leydig cells, macrophages, blood vessels, lymphatics, and connective tissue. The basement membrane of the tubules is lined by Sertoli cells and spermatogonia. Germ cells are visible in all stages of spermatogenesis. More than 15 condensed, oval spermatids per round tubule should be visible. Normal findings are typically found in azoospermic men with ductal obstruction.

Hypospermatogenesis

In this condition, seminiferous tubules contain a reduced number of all germinal elements. Disorganization of the germinal epithelium may be present in places with immature germ cells in the lumen. The interstitium and Leydig cells are normal. Diffuse hypospermatogenesis may manifest clinically with oligospermia or azoospermia.

Maturation arrest

These testes display a normal spermatogenesis proceeding up to a specific stage of development but no further. The arrest may be early (primary or secondary spermatocyte) or late (round spermatid). Mixed patterns are occasionally seen and some cases of late maturation arrest may be difficult to differentiate from normal spermatogenesis. A "touch prep" or "wet prep" of testicular tissue may help to evaluate complete spermatogenesis during testis biopsies. Most patients with maturation arrest have non-obstructive azoospermia.

Sertoli cell only syndrome

Also known as germinal aplasia, this condition is apparent histologically as a complete absence of germ cells. Seminiferous tubule diameter is reduced and the interstitium may be minimally altered or demonstrate Leydig cell hyperplasia. The Sertoli cells are easily identified by their basal location in the seminiferous tubules, and the single prominent nucleolus in the nucleus of each cell. Clinically, these patients typically have bilateral atrophic, soft testicles and elevated levels of FSH.

Sclerosis

Seminiferous tubules and the surrounding interstitium are sclerotic and hyalinization may be apparent. Germ cells are absent and Leydig cells may be present in hypertrophic nodules. On physical exam, these testes are usually small and firm.

Evaluation algorithm

Men presenting for infertility evaluation will generally fall into one of four groups based upon their semen analysis results: (1) all parameters normal; (2) azoospermia; (3) abnormalities in all semen parameters; (4) isolated problems restricted to one parameter. Categorizing patients in this manner helps guide treatment and evaluation.

Normal

If all semen parameters are normal, a thorough evaluation of the female partner is necessary. If her evaluation reveals no abnormalities or identifies abnormalities that are successfully treated, then one may consider a post-coital test or antisperm antibody evaluation. If these are normal, one can consider more sophisticated testing of sperm function. These men are those with "idiopathic infertility". Though historically the SPA assay may be used to direct people directly to ICSI versus IVF or IUI, with the current widespread application of ICSI this test may not be as widely used.

Azoospermia

If an initial semen analysis shows a complete absence of sperm, the diagnosis should be confirmed by centrifuging the specimen and examining the pellet. If even a few sperm are found in the spun pellet, then complete obstruction has been ruled out and one can consider evaluation of causes of oligospermia. In cases of true azoospermia, hormonal evaluation is the mandatory next step and gives essential information to guide further work-up. At a minimum, an FSH and testosterone should be obtained. Even in cases with a clear etiology for the azoospermia, including previous vasectomy and congenital bilateral absence of the vas, hormonal profiling may give useful information in counseling patients regarding reproductive outcomes.

A low FSH and LH combined with a reduced serum T level is indicative of hypogonadotropic hypogonadism. The condition may be congenital (e.g. Kallman's syndrome), acquired (e.g. pituitary tumor), or idiopathic. Imaging of the pituitary with MRI along with further hormonal testing is required. PRL levels should also be obtained, but evaluation of adrenocorticotropic hormone, thyroid stimulating hormone, and growth hormone is rarely indicated for the infertile male. High circulating PRL levels decrease gonadotropin release and also may have direct detrimental effects on the testes. Idiopathic elevations in PRL usually respond to bromocriptine administration.

Pituitary tumors are usually managed medically with oral bromocriptine or cabergoline. Resistant or symptomatic macroadenomas may require surgical management or radiation. Deficiencies in GnRH or gonadotropins are managed with either hCG and FSH or clomiphene citrate and FSH for those desiring fertility. Testosterone should not be used in this instance because of its suppression of spermatogenesis.

If FSH, LH, and T levels are normal, retrograde ejaculation, failure of emission, or obstruction should be considered as a cause for the azoospermia. Occasionally, aspermia can result from failure of seminal emission (anejaculation). For these men, semen does not enter the urethra or bladder following climax despite an absence of ejaculatory duct obstruction. This results from complete functional failure of the entire ejaculatory mechanism. Retrograde ejaculation usually has an obvious cause such as diabetes or prior retroperitoneal surgery (e.g. RPLND for testicular cancer). The prostate and bladder neck are densely populated with alpha-adrenergic receptors. Failure of the bladder neck to close during emission results in retrograde flow of semen into the bladder instead of antegrade out the urethra. This abnormality is diagnosed by finding sperm in the urine on postejaculatory urinalysis (greater than 10 per HPF, or more than half of the total volume of emitted sperm). Initial treatment is with sympathomimetic agents which help to close the bladder neck prior to emission and ejaculation. If unsuccessful, sperm may be retrieved from a post-ejaculatory urine specimen by centrifugation and used for insemination (e.g. IUI). However, urine is very toxic to sperm. Therefore, the post-ejaculatory urine should be promptly centrifuged to minimize contact of sperm with urine. Alternatively, the patient may be catheterized immediately before ejaculation, the bladder filled with buffer and the post-ejaculatory urine used to extract spermatozoa for IUI. Failing treatment with sympathomimetics or in cases of anejaculation, penile vibratory stimulation or electroejaculation may be required.

If no sperm are found in the post-ejaculatory urine, evaluation of the ejaculatory ducts and seminal vesicles should be done. Suspicion for ejaculatory duct obstruction should be high in a patient with low-volume (< 1 ml) acidic ejaculate. Visualization of dilated seminal vesicles (> 1.5 cm) helps corroborate the diagnosis. Prior to treatment, confirmation of the presence of vasa in the scrotum (by physical exam) and retroperitoneum (by transrectal ultrasound) is necessary. Fine needle aspiration of the seminal vesicles has also been described to confirm the diagnosis of ejaculatory duct obstruction [23]. Ejaculatory duct obstruction may be treated endoscopically while congenital bilateral absence of the vas requires sperm retrieval and assisted reproduction.

Azoospermic patients with normal FSH, palpable vasa, and no evidence of ejaculatory duct obstruction should undergo testis biopsy. If quantitatively limited spermatogenesis is found (less than 10–15 mature spermatids per tubule), TESE-ICSI, adoption and donor insemination are options. If biopsy results are normal, exploration for obstruction, beginning with sampling of the intravasal fluid and vasography, is indicated. Points of focal obstruction can often be repaired with microsurgical vasovasostomy or vasoepididymostomy. If no sperm are present in the vasal fluid and the testis biopsy is normal, then a diagnosis of epididymal obstruction is present. Epididymal blockage can frequently be successfully bypassed by microsurgical vasoepididymostomy. These procedures require an operating microscope and microsurgical training for the best results. With modern techniques, motile sperm are seen in up to 67% of patients with the two-suture longitudinal suture technique [24]. To avoid the need for subsequent sperm retrieval procedures if the microsurgical reconstruction is unsuccessful, sperm retrieval and cryopreservation should be considered during the reconstructive procedure. Another therapeutic option in obstructive azoospermia, especially if the obstruction is beyond repair, is retrieval of spermatozoa through microsurgical epididymal sperm aspiration for subsequent IVF and ICSI [25]. This approach is a primary treatment option for patients with congenital absence of the vas.

Diffuse semen abnormalities

Many patients present with abnormalities involving all semen parameters including oligospermia (densities less than 20 million sperm per ml), decreased motility, and abnormal morphology. Repeat analysis is necessary since even transient fevers or illness over the last few months may cause a transient decrease in all semen quality. For men with impaired semen quality, an appropriate search for correctable etiologies is necessary. This includes hormonal abnormalities, varicoceles, antisperm antibodies, heat/environmental factors, infections, sexual dysfunction, certain prescription medications and toxins that can affect sperm quality. Those with severe oligospermia (< 10 million per ml) should have a hormone evaluation (FSH and testosterone).

Barring recent illness, varicoceles are the most common cause of diffuse defects in semen parameters. They can be diagnosed on physical exam of the spermatic cord as mentioned earlier. Scrotal ultrasound can be used to confirm the diagnosis and may also be helpful in cases where physical exam proves difficult (e.g. morbid obesity). Varicoceles can be surgically corrected via a number of approaches, including retroperitoneal, inguinal, and subinguinal. Improved semen parameters are seen in approximately 70% of patients. However, not all varicoceles cause infertility and need to be repaired. But if a man has a clinically detectable varicocele, semen abnormalities and subfertility, then treatment may increase the chances of conception if the female partner is normal. However, if no cause is found this is "idiopathic subfertility". Empirical therapy with antiestrogens such as clomiphene citrate, either alone or in combination with supplemental gonadotropins, has been attempted with inconsistent results. These patients often require assisted reproductive techniques (IUI or IVF-ICSI).

Single parameter abnormalities

Low sperm motility with impaired forward progression (asthenospermia) is the most common isolated semen parameter abnormality. This problem is often due to antisperm antibodies and evidence of agglutination may be present. The microscopic finding of two sperm joined head to head or tail to tail (dimers) is almost pathognomonic for the presence of antibodies. The diagnosis is ultimately made using the previously described direct immunobead assays. Treatment with immunosuppressive steroids has been reported but results have been inconsistent and this approach remains controversial because of the risk of aseptic necrosis of the head of the femur associated with steroid administration. Semen processing followed by assisted reproduction including ICSI is the most commonly pursued therapeutic option.

Poor motility may also be caused by genital tract infection. The presence of leukocytes in the semen along with positive urine culture results is diagnostic of a genital tract infection. Any suggestion of infection should be managed with antibiotics prior to embarking on a more involved and expensive work-up or treatment course. The choice of antibiotics is important and may affect sperm production. Nitrofurantoin and sulfa drugs have been shown to be toxic to the testis or sperm themselves. Fluoroquinolones (e.g. ciprofloxacin) and tetracyclines (e.g. doxycycline) are generally considered to be safe and effective for most pathogens in the genitourinary tract.

Patients with low-volume ejaculates (less than 1 ml) should be evaluated for ejaculatory duct obstruction or malformation of the vas/seminal vesicles. Partial ejaculatory duct obstruction or severe hypoandrogenic states also can result in isolated low semen volume on rare occasions. High-volume ejaculates result in sperm dilution with an indeterminate effect on fertility. High semen volumes should only be treated if the post-coital test is abnormal. Mechanical concentration by centrifugation or use of a split ejaculate can be performed and are relatively straightforward.

Isolated problems with sperm density can be managed with semen processing and IUI or other assisted reproductive techniques once treatable conditions have been ruled out. Accumulation of poor-quality ejaculates by freezing samples over time may be limited by the low freeze-thaw survival rate observed for sperm with poor motility. Nonspecific epididymal dysfunction or partial obstruction may occur as well and diagnosis is difficult.

Hyperviscosity as an isolated problem should also only be treated if the post-coital test is poor. Oral treatment with vitamin C (250 mg/day), mucolytics (guaifenesin) or sperm processing followed by IUI are treatment options.

Conclusions

The assessment of the male partner is an essential component of the work-up of the infertile couple. With up to 60% of infertility cases involving a male factor, lack of an adequate male work-up is unacceptable. The modern practitioner of male reproductive medicine must have a strong understanding of the indications, risks, benefits, and costs of the staggering array of tests available. With a thorough understanding of the proper work-up algorithm, there is less unnecessary testing, which will benefit patients both financially and emotionally.

Acknowledgements

Dr. Hsiao is supported by a grant from the Frederick J. and Theresa Dow Wallace Fund of the New York Community Trust.

References

1. Agarwal A, Deepinder F, Cocuzza M, Short RA, Evenson DP. Effect of vaginal lubricants on sperm motility and chromatin integrity: a prospective comparative study. *Fertil Steril* 2008; **89**(2): 375–9.

2. Kogan S. Cryptorchidism. In Kelalis PP, King LR, Belman AB, eds. *Clinical Pediatric Urology*, 2nd edn. Philadelphia: Saunders, 1985.

3. Nagler HM, Deitch AD, deVere White R. Testicular torsion: temporal considerations. *Fertil Steril* 1984; **42**(2): 257–62.

4. Ramasamy R, Ricci JA, Palermo GD, *et al.* Successful fertility treatment for Klinefelter's syndrome. *J Urol* 2009; **182**(3): 1108–13.

5. Jeyendran RS, Van der Ven HH, Perez-Pelaez M, Crabo BG, Zaneveld LJ. Development of an assay to assess the functional integrity of the human sperm membrane and its relationship to other semen characteristics. *J Reprod Fertil* 1984; **70**(1): 219–28.

6. Chan SY, Fox EJ, Chan MM, *et al.* The relationship between the human sperm hypoosmotic swelling test, routine semen analysis, and the human sperm zona-free hamster ovum penetration assay. *Fertil Steril* 1985; **44**(5): 668–72.

7. Homyk M, Anderson DJ, Wolff H, Herr JC. Differential diagnosis of immature germ cells in semen utilizing monoclonal antibody MHS-10 to the intra-acrosomal antigen SP-10. *Fertil Steril* 1990; **53**(2): 323–30.

8. Kim ED, Gilbaugh JH 3rd, Patel VR, Turek PJ, Lipshultz LI. Testis biopsies frequently demonstrate sperm in men with azoospermia and significantly elevated follicle-stimulating hormone levels. *J Urol* 1997; **157**(1): 144–6.

9. Baker HWG, Burger HG, de Kretser D. Relative incidence of etiologic disorders in male infertility. In Santen RJ, Swerdloff RS, eds. *Male Reproductive Dysfunction: Diagnosis and Management of Hypogonadism, Infertility, and Impotence*. New York: Marcel Dekker, 1986. p. xvii, 613 p., viii p. of plates.

10. Ramasamy R, Lin K, Gosden LV, *et al.* High serum FSH levels in men with nonobstructive azoospermia does not affect success of microdissection testicular sperm extraction. *Fertil Steril* 2009; **92**(2): 590–3.

11. Mak V, Jarvi KA. The genetics of male infertility. *J Urol* 1996; **156**(4): 1245–56; discussion 56–7.

12. Hopps CV, Mielnik A, Goldstein M, *et al.* Detection of sperm in men with Y chromosome microdeletions of the AZFa, AZFb and AZFc regions. *Hum Reprod* 2003; **18**(8): 1660–5.

13. Mortimer D, Aitken RJ, Mortimer ST, Pacey AA. Workshop report: clinical CASA – the quest for consensus. *Reprod Fertil Dev* 1995; **7**(4): 951–9.

14. Rumke P, Van Amstel N, Messa EM, Rezemar PD. Prognosis of fertility in men with sperm agglutins in the serum. *Fertil Steril* 1973; **24**: 35.

15. Swanson RJ, Mayer JF, Jones KH, Lanzendorf SE, McDowell J. Hamster ova/human sperm penetration: correlation with count, motility, and morphology for in vitro fertilization. *Arch Androl* 1983; **10**: 69.

16. Smith RG, Johnson A, Lamb D, Lipshultz LI. Functional tests of spermatozoa. Sperm penetration assay. *Urol Clin North Am* 1987; **14**(3): 451–8.

17. Corson SL, Batzer FR, Marmar J, Maislin G. The human sperm-hamster egg penetration assay: prognostic value. *Fertil Steril* 1988; **49**(2): 328–34.

18. Burkman LJ, Coddington CC, Fraken DR, *et al.* The hemizona assay (HZA): development of a diagnostic test for the binding of human spermatozoa to the human hemizona pellucida to predict fertilization potential. *Fertil Steril* 1988; **49**: 688.

19. Talbot P, Chacon RS. A triple-stain technique for evaluating normal acrosome reactions of human sperm. *J Exp Zool* 1981; **215**(2): 201–8.

20. Cross NL, Morales P, Overstreet JW, Hanson FW. Two simple methods for detecting acrosome-reacted human sperm. *Gamete Research* 1986; **15**: 213.

21. Benchaib M, Lornage J, Mazoyer C, *et al.* Sperm deoxyribonucleic acid fragmentation as a prognostic indicator of assisted reproductive technology outcome. *Fertil Steril* 2007; **87**(1): 93–100.

22. Muriel L, Garrido N, Fernandez JL, *et al.* Value of the sperm deoxyribonucleic acid fragmentation level, as measured by the sperm chromatin dispersion test, in the outcome of in vitro fertilization and intracytoplasmic sperm injection. *Fertil Steril* 2006; **85**(2): 371–83.

23. Jarow JP. Transrectal ultrasonography in the diagnosis and management of ejaculatory duct obstruction. *J Androl* 1996; **17**(5): 467–72.

24. Schiff J, Chan P, Li PS, Finkelberg S, Goldstein M. Outcome and late failures compared in 4 techniques of microsurgical vasoepididymostomy in 153 consecutive men. *J Urol* 2005; **174**(2): 651–5; quiz 801.

25. Schlegel PN, Palermo GD, Alikani M, *et al.* Micropuncture retrieval of epididymal sperm with in vitro fertilization: importance of in vitro micromanipulation techniques. *Urology* 1995; **46**(2): 238–41.

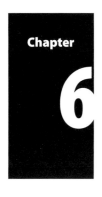

Ultrasound in the investigation of the subfertile female

Marion Dewailly, Edouard Poncelet and Didier Dewailly

The pelvic ultrasound (U/S) examination is now essential first-line investigation of female infertility. It allows the detection of ovarian functional disorders, where it became one of the key tests in the approach of ovulation disorders. U/S also allows the diagnosis of certain organic abnormalities responsible for infertility or can detect indirect signs of organic etiologies leading to complementary investigations, particularly magnetic resonance, hysterosonography, and hysteroscopy.

Technical aspects and recommendations

Women with regular cycles should undergo investigation at the start of the follicular phase (days 3 to 5 of the cycle). Women with oligoamenorrhea may be investigated either at any time, or between 3 and 5 days after progestin-induced withdrawal bleeding. For the study of leiomyomas and uterine malformations, it may be interesting to scan the patient during the luteal phase.

2D ultrasonography

The transabdominal route should always be the first step of pelvic sonographic examination, followed by the transvaginal route, except in virgin or refusing patients. Of course, a full bladder is required for visualization of the ovaries. However, one should be cautious that an overfilled bladder can compress the ovaries, yielding a falsely increased length. The main advantage of this route is that it offers a panoramic view of the pelvic cavity. Therefore, it allows the ruling out of associated uterine or ovarian abnormalities with an abdominal component. Indeed, lesions extending into the abdomen could be missed by using the transvaginal approach exclusively. The abdominal route also allows examination of the urinary tract, which may be helpful in some situations.

Next, the transvaginal examination can be performed, with an empty bladder, using high-frequency probes (> 6 MHz), which have a better spatial resolution but less examination depth. This allows a precise analysis of the pelvic organs. The ultrasonographer must provide a complete analysis of the uterus (size, general morphology, myometrial homogeneity, endometrial thickness and homogeneity) and of the ovaries (volume or area, antral follicle count [AFC]; see below).

3D ultrasonography

The 3D ultrasound is a diagnostic tool complementary to the 2D mode, fast and efficient, feasible during a traditional examination or during hysterosonography. In practice,

The Subfertility Handbook: A Clinician's Guide, Second Edition ed. Gab Kovacs. Published by Cambridge University Press. © Cambridge University Press 2011.

examination begins by a conventional 2D assessment of the pelvis and then the target organ is placed in the center of the screen, oriented along its long axis (uterus in longitudinal plane for example) with optimization of the depth, focus, and gain. The window of 3D acquisition is set by adjusting its size manually. An acquisition volume is then performed, the patient being in apnea and the examiner's hand being still for a few seconds to avoid artifact kinetics. According to the machine, the scanning of the region of interest can be done manually or automatically, the latter seeming better. The 3D acquisition can be replayed and reworked on the ultrasound machine directly or secondarily on any computer.

The volume thus acquired will then be processed by the machine, which will yield views with multiplanar reconstruction (MPR) in all planes of volume, as in cross-sectional imaging such as CT or MRI, allowing for navigation in the volume. Tomographic ultrasound imaging can also be obtained, generating a series of cuts in a given plane with a presentation style "plate" as with CT or MRI. Videos can be obtained, scrolling the different cuts in 2D mode or in volume rendering. The reading of the acquired volume in mode "cinema" is helpful to re-interpret the images, to get a second opinion, and also for correlation with data obtained by cross-sectional imaging techniques. Software adaptable to 3D ultrasound is now available, allowing automatic volume calculation or counting of follicles, but their value in clinical practice needs to be evaluated (Figure 6.1).

Other advantages of this technique, especially for the study of the ovaries, is that the 3D probe provides an excellent 2D spatial resolution and that it widens the field of view over 180°. This allows visualization of the lateral pelvis (even blocked by vaginal access) through the modification of firing angles.

The 3D ultrasound is particularly interesting for the study of uterine malformations since it is possible to reconstruct the image in different planes. In particular, the frontal plane, which is not accessible by the 2D mode, is very useful for the study of uterine malformations. It is also useful in conjunction with hysterosonography.

Doppler study

Color or power Doppler can help the diagnosis by showing vessels inside a lesion (myomas, polyps, ovarian inclusion). Pulsed Doppler allows assessment of the uterine artery resistance through determination of the resistance index (RI) and pulsatility index (PI).

Hysterosonography or saline infusion sonography (SIS)

Hysterosonography consists of conducting an ultrasound after filling the uterine cavity with saline or contrast fluid. This examination allows the study of the uterine cavity (with use of saline) but also allows assessment of tubal patency (use of contrast fluid and Doppler mode). It is an alternative to hysterosalpingography. In practice it is performed in the first part of the cycle; a catheter is placed at the cervix in the same way as during a hysterosalpingography. Then the ultrasound study is performed with a high-resolution transvaginal probe, before and after intra-cavitary injection of saline or contrast fluid.

Various studies have shown that hysterosonography is highly efficient in the diagnosis of intra-cavitary disease (sensitivity: 95–100%), in particular for the differential diagnosis between intra-cavitary myoma and polyp and for the assessment of intra-uterine synechia (see below) [1]. Tubal patency can also be confirmed when a flow at color or energy Doppler is seen in the fallopian tubes after injection of contrast fluid. The sensitivity and specificity of sonosalpingography in this indication are respectively 90–95% and 80–85%. In comparison

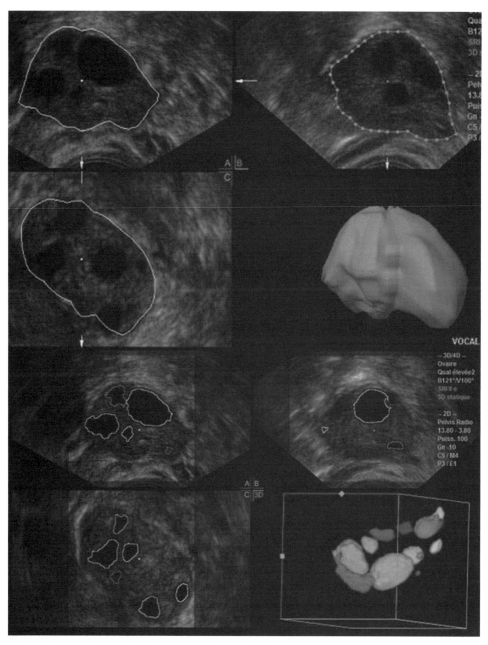

Figure 6.1 Software developed for automatic detection of follicles. See color plates.

to hysterosalpingography, it has the advantage of not being irradiating and gives information at the same time about the morphology of myometrium and ovaries. However, in the case of tubal occlusion, it does not describe the internal tubal morphology, nor does it indicate the level of the obstacle. So far, it has not replaced hysterosalpingography in the routine clinical work-up.

Ovarian disorders

Ultrasonography is now a must in the investigation of ovulation disorders, along with clinical findings and hormonal assays. It allows estimation of the ovarian function, mainly estrogen secretion, through measurement of the endometrial thickness: endometrial atrophy or severe hypotrophy (thickness < 5 mm) indicates hypoestrogenism. It also contributes greatly to the diagnosis of ovulation disorders, in particular polycystic ovary syndrome (PCOS) and primary ovarian failure (POF), along with the clinical/biological data.

PCOS

PCOS is an ovarian dysfunction syndrome of which the main features are hyperandrogenism and an ultrasound appearance of polycystic ovaries (PCO). Its prevalence among women of reproductive age is about 10%. Clinical signs may include irregular menstruation, signs of androgen excess, and obesity. The syndrome now includes a broader spectrum of signs and symptoms of ovarian dysfunction than that set out in the original criteria [2]. It is now agreed that women with regular menstrual cycles and hyperandrogenism and/or PCO at ultrasound are in fact presenting with this syndrome. In addition, the majority of authors now agree that women with this syndrome may present an appearance of PCO at ultrasound without any sign of androgen excess, although with indicators of ovarian dysfunction [2].

Therefore, the Rotterdam classification [3] should be used to define PCOS. It requires at least two of the following three criteria, providing that all other diagnoses have been ruled out:

- menstrual cycle anomalies (amenorrhea, oligomenorrhea or long cycles)
- clinical and/or biochemical hyperandrogenism
- ultrasound appearance of PCO (Figure 6.2).

According to the literature review dealing with all available imaging systems and to the discussion at the joint ASRM/ESHRE consensus meeting on PCOS held in Rotterdam, 1–3 May 2003, the current consensus definition of PCO is the following: either 12 or more follicles measuring 2–9 mm in diameter and/or increased ovarian volume (> 10 cm^3) [4].

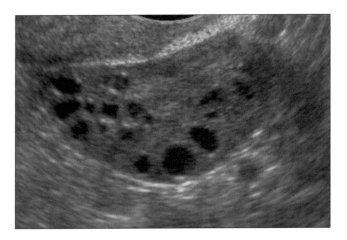

Figure 6.2 Polycystic ovary: enlarged ovary containing multiple follicles less than 10 mm in diameter.

The priority was given to the ovarian volume and to the follicle number because both have the advantage of being physical entities that can be measured in real-time conditions and because both are still considered as the key and consistent features of PCO.

Increased ovarian volume

Many studies have reported an increased mean ovarian volume in a series of patients with PCOS (reviewed in Ref. 4). However, the upper normal limit of the ovarian volume suffers from some variability in the literature (from 8 to 15.6 cm^3). The consensual volume threshold to discriminate a normal ovary from a PCO is 10 cm^3. It has been empirically retained by the expert panel for the Rotterdam consensus, as being the best compromise between the studies that were available at that time [4]. However, none of them had used an appropriate statistical appraisal of sensitivity and specificity of the volume threshold. This prompted us to recently revisit this issue through a prospective study including 154 women with PCOS compared to 57 women with normal ovaries [5]. The receiver operating characteristic (ROC) curves indicated that a threshold at 10 cm^3 yielded a good specificity (98.2%) but a weak sensitivity (39%). Setting the threshold at 7 cm^3 offered the best compromise between specificity (94.7%) and sensitivity (68.8%). Then, in our opinion, the threshold at 10 cm^3 should be lowered in order to increase the sensitivity of the ovarian volume for the definition of PCO.

Increased follicle number

The polyfollicular pattern (i.e. excessive number of small echoless regions less than 10 mm in diameter) is strongly suggestive, since it is in perfect correlation with the label of the syndrome (i.e. "polycystic"). It is now broadly accepted that most of these cysts are in fact healthy oocyte-containing follicles and are not atretic.

The consensus definition for a PCO is one that contains 12 or more follicles of 2–9 mm diameter. Again, the expert panel for the Rotterdam consensus considered this threshold as being the best compromise between the most complete studies, including the one in which we compared 214 patients with PCOS to 112 women with normal ovaries (reviewed in Ref. 3). By ROC analysis, an antral follicle count (AFC) of ≥ 12 follicles of 2–9 mm diameter yielded the best compromise between sensitivity (75%) and specificity (99%) for the diagnosis of PCO. However, the continuing improvement in picture resolution will lead to reconsideration of these thresholds when using the newest machines, since follicles less than 2 mm in diameter can now be detected and counted.

The Rotterdam consensus did not address the difficult issue of multifollicular ovaries (MFO). This concept is highly disputed. First, there is no consensual U/S definition for MFO, although they have been described a long time ago as ovaries in which there are multiple (≥ 6) follicles, usually 4–10 mm in diameter, with normal stromal echogenicity (reviewed in Ref. 6). Second, no histological data about MFO are available. The presence of MFO has been reported during puberty and in women recovering from hypothalamic amenorrhea but the question remains whether MFO are a distinct entity or are simply PCO in a peculiar clinical context. We recently revisited the ovarian follicular pattern in a group of women with hypothalamic amenorrhea. About 40% had an AFC higher than 12 (unpublished personal data). In agreement with others' opinion [7], we hypothesize that these women truly have PCO but not PCOS because the clinical and biological expression of PCOS, mainly hyperandrogenism, has been switched off by the chronically suppressed LH levels due to their secondary and superimposed hypothalamic dysfunction. Once these patients recover from their HA (or under pulsatile GnRH or gonadotropin administration), they resume their PCOS features [7].

Other criteria, other techniques, and other definitions

External morphological signs of PCO

At its beginning in the 1970s, the weak resolution of U/S abdominal probes allowed detection exclusively of the external morphological ovarian features that were used as the first criteria defining PCO:

- the length, whose upper limit is 4 cm, is the simplest criterion, but this uni-dimensional approach may lead to false-positive results when a full bladder compresses the ovary (with the transabdominal route) or false-negative results when the ovaries are spheric, with a relatively short length;
- because of the increased ovarian size and the normal uterine width, the uterine width/ovarian length (U/O) ratio is decreased (< 1) in PCO;
- PCO often display a spherical shape in contrast to normal ovaries which are ellipsoid; this morphological change can be evaluated by the sphericity index (ovarian width/ovarian length), which is higher than 0.7 in PCO.

These parameters are less used nowadays because of their weak sensitivity.

The ovarian area

It is less used than the volume and was not retained in the consensus definition but, in our recent study revisiting the ovarian volume [5], the diagnostic value of the ovarian area (assessed by the ROC curves) was slightly better than the ovarian volume (sensitivity 77.6%, specificity 94.7% for a threshold at 5 cm^2/ ovary). We also observed that the measured ovarian area (by outlining by hand the ovary or by fitting an ellipse to the ovary) was more informative than the calculated ovarian area (by using the formula for an ellipse: length × width × π/4). Indeed, ovaries are not strictly ellipsoid and this can explain why the diagnostic value of the former was better than the latter.

Increased stroma

Stromal hypertrophy is characterized by an increased component of the ovarian central part, which seems to be rather hyperechoic (Figure 6.1). In our and in others' opinion [4], the stromal hypertrophy is highly specific of PCO. However, in the absence of a precise quantification, it remains a subjective sign.

Fulghesu et al. [8] proposed the ovarian stroma/total area ratio as a good criterion for the diagnosis of PCOS. The ovarian stromal area was evaluated by outlining with the caliper the peripheral profile of the stroma, identified by a central area slightly hyperechoic with respect to the other ovarian area. Although highly specific, this parameter is not easy to register in routine practice and its superiority over the AFC has not been established.

The estimation of stromal hyperechogenicity is also highly subjective, mainly because it depends on the settings of the ultrasound machine. Conversely, ovarian volume or area correlates well with ovarian function and is both more easily and more reliably measured in routine practice than ovarian stroma. Thus, in order to define the polycystic ovary, neither qualitative nor quantitative assessment of the ovarian stroma is required.

Follicle distribution

In PCO, the follicle distribution is predominantly peripheral, with typically an echoless peripheral array. At the Rotterdam meeting, this subjective criterion was judged to be too inconstant and subjective to be retained for the consensus definition of PCO [4].

3D Ultrasound

The 3D U/S has been initially proposed to avoid the difficulties and pitfalls in outlining or measuring the ovarian shape (reviewed in Ref. 9). From the stored data, the scanned ovarian volume is displayed on the screen in three adjustable orthogonal planes, allowing the three dimensions and subsequently the volume to be more accurately evaluated.

The superiority of 3D over 2D ultrasound to determine accurately the AFC is not evident, but the literature is still scarce about this issue. To our knowledge, there is so far no study comparing both techniques in the same groups of patients and controls. Our preliminary results indicate no significant difference (unpublished personal data). In a study including small numbers of patients and controls [10], the threshold of AFC discriminating between PCO and normal ovaries was set at 20 with 3D U/S, hence clearly higher than the "Rotterdam" threshold. Whether this is due to the 3D technique specifically or to the higher resolution of those new machines impacting both on 2D and 3D data has still to be investigated.

So far, the main interest of 3D U/S resides essentially in the possibility to re-analyse the data on the saved volumetric acquisitions. The follicle count can be done retrospectively by "navigating" within the ovary in three planes. This is helpful in the case of discordance between U/S and clinical/biological data. Some software allows an automatic count of the follicles on the volumetric acquisitions but for the moment they are not reliable enough for follicles smaller than 10 mm.

Ovarian Doppler ultrasonography

Doppler allows detection of the vascularization network within the ovarian stroma. Power Doppler is more sensitive to the slow flows and shows more vascular signals within the ovaries, but it does not discriminate between arteries and veins. The combination of 3D and power Doppler ultrasound ("3D power Doppler angiography") allows closer examination of the vascularity of PCO [9]. The blood flow is more frequently visualized in PCOS than in normal patients in early follicular phase and seems to be increased. However, the study of the ovarian vascularization with both the 2D and 3D techniques is still highly subjective. Therefore, a significantly increased ovarian stromal vascularization was not found in all PCOS populations with the 3D ultrasound technique [9].

Some data indicate that Doppler blood flow may have some value in predicting the risk of ovarian hyperstimulation during gonadotropin therapy. Increased stromal blood flow has also been suggested as a more relevant predictor of ovarian response to hormonal stimulation than parameters such as ovarian or stromal volume, but the evidence is still scarce in the literature (reviewed in Ref. 10).

To summarize, no data support so far any diagnostic usefulness of ovarian Doppler in PCO.

Premature ovarian failure (POF) and poor responders to controlled ovarian hyperstimulation (COH)

POF is due to a premature exhaustion of the pool of primordial ovarian follicles. This may happen before puberty, such as in Turner's syndrome, leading to primary amenorrhea and pubertal delay. When occurring after puberty, the clinical picture is typically a secondary amenorrhea with hot flushes. However, many attenuated and intermittent forms can be

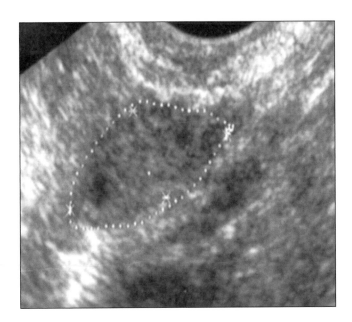

Figure 6.3 Premature ovarian failure: small ovary containing a few follicles.

observed [11], especially at the beginning of the disease. Many authors designate a poor response to controlled ovarian hyperstimulation (COH) as sub-clinical POF, although the link between these two states is not fully demonstrated. A poor response to COH is defined by less than three mature follicles and/or insufficient rise in estradiol serum levels (< 500 pg/ml) during COH and/or less than four oocytes at follicle puncture.

U/S is useful for the diagnosis of POF and for predicting a poor response to COH since it detects earlier than the FSH assay the decline in the follicle pool [12]. However, the U/S definition for POF is not agreed. The most frequently used is either an ovarian volume < 3 cm^3 (or area < 2.5 cm^2) and/or a AFC < 5 (cumulating both ovaries) (Figure 6.3). The threshold for AFC will certainly have to be raised in the future, with the advent of high-resolution devices allowing detection of small follicles < 2 mm. It has been emphasized that AFC is more accurate when only follicles < 7 mm are counted, especially for predicting a poor response to COH within the frame of IVF. The ovarian volume is not a good predictor for low response to COH [13].

Other U/S signs of POF are endometrial atrophy, increased resistance of uterine arteries (with a PI > 3), and stagnation of follicle growth on consecutive U/S during the same cycle.

Uterine abnormalities

U/S is highly sensitive in detecting those lesions that are responsible for infertility through interference with egg migration and implantation and/or with sperm progression, such as fibroids, polyps, synechiae, or malformations [14]. Conversely, it is less sensitive than laparoscopy in detecting mild pelvic adhesions or peritoneal endometriosis. However, the role of the latter in female infertility is highly questionable. Therefore, many authors now propose avoiding laparoscopy when U/S is negative in an infertile woman who has patent fallopian tubes at hysterography.

Fibroids (leiomyomas)

Fibroids are better detected and analysed in the luteal than in the follicular phase. Most often, they appear as a hypoechoic heterogeneous mass, with peripheral crown vascularization at color Doppler. It is very important to accurately measure their size, location and vascularization [15] . This can be optimized with 3D U/S and/or with hysterosonography. MRI can be necessary in difficult cases.

Their prevalence is high in infertile women, especially in Africans [15] , but also in fertile women, although less. Only those that are intra-cavitary or in a submucosal location, that distort the endometrium, that measure 5 cm or more and that are close to the isthme or the tube ostium should be considered as having an effect on fertility [16]. Otherwise, they should not be considered as responsible for infertility and there is no evidence that removing them will improve the outcome. For those fibroids that can affect fertility (submucosal location), it is important to detect contraindications to endoscopic treatment, in particular an insufficient thickness (less than 5 mm) of normal myometrium in the periphery of the lesion and a size greater than 5 cm.

Hysterosonography can be useful to distinguish the intra-cavitary component of a leiomyoma (Figure 6.4) [16].

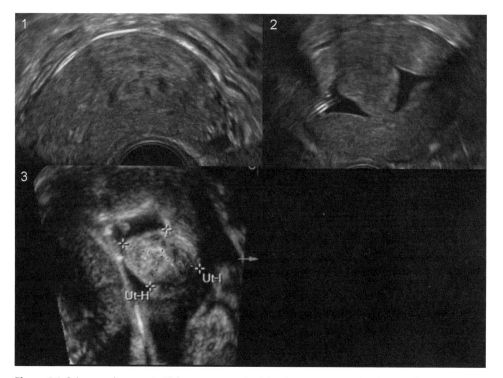

Figure 6.4 Submucosal myoma in 3D hysterosonography: (1) without preparation: localization of the myoma difficult to specify; (2) after filling: good display of intramural and intra-cavitary components (2D image); (3) reconstruction in the coronal plane (3D). See color plates.

Adenomyosis

Adenomyosis is defined by the presence of ectopic endometrial tissue within the myometrium. U/S signs of adenomyosis are enlarged uterus, with thickening of the myometrium; heterogeneous lesions with poorly defined borders within the myometrium [14]; presence of submucosal cysts in the internal part of the myometrium which are either anechoic or hyperechoic (Figure 6.5). At Doppler, blood supply is more penetrating than in fibroids. MRI can help but sometimes the diagnosis remains difficult [15]. For this reason, the role of adenomyosis in infertility has never been well demonstrated.

Synechiae (intra-uterine adhesions)

They are often secondary to infection or uterine trauma by surgery or curettage. U/S is seldom sufficient to make the diagnosis. It may show a hypo- or hyperechoic endometrial lesion with calcifications in some instances [17] (Figure 6.6). Hysterography and hysterosonography [14] are better tests.

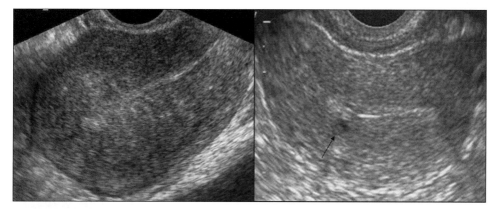

Figure 6.5 Adenomyosis with globular uterus, thickening of the junctional zone, sub-endometrial cysts (→), and hyperechoic striations in the inner part of the myometrium.

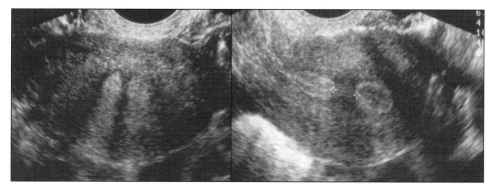

Figure 6.6 Uterine synechia: interruption of the uterine cavity by a hypoechoic image with posterior attenuation (calcification likely).

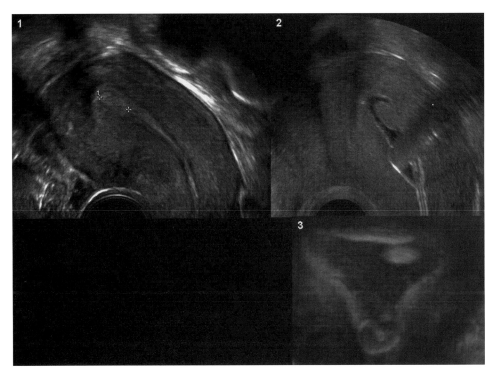

Figure 6.7 Polyp in 2D ultrasound (1), hysterosonography 2D (2) and coronal 3D reconstruction (3): intra-cavitary hyperechoic lesion, better visualized after filling the uterine cavity.

Polyps

Although they are quite frequently encountered in infertile women (10–15%), their role in infertility is still under discussion. They are better visualized in the first part of the cycle. They appear as hyperechoic round or oval lesions within the uterine cavity, sometimes cystic [17]. It is sometimes difficult to distinguish between a polyp and a submucosal fibroid. Doppler may help by showing a thin and single vessel axis but here again, hysterosonography is much more informative (Figure 6.7) [16].

Congenital malformations of the uterus

They are due to abnormal development of the Müllerian ducts during fetal life. They are seldom the sole cause of infertility and are more often associated with tubal abnormalities or endometriosis. Actually, they are more often involved in repeated spontaneous abortion than in infertility [18].

Their precise characterization often requires the use of MRI but ultrasound can detect some suggestive signs. It should be conducted in the second part of the cycle when the endometrium is hyperechoic and allows a good visualization of the uterine cavity and it will always be associated with renal ultrasound for detecting urinary malformations, which are frequently associated.

The main defects encountered are:

- bilateral incomplete uterine agenesis (Rokitansky-Kuster-Hauser syndrome): it is rarely found in investigation of infertility but rather is diagnosed because of primary non-endocrine amenorrhea;

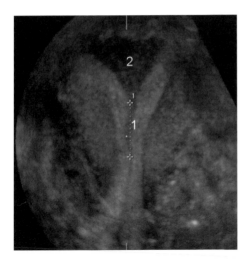

Figure 6.8 Septate uterus in 3D, with partition having a fibrous portion (1) and a muscular portion (2). Coronal reconstruction. See color plates.

- unicornuate uterus (unilateral agenesis), the ultrasound findings for which are a significant uterine latero-deviation, ellipsoid-shaped uterus, ipsilateral renal agenesis, which is often associated; and sometimes the presence of a contralateral rudimentary tube and/or horn, unconnected to the cervix (pseudo-unicornuate uterus); it is important to detect and to remove a pseudo-horn before considering pregnancy because the egg can establish itself in the pseudo-horn with a risk of cataclysmic rupture;
- bicervical bicornuate uterus with blind hemi-vagina; rarely found in investigation of infertility, diagnosed because of dysmenorrhea (menstrual retention);
- bicornuate unicervical uterus, when imaging shows two divergent horns forming an angle greater than 60°, separated by more than 4 cm; sign of the "bladder V" (the posterior bladder wall creeping between the two horns); presence of a myometrial fundal notch larger than 1 cm; crown vascularization of each horn in color Doppler mode;
- septate uterus, the differential diagnosis of which is bicornuate uterus and is sometimes difficult. In the former, the following signs are observed: two slightly divergent cavities with angle less than 60° and with a distance between horns less than 4 cm; presence of a hypoechoic septum; no fundal notch or presence of a small notch less than 1 cm (Figure 6.8); single crown peripheral vascularization in color Doppler mode; no association with renal malformations. An additional MRI is often necessary in order to better characterize the signal tissue between the two cavities, which will be fibrous in the case of septate uterus and myometrial if bicornuate uterus. The septate uterus is responsible for subfertility due to impaired implantation on the fibrous septum. Pregnancy rate is increased and abortion rate is decreased after endoscopic resection of the septum;
- arcuate uterus (septate uterus fundus), which corresponds to a minor form of septum, without proven consequences for reproduction;
- uterine anomalies related to DES, the diagnosis of which is made by hysterosalpingogram rather than by U/S, and include uterine hypoplasia, T-shaped uterus and annular stenosis of body or horns.

The 3D ultrasound can help in the diagnosis of uterine malformations [19]. First, it allows a better study of the fundus through the reconstructions in the coronal plane of the uterus [18].

It thus allows accurate measuring of the length of one wall and the fundal myometrial thickness. It also allows one to search for a rudimentary horn in the case of unicornuate uterus and to specify whether there are one or two cervixes in the case of bicornuate uterus, which is particularly difficult when the uterus is in an intermediate position. Lastly, it calculates the cavity volume for hypoplastic, uni- or bicornuate uterus.

Tuboperitoneal etiologies

Tubal obstructions

The majority of tubal obstructions are secondary to sexually transmitted infections, particularly gonorrhea and chlamydia. They are also due to postoperative adhesions and lesions of endometriosis. Beside hysterosonography (see above), conventional U/S is a bad test for the study of tubal patency and hysterosalpingography remains the modality of choice. Indeed, a normal U/S does not in any case eliminate a tubal obstruction. However, U/S allows investigation of a tubal obstruction especially when viewing a hydrosalpinx due to fluid dilatation of the tube upstream of a distal stenosis. It looks like a tubular lateral or retro-uterine anechoic or finely echogenic image with incomplete septa (kinking) and/or pseudo-vegetation of the same size, not hypervascularized on Doppler (which allows differentiation of cysts with endo-cystic vegetations) [16].

Peritoneal factors

They are to be looked for when there is a history of abdomino-pelvic surgery, peritonitis, severe genital infection or endometriosis contributing to the formation of adhesions that limit tubal motility. The gold standard for their exploration is laparoscopy, which furthermore allows therapeutic procedures.

They may, however, be apparent on U/S when peritoneal pseudocysts or macropolycystic ovaries are observed. The peritoneal pseudo-cysts present as pelvic fluid masses without a well-defined wall, not creating a mass effect but grinding on adjacent structures. They can be depressed by abdominal palpation. Macropolycystic ovaries should not be confused with PCO, which has a radically different context. They have no pathogenic role in infertility on their own and are not responsible for dysovulation. But there is a statistical association between macropolycystic ovaries and infertility, occurring in the same context as peritoneal causes of infertility with which they are frequently associated. Sonographically, they consist of enlarged ovaries with polycyclic contours, containing multiple cysts larger than 15 mm, frequently asymmetric and varying from one cycle to another.

Pelvic endometriosis

Endometriosis is defined by the presence of ectopic endometrium outside the uterine cavity. There are different forms of endometriosis: peritoneal endometriosis, the diagnosis of which is not accessible by imaging and is done by laparoscopy; ovarian endometriosis (endometriomas); sub-peritoneal endometriosis (deep) with posterior lesions (90%) (torus uterinum and utero-sacral ligaments, rectum and/or sigmoid, Douglas cul-de-sac, vagina and recto-vaginal wall) and/or with anterior lesions (less frequent): bladder-uterus cul-de-sac and/or bladder.

Endometriosis is a common disorder affecting 10% of women during their reproductive years. Endometriotic lesions are found in 40% of patients consulting for infertility, but the direct causal link is still debated. The mechanisms discussed are disorders of ovulation by ovarian parenchyma destruction and interference with follicular development associated with the presence of endometriomas, adhesion formation, development of local inflammation and angiogenic factors.

U/S is a very good first-line tool for the diagnosis of endometriomas and sub-peritoneal locations [20]. It will be supplemented by MRI in order to establish a complete lesion mapping before surgical management. The examination always begins with a study by the abdominal route including the systematic study of the urinary tract. It is then supplemented via the endo-vaginal route with exploration of the posterior wall of the vagina during the withdrawal of the probe at the end of examination. The U/S symptoms of endometriosis are variable depending on the different locations [20].

1. Ovarian lesions: endometriomas (the most common location): fluid lesion, rounded, finely echogenic, homogeneous with an inconstantly sloping sedimentation level (Figure 6.9). The walls may contain thin hyperechoic punctuations. Other signs are: moderated posterior strengthening, no vascular flow at Doppler and frequent bilaterality.
2. Tubal lesions, the diagnosis of which is primarily done by hysterosalpingography. The only nonspecific sonographic sign may be hydrosalpinx. Sometimes a nodule, isoechoic to the myometrium, can be observed in the axis of the uterine horns.
3. Sub-peritoneal endometriosis, direct signs of which are: hypoechoic nodule or thickening, more or less retractile, regular or irregular, sometimes associated with anechoic cystic or hyperechoic hemorragic lesions (Figure 6.10). Indirect signs are: uterine retroflexion, retro-uterine position of the ovaries which are adherent to one another (kissing ovaries), hydrosalpinx, anterior attraction of the recto-sigmoid with a triangular appearance of the digestive tract, and uretero-hydronephrosis.

U/S is very useful for the diagnosis of gastrointestinal (GI) damage, particularly recto-sigmoid, with the typical thickening of the hypoechoic muscularis. In one study comparing U/S to MRI [20], sensitivities for detecting lesions in utero-sacral ligaments, vagina, and GI were 78.3% vs. 84.4%, 46.7% vs. 80% and 93.6% vs. 87.3%, respectively.

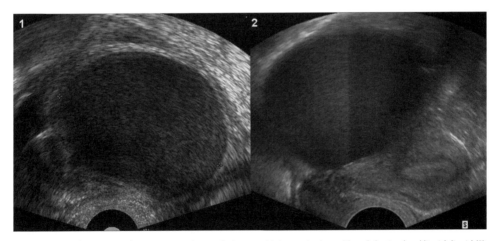

Figure 6.9 Endometrioma: homogeneous hypoechoic cyst with internal echoes (1) and sloping level liquid–liquid (2).

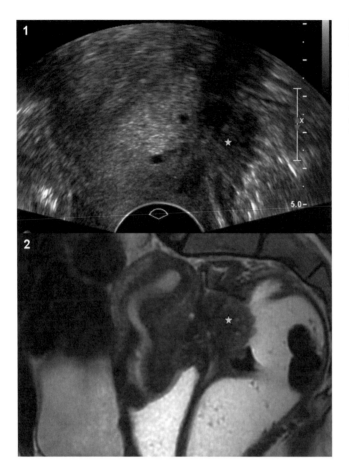

Figure 6.10 Sub-peritoneal endometriosis with uterus in intermediate retroreflected position and with hypoechoic posterior fibrous lesion (*) between the uterus and the recto-sigmoid and with associated external adenomyosis with fluid spots on ultrasound (1) and MRI (2) (sagittal view).

Conclusion

More than ever, the use of pelvic U/S to investigate the subfertile female needs a close collaboration between the gynecologist and the radiologist. U/S has not yet replaced hysterography for evaluation of tubal patency but it provides much other useful information, adding to that obtained by clinical examination. New developments such as hysterosonography and 3D U/S are starting to be used and will certainly reinforce the pivotal role of U/S. The new machines allowing spatial reconstruction will make even more essential the input of the radiologist, who is more familiar with cross-sectional imaging than the gynecologist.

References

1. Radić V, Canić T, Valetić J, Duić Z. Advantages and disadvantages of hysterosonosalpingography in the assessment of the reproductive status of uterine cavity and fallopian tubes. *Eur J Radiol* 2005; **53**: 268–73.

2. Norman RJ, Dewailly D, Legro RS, Hickey TE. Polycystic ovary syndrome. *Lancet* 2007; **370**: 685–97.

3. The Rotterdam ESHRE/ASRM-sponsored PCOS consensus workshop group. Revised 2003 consensus on diagnostic criteria and

long-term health risks related to polycystic ovary syndrome (PCOS). *Human Reprod* 2004; **19**: 41–7.

4. Balen AH, Laven JS, Tan SL, Dewailly D. Ultrasound assessment of the polycystic ovary: international consensus definitions. *Hum Reprod Update* 2003; **9**: 505–14.

5. Jonard S, Robert Y, Dewailly D. Revisiting the ovarian volume as a diagnostic criterion for polycystic ovaries. *Hum Reprod* 2005; **20**: 2893–8.

6. Porter MB. Polycystic ovary syndrome: the controversy of diagnosis by ultrasound. *Semin Reprod Med* 2008; **26**: 241–51.

7. Wang JG, Lobo RA. The complex relationship between hypothalamic amenorrhea and polycystic ovary syndrome. *J Clin Endocrinol Metab* 2008; **93**: 1394–7.

8. Fulghesu AM, Ciampelli M, Belosi C, *et al.* A new ultrasound criterion for the diagnosis of polycystic ovary syndrome: the ovarian stroma/ total area ratio. *Fertil Steril* 2001; **76**: 326–31.

9. Lam PM, Raine-Fenning N. The role of three-dimensional ultrasonography in polycystic ovary syndrome. *Hum Reprod* 2006; **21**: 2209–15.

10. Allemand MC, Tummon IS, Phy JL, *et al.* Diagnosis of polycystic ovaries by three-dimensional transvaginal ultrasound. *Fertil Steril* 2006; **85**: 214–19.

11. Nelson LM, Covington SN, Rebar RW. An update: spontaneous premature ovarian failure is not an early menopause. *Fertil Steril* 2005; **83**: 1327–32.

12. Knauff EA, Eijkemans MJ, Lambalk CB, *et al.* Anti-Mullerian hormone, inhibin B, and antral follicle count in young women

with ovarian failure. *J Clin Endocrinol Metab* 2009; **94**: 786–92.

13. Broekmans FJ, Kwee J, Hendriks DJ, Mol BW, Lambalk CB. A systematic review of tests predicting ovarian reserve and IVF outcome. *Hum Reprod Update* 2006; **12**: 685–718.

14. Steinkeler JA, Woodfield CA, Lazarus E, Hillstrom MM. Female infertility: a systematic approach to radiologic imaging and diagnosis. *Radiographics* 2009; **29**: 1353–70.

15. Bazot M, Deux JF, Dahbi N, Chopier J. Myometrium diseases. *J Radiol* 2001; **82**: 1819–40.

16. Van Voorhis BJ. Ultrasound assessment of the uterus and fallopian tube in infertile women. *Semin Reprod Med* 2008; **26**: 232–40.

17. Robert Y, Launay S, Lemercier E, *et al.* Imaging of the endometrium. *J Radiol* 2001; **82**: 1795–814.

18. Puscheck EE, Cohen L. Congenital malformations of the uterus: the role of ultrasound. *Semin Reprod Med* 2008; **26**: 223–31.

19. Salim R, Woelfer B, Backos M, Regan L, Jurkovic D. Reproducibility of three-dimensional ultrasound diagnosis of congenital uterine anomalies. *Ultrasound Obstet Gynecol* 2003; **21**: 578–82.

20. Bazot M, Lafont C, Rouzier R, *et al.* Diagnostic accuracy of physical examination, transvaginal sonography, rectal endoscopic sonography, and magnetic resonance imaging to diagnose deep infiltrating endometriosis. *Fertil Steril* 2009; **92**: 1825–33.

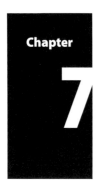

Chapter 7

Treatment options for male infertility

Robert I. McLachlan and Gab Kovacs

Introduction: the importance of assessment of the male partner

Male reproductive dysfunction is the sole or contributory cause in half of infertile couples. Remarkable advances in ART, particularly intracytoplasmic sperm injection (ICSI), now provide fertility in previously sterile men. Such powerful technology does not remove the clinician's obligation to fully evaluate infertile men because, for example, natural fertility may be restorable, and, even when treatment is not possible, providing the man with a reason for his infertility will assist him in coming to terms with his disability. In addition, some health issues are more prevalent in infertile men and must be sought (e.g. androgen or gonadotropin deficiency, testicular cancer) and the opportunity taken to assess and improve general and sexual health. A diagnosis will allow consideration of medical and surgical therapies that permit natural pregnancy. Natural fertility should always be the prime goal so that basic discussions should occur with the couple about the physiology of conception and the timing of intercourse and include preconception counseling of both partners to optimize their health. (See also Chapters 2 and 3.) The effects of the stress of infertility on the couples' individual and relationship health must be considered and counseling offered as indicated: most fertility programs have specialist staff available for this purpose (Chapter 19).

Fertility practices are often staffed by gynecologists yet a process must be in place that facilitates full evaluation of the man on site or through collaborative arrangements. He should undergo medical assessment including a general and reproductive history and examination focused on the state of virilization and external genitalia (testis size and texture, epididymides and vasa) [1].

Causes of male infertilty

The five common diagnostic categories are outlined in descending order of importance:

1. Primary spermatogenic failure is a collective term for a diverse range of disorders affecting spermatogenesis that lead to the generation of inadequate numbers of motile and/or functional sperm. It affects about 5% of all men and accounts for over half of male infertility. Most cases are unexplained (idiopathic) but increasingly genetic factors are being recognized, including karyotypic anomalies (numerical, structural) and Y chromosomal deletions [2]. Alternatively damage may arise from drug, chemo- or radiotherapy, infection or other vascular insults. Our ignorance of the pathophysiology has two consequences:

The Subfertility Handbook: A Clinician's Guide, Second Edition ed. Gab Kovacs. Published by Cambridge University Press. © Cambridge University Press 2011.

- a lack of effective treatments and a heavy reliance on ART to circumvent poor sperm number, motility or function
- the promotion of empirical therapies based on thin or quasi-scientific premises. In most part these are both harmless and useless yet fill that need, felt by patient and clinician alike, "to do something".

2. Obstruction accounts for about 25% of cases and may arise at any point in the tract as a result of infection, trauma, surgery, vasectomy or congenital bilateral absence of the vas.
3. Erectile, ejaculatory or other sexual dysfunction of diverse etiologies (neurovascular, anatomical, psychogenic) that prevent frequent ejaculatory vaginal intercourse.
4. Hypogonadotropic hypogonadism (HH) due to hypothalamo-pituitary disease is rare but diagnosis is vital and gonadotropin replacement therapy restores fertility. Anabolic steroid-induced HH suppresses fertility and has a protracted recovery phase upon drug cessation.
5. Sperm antibodies: these may be directed to fertility-critical determinants on sperm membranes and impair motility, vitality and/or function. They may arise following trauma, surgery (especially vasectomy) or infection but are often idiopathic.

Management overview

Spontaneous conception may occur in many couples with male factor subfertility [1]. In counseling patients, the severity of the male's reproductive problem, the duration of unprotected intercourse, and its frequency and timing, and the female partner's age and reproductive status are all important variables. In other cases, it is evident that fertility will not occur (male sterility) and advice on alternatives (donor insemination, adoption, child-free existence) will dominate discussion. Depending on the couple's age, reproductive history and attitude, some couples are happy to delay treatment in the hope that they will conceive while others will express a wish for immediate intervention.

There is a substantial background rate of spontaneous conception in subfertile men (Figure 7.1) such that about 30% of couples with sperm densities of 1–5 million/ml as the only apparent fertility issue achieved pregnancy over a two- to three-year period. For any proposed treatment to be regarded as effective, it ought "lift" the life table curve up toward that of normally fertile couples, i.e. it ought improve the proportion and speed at which pregnancy occurs relative to placebo. Many extravagant claims for effective treatment in idiopathic male infertility have been made in the absence of these critical placebo-controlled randomized controlled trial (RCT) data. Clinicians must continually monitor the field for new information. There are also some emerging treatments for which one or more trials have failed to find a benefit but supportive evidence may emerge from further studies of larger numbers or through utilizing meta-analysis.

In considering the evidence for any treatments, several points must be made.

- Semen parameters are highly variable and remarkable "spontaneous recoveries" are common and readily misinterpreted as treatment effects.
- Single-limb trials cannot control for placebo effect and for the tendency for a group, having been selected based on a low value, to have a higher value upon re-analysis ("regression to the mean" effect).
- Pregnancy rates must be assessed by rigorous statistical methods such as life table analysis. The impact of variables on pregnancy outcome and therapeutic trials can be assessed by regression analysis with censored data. Couples are rightfully concerned

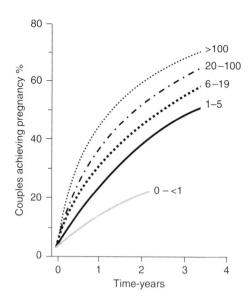

Figure 7.1 Prospects of pregnancy among couples as a function of baseline sperm density (shown in million/ml). Note the slower rate and declining proportion of couples falling pregnant as sperm density falls and that the monthly chance of pregnancy falls progressively as time passes. Nonetheless a considerable proportion of those < 5 million/ml achieve a pregnancy over several years. In counselling couples it must be recognized that female age and reproductive potential have additional effects.

Modifed after Baker HWG. Male infertility. Chapter 171. In DeGroot LJ, Jameson JL, chief eds. *Endocrinology*, 4th edn. Philadelphia, PA: W. B. Saunders, 2001; 2308–28.

about pregnancy outcome, not marginally significant improvement in surrogate fertility markers such as semen parameters.

- Meta-analysis is a popular approach to distilling inconclusive or contentious studies yet differences in study populations, treatment, design, and endpoints may be problematic and individual well-designed and powered studies are preferred.

Accordingly treatments can be considered in two classes; empirical or evidence-based.

Empirical treatments

These approaches variably feature an intrinsically appealing rationale and/or anecdotal or weak evidential support. Most hopefully do no harm nor excessively burden the patient (including cost). Their widespread use is clear evidence that they fill the need felt by both doctor and patient to "do something". It may be that true efficacy exists but has not yet been revealed by systematic study. In male subfertility, the use of empirical therapies often fills a period of "wishful waiting" until natural conception intervenes to spare the couple the cost and burden of ART. However, it should be made clear to patients that any such treatment has not yet been shown to be effective and that in some cases a delay in undertaking effective treatment may in the long term hinder their chances, especially when female reproductive aging is a factor.

Evidence-based interventions

Few treatments for male infertility have met this standard of proof. Yet there are examples based on firm theoretical grounds and supported by clinical data or placebo-controlled RCTs. Nowadays even "effective" treatments that are burdensome, expensive or with a low success rate need also to be viewed in a cost-effectiveness comparison with modern ART approaches.

The appropriateness of treatment choice may in part depend on non-scientific factors such as:

- prevailing healthcare system: public versus private healthcare and insurance considerations
- psychosocial and demographic factors that may for example direct patients toward ART despite evidence for other therapies. Post-vasectomy infertility is a good example; reversal surgery outcomes are dependent on clinical factors (type and time since the procedure, female partner's age and fertility potential), available surgical vs. ART expertise and applicable health system and costing. Cost-effectiveness calculations will differ from country to country. Ultimately there may be "no right answer" but rather the clinician must fully inform the couple to ensure their choice is well informed.

Non-ART treatments

Effective medical interventions

Gonadotropin therapy

In gondatropin deficiency due to hypothalamic/pituitary disease, human chorionic gonado-tropin (hCG) treatment (as an LH substitute) will increase intra-testicular androgen levels and concomitant FSH treatment will stimulate Sertoli cell activity. Together these frequently initiate (in congenital disorders) or restore (in adult-onset cases) spermatogenesis. This process may take 6–24 months and spontaneous conception usually occurs when sperm density increases to around 5 million/ml. In the minority in whom sperm output remains low, ICSI provides a back-up option. The treatment protocols are well described elsewhere [3].

In idiopathic male infertility, RCT data do not suggest a benefit to combined gonado-tropin therapy relative to placebo [4]; very limited and unconfirmed data stemming from studies with significant design deficiencies suggest a role for FSH treatment (whether baseline FSH levels are normal or elevated). Despite the appealing notion that elevating gonadotropin levels will "drive spermatogenesis harder", this seems unlikely to improve intrinsically defective spermatogenesis. Further research is required to define the phenotype of suitable candidates, if any.

Immunosuppression and sperm antibodies

High-dose glucocorticoid therapy in severe sperm autoimmunity has been shown to improve pregnancy outcomes but is associated with both reversible (Cushingoid features, hyper-tension, myopathy) and irreversible (aseptic necrosis of the femoral heads) side effects and with rare exception has been superseded by ICSI (see below).

Genitourinary infection

In the setting of confirmed infection, appropriate antibiotic treatment may improve fertility and prevent permanent damage to the spermatogenesis and excretory ducts.

Withdrawal of drugs

Chemotherapeutic agents used in oncology or renal practice can temporarily or permanently impair spermatogenesis, making sperm cryopreservation a key consideration before treatment.

Reversible suppression in fertility may occur due to exogenous sex steroid use that suppresses gonadotropin levels, or that directly effects spermatogenesis, such as salazopyrine used in the management of inflammatory bowel disease. Finally, many drugs impair libido or sexual function. Consideration of the ongoing need for these agents is essential during evaluation.

Approaches of uncertain efficacy

Varicocele ligation/occlusion

The role of varicocele in infertility and the impact of intervention are highly contentious. Appearing around puberty, they represent a failure of venous valve structures to prevent orthostatic pressure backflow, leading to position-dependent varicosity of the pampiniform plexus. This results in interference of the countercurrent heat exchange that relies upon scrotal evaporative cooling of the venous blood so as to reduce the intra-testicular temperature by 2°C below core body levels. Potential mechanisms for the association with poor semen quality and varicocele include increased scrotal temperature (including that of the contralateral "unaffected" testis), higher rates of germ cell apoptosis, reactive oxygen species generation and sperm DNA damage.

These considerations and varicocele's high prevalence has led to many large single-limb trials reporting improved semen quality and fertility. Yet these studies often suffer from design flaws as discussed above. An unquestioning acceptance that "varicocele causes infertility and thus treatment must improve fertility" is a simplistic approach to a complex issue and a solid evidence base is lacking. Several facts "get in the way of a good story".

- varicoceles are more prevalent in infertile men yet are present in approximately 10% of fertile men
- most men with varicoceles are subfertile (not azoospermic) and have a significant spontaneous pregnancy rate; there are very few RCT data addressing the key question, "are fertility outcomes improved relative to no intervention?"
- overall the fertility outlook seems similar with or without intervention [5].

Conducting an RCT with the power to determine fertility outcomes is exceedingly difficult for many reasons: (i) couples are not willing to accept non-intervention, or wish to move expeditiously to ART treatment; (ii) background rates of conception are significant and few investigators have the resources to conduct adequately powered studies. In a recent Cochrane review [5], eight RCTs reporting pregnancy rates and data in treated (surgical or embolization) and untreated groups were examined; the odds ratio for pregnancy was 1.10 (95% CI 0.73–1.68), indicating no benefit of varicocele treatment over expectant management in subfertile couples in which varicocele was the only abnormal finding.

Interventions for varicoceles include microsurgical ligation of the veins within the scrotum or higher in the inguinal canal, with care to leave the arterial supply and vas undamaged. An alternative approach is transvenous embolization of the (usually left) testicular vein using coils. The initial success rate is similar but higher relapse rates over time may occur with the embolization approach because of collateral veins in the scrotum; this potential disadvantage may be offset by the lower cost and morbidity of the radiographic approach.

In conclusion, two opposing views are prevalent; that varicocele removal has either no role in fertility management or that it is a major reversible cause of poor semen quality that demands treatment. Some clinicians sit uncomfortably in the middle trying to "pick candidates" based on selection criteria of doubtful veracity. Any discussion of treatment for asymptomatic varicoceles associated with idiopathic infertility must include the fact that a significant fertility benefit is unproven [6].

Potential groups worthy of further consideration for intervention include:

- late adolescent or early adult before ipsilateral testis size is compromised
- bilateral varicocele or a unilateral varicocele associated with a contralateral atrophic (or absent) testis in which setting improvement in testicular function might significantly improve overall sperm output.

Intervention may be warranted for symptomatic varicocele (discomfort, pain). Intervention is not likely to be of benefit in non-obstructive azoospermia, especially with an elevated FSH, nor in non-clinically apparent varicoceles seen only on ultrasound.

Lifestyle interventions

Positive health benefits can flow from correction of poor lifestyle factors (e.g. smoking or other social drugs, excessive alcohol intake, sedentary lifestyle and obesity) yet for most men with spermatogenetic disorders a return of semen parameters and fertility to normal is unlikely. Nonetheless the opportunity to impart general health advice is warranted as the presentation with male infertility presents a window of opportunity to address these matters.

Antiestrogens

By impairing estrogen-mediated gonadotropin feedback, treatment with agents such as tamoxifen and clomiphene citrate elevates serum FSH, LH and testosterone levels. However, again, whether this improves spermatogenic outcome is controversial [7].

Antioxidants

Oxidative stress may damage sperm DNA and antioxidant therapy has been proposed to improve DNA quality and fertility outcome. Yet the few supportive data that exist are conflicting and placebo-controlled RCT studies, adequately powered to assess live birth rates, are required and should involve carefully selected patients exhibiting consistently high levels of sperm DNA damage.

Nutritional supplements

Many preparations are commercially promoted and include vitamins, herbal extracts, and minerals. Usage of such "natural therapies" is high and while there is little/no evidence of efficacy coming from RTCs, at best one hopes they are harmless, although some may contain contaminants and be potentially harmful.

Historical and disproven treatments

Androgens

Temporary suppression of gonadotropin levels and thus spermatogenesis was once thought to be followed by a rebound in sperm production upon cessation. This approach has no place in the management of the infertile male. Similarly androgen treatment does not improve sperm quality through improvement in epididymal maturation as once proposed.

Antibiotics and anti-inflammatory drugs

These have no role in the absence of documented infections or inflammations in the accessory sex organs.

Scrotal temperature

Elevation of testicular temperature is recognized to impair semen quality. This has been extrapolated to propose the wearing of loose underwear and various methods of scrotal cooling as treatments for idiopathic male infertility, yet the data are inconsistent and this approach is not practical [8].

Assisted reproductive treatments

Overview

For most men with poor semen quality or azoospermia, evidence-based treatments to improve natural fertility are not available. Fortunately ART provides an effective means of bypassing their reproductive limitations and achieving a healthy pregnancy. The ability to provide ART as a treatment option for male infertility is essential in fertility practice.

Intracytoplasmic sperm injection (ICSI) has revolutionized management by permitting pregnancy whenever sperm (of almost any quality) can be located in the semen or genital tract, including from the seminiferous tubules [9]. For men with milder fertility impairments, conventional IVF, wherein motile sperm are incubated with mature oocytes, provides similar fertilization and pregnancy outcomes. Accordingly ICSI is not recommended for all male factor cases as it involves additional interventions and costs and, despite reassuring data thus far, less is known of its long-term safety. Nonetheless in most ART programs, ICSI accounts for the majority of male factor cycles and has genuinely "levelled the playing field" for fertility outcomes relative to other etiologies such as idiopathic infertility or female tubal obstruction. These issues are discussed in detail in Chapter 11.

Artificial insemination (AIH) using the partner's fresh or frozen semen has a limited place as pregnancy outcome appears no greater than those occurring naturally unless there is an associated female factor [10]. In our opinion, it is not a particularly useful first intervention as its success rate is significantly less than for IVF/ICSI yet it still involves considerable monitoring and cost, and additionally it has a higher risk of high multiple pregnancy. Notable exceptions are couples with sexual or ejaculatory difficulties in whom vaginal intercourse is not occurring and AIH may be useful. The possible role of AIH is discussed fully in Chapter 9.

Unfortunately there are men in whom viable sperm cannot be located, or who have genetic disorders that make normal embryonic development impossible: for such couples, a sensitive discussion of donor insemination may be appropriate.

Evaluation of semen quality for ART

Semen testing is best performed by the ART facility rather than a general pathology laboratory as it will probably provide a more thorough and informative assessment. Semen is best collected on site in appropriate facilities in order to avoid temperature-related motility artifacts during transportation. Poor semen quality should be confirmed with repeat analysis 4–6 weeks later.

For men with severe oligospermia (< 1 million/ml), cryopreservation of the sample for future use should be considered as sperm output can fluctuate; azoospermia or only immotile sperm may be found on the day of egg collection, in which case having a cryopreserved back-up sample avoids the need for surgical recovery attempts.

Very poor motility and vitality can sometimes be a reflection of infrequent ejaculation: relatively short periods of abstinence (1–2 days) should be encouraged to ensure that motile sperm of optimal vitality are available. As ICSI only needs a few sperm, sperm quality (particularly vitality and thus DNA integrity) maximizes the potential for healthy embryonic development. While conventional IVF might be planned based on prior semen samples, there is always the possibility of a poorer-quality sample on the day of egg collection, necessitating a change to ICSI; thus ART programs need to have that flexibility.

Finally, some men find the collection of semen at the time of egg collection very stressful; if practicable such men may collect the sample at home and/or use PDE5 inhibitors to maintain an adequate erection. If there is performance anxiety about producing on the day of oocyte collection, semen can be collected in advance and cryostored.

Sperm preparation for conventional IVF and ICSI

There is a range of sperm preparation procedures. Briefly, in our unit, raw semen is subjected to gradient separation using a proprietary gel material followed by several cycles of centrifugation and pellet resuspension in media, with the final concentration and motility being assessed using a Makler chamber. The appropriate number of motile sperm are then incubated for IVF or a small number selected for ICSI.

In a man who has been assessed as suitable for IVF or ICSI, on the day of egg collection the initial sample may be incomplete or of inadequate quality for the purpose; a second sample is sometimes requested, and may provide adequate sperm for ICSI without having to resort to surgery.

Indications for using ICSI include the availability of insufficient progressively motile sperm after sperm preparation, elevated levels of abnormal sperm morphology (> 90–95% using strict criteria: a surrogate marker of impaired sperm function), sperm autoimmunity affecting the head and/or mid-piece, and when using epididymal or testicular sperm as these do not show the normal sperm/oocyte interaction required for successful IVF.

Surgical sperm isolation for ICSI

Successful testicular sperm extraction (TESE) for ICSI provides a means to fatherhood for many previously sterile men. A range of surgical approaches to sperm recovery have been described. In addition to loss of testicular mass and infection risk, all carry some risks of damaging the testicular blood supply, which is tenuous due to a lack of collateral supply. There is the potential for hemorrhage within the inelastic tunica albuginea causing tamponade and ischemic damage or atrophy.

All men must be made aware of the small but tangible risk of permanent testicular dysfunction, especially androgen deficiency, particularly those with only one testis and/or spermatogenic disorders in whom overt or incipient androgen deficiency often preexists [11]. Clinical and biochemical assessment of androgen status should be performed before and several months after surgery, especially before repeat surgeries.

The clinical settings wherein mature spermatids are surgically isolated for ICSI include the following.

Obstructive azoospermia (OA)

In non-surgically remediable obstructive azoospermia of any cause, fine-needle aspiration (FNA) testicular biopsy, usually under local anesthesia, provides a safe, quick, reliable, and cost-effective means of isolating mature spermatids for ICSI. Despite its higher cost, some advocate microsurgical epididymal sperm aspiration (MESA) in vasal or epididymal obstruction as it may allow collection of large numbers of sperm for cryopreservation and thereby avoid further surgery [12]. Percutaneous epididymal sperm aspiration (PESA) is a simple, low-cost approach to recovery in these setting [13]. However, in both MESA and PESA, as a result of epididymal stagnation, poor sperm vitality and DNA integrity may be as problem. When using PESA, usually in the setting of a previous vasectomy, if we find poor sperm vitality we move to FNA to obtain fresh testicular sperm. Overall we find FNA to provide sperm in 99% of OA cases and to be preferred over MESA despite the need for repeated procedures if subsequent cycles are needed.

Spermatogenic failure

In men with severe spermatogenic problems, extreme oligospermia with only non-motile/non-vital sperm present or azoospermia (often called "non-obstructive azoospermia", NOA) testicular biopsy of some type will be required (see below). A fresh semen sample on the day of egg collection should be performed as occasionally it may provide sperm for ICSI without having to resort to surgery.

Our broad approach has been to attempt a FNA involving multiple passes through the testis followed, if needed, by an open testicular biopsy. FNA may not be possible with very small and soft testes due to difficulty in passing through the tunica and open biopsy is required from the outset. Unless contraindicated, both testes are biopsied. Overall we find sperm on FNA in over 50% of NOA cases but open biopsy will go to provide sperm in half the remaining cases. A recent report has confirmed the utility of sequential testicular sperm aspiration followed by open TESE if needed [14].

Sexual dysfunction and ejaculatory disorders

Various less invasive options must first be considered in men with complete erectile or ejaculatory failure, for example those with vascular disease or diabetic autonomic neuropathy (PDE5 inhibitors), retrograde ejaculation (isolation of post-orgasmic urine for AIH) or spinal cord injury (vibro- or electroejaculation). Increasingly the excellent outcomes from FNA/ICSI are regarded as a cost-effective alternative, particularly if advancing female age or confounding factors are also present.

Outlook for surgical sperm recovery in spermatogenic failure

In NOA or when only exceedingly poor-quality semen is available, testicular sperm provides a good prospect for pregnancy. Overall in NOA there is an approximately 50% chance of recovering sperm from testicular biopsy. A few prognostic factors can help identify candidates who will ultimately be successful.

1. Testicular histology is the best predictor: the finding of hypospermatogenesis (the presence of all germ cell forms including spermatids even in the minority of tubules) carries a good prospect (> 90%) of sperm recovery whilst Sertoli-only cell syndrome (present in every tubule in a diagnostic biopsy) is still associated with a 25% prospect of sperm recovery, presumably due to tubule heterogeneity that has not been reflected in the diagnostic biopsy. The least common histological pattern is germ cell arrest at the primary spermatocyte stage; this condition effects all tubules in the biopsy and is associated with a poor chance of recovery at TESE, presumably because it reflects a global genetically based abnormality in meiosis. Occasionally there is a mixed pattern with and between testes, in which case the prognosis is reflected by the most favorable pattern [15].

2. Y chromosome microdeletions affect about 5% of severely infertile men. The subgroup with the most extensive deletion involving the AZFa and AZFb regions in addition to the common AZFc are associated with a very poor chance of sperm recovery and realistically point to donor insemination as the viable alternative [16].
3. Chemotherapy or radiotherapy: previous cancer treatment may affect the prospects for sperm recovery depending upon the drugs used, the dosage, and duration, such that one must be circumspect about the prospects. Nonetheless reasonable sperm recovery rates have been reported but prognostication for individual patients is difficult [17].

Factors which are surprisingly not predictive in any clinically useful way are testicular size, serum FSH, and the diagnosis of Klinefelter's syndrome (KS). Indeed in KS, sperm have been isolated in up to 70% of non-mosaic cases by open testicular biopsy, indicating that often tubules are present in which a normal 46XY spermatogonial cell lineage is present or that there is extrusion of the additional X during meiosis [18]. The prospects of sperm aneuploidy are increased in Klinefelter's syndrome but the majority of spermatids have a normal complement that is usually reflected in the birth of offspring with a normal sex chromosomal complement [19]. Nonetheless all such couples require counseling with consideration for PGD or amniocentesis.

Methods for surgical sperm isolation

Fine-needle aspiration (FNA).

This simple procedure involves instillation of 5 ml of lignocaine around the spermatic cord to provide testicular anesthesia followed by needle aspiration (or punch biopsy) to obtain small fragments of seminiferous tubule for diagnosis analyses and/or sperm retrieval. It carries a small risk of serious vascular damage (around one in several hundred) due to the transection of the sub-tunical artery about which patients must be advised and observed after the procedure; a Doppler ultrasound should be performed in the setting of marked swelling or pain. In our experience multiple needle aspiration biopsies can be safely performed over time if required with little risk of a serious adverse event.

Open testicular biopsy

This is usually performed under general anesthesia, and can be performed using either

- random, multi-site biopsy (two or three sites per testis) removing ≈250 mg of tubule tissue for mincing and isolation of sperm from amongst various cell types and debris , or
- the microdissection procedure ("micro-TESE") described by Schlegel and Li [20] in which the thicker seminiferous tubule segments that are more likely to contain sperm are directly visualized using an operating microscope.

Micro-TESE has been reported in several studies to have a somewhat higher sperm recovery rate (≈65% vs. 50%), particularly in Klinefelter's, when the small testis size allows excellent visualization of tubule lobules. However, it requires a higher degree of technical skill and added cost, and many programs continue to achieve reasonable results with random biopsy.

All operative procedures may transiently impair sperm production and repeat operations should not occur within 4–6 months [21]. Androgen status and testis size must be checked prior to all procedures. For new patients in whom androgen deficiency is already evident testosterone treatment should be deferred until either ejaculated sperm has been cryopreserved or the patient has undergone his TESE attempt because testosterone administration will suppress gonadotropins and may obliterate any residual spermatogenesis. This is an important issue for counseling and must be addressed immediately upon completion of the ART attempts. Repeated open testicular biopsy increases the risk of hypogonadism due to acute surgical complications and of the long-term loss of testicular tissue.

ART outcomes in male infertility

Fertilization, embryonic development, implantation rates and live birth rates are on the whole similar for male factor infertility as compared to other forms of infertility. There are a couple of exceptions particularly when sperm vitality and motility is poor, in which setting all of these results can be impaired. As mentioned above genetic abnormalities are more common in severely infertile men, in particular chromosomal abnormalities (sex chromosome aneuploidy, translocations and inversions) which carry high rates of embryonic abnormalities, miscarriage, and increased live birth rates with anomalies. Overall ICSI offspring have a 2–3-fold higher rate of chromosomal aneuploidies (some hereditary, some de novo) compared to the age-matched population. Some of these are benign with no consequence but others can be significant and genetic counseling is an important part of ART management.

As a general guideline we would recommend the following [2]:

1. karyotypic analysis of the male when sperm density is < 10 million/ml
2. Y chromosome microdeletion analysis with sperm densities of < 5 million/ml; this cut off captures the vast majority of men with this problem
3. cystic fibrosis gene screening should be performed on all men with bilateral genital absence of the vas or unexplained epididymal obstruction or any other structural anomalies affecting the Wolffian duct derivatives, e.g. asymmetric deficiencies in the vas or absence of the seminal vesicles. This is because there is a high rate of heterozygosity or compound heterozygosity for CFTR mutations [22]. If combined with a female partner also carrying a CFTR mutation it would carry the risk of clinical CF. Given the above circumstances genetic counseling and consideration of a PGD (for example sex selection in the case of the Y-chromosome deletion or PGD in the setting of balanced autosomal translocation) are now an important part of practice [23].

References

1. Baker G. Clinical management of male infertility. In de Groot L, McLachlan R, eds. www.ENDOTEXT.org, Chapter 7. South Dartmouth, MA: MDTEXT.COM.Inc.

2. McLachlan RI, O'Bryan MK. State of the art for genetic testing of infertile men. *J Clin Endocrinol Metab* Rapid Electronic Publication first published on 20 Jan 2010.

3. Hayes F, Pitteloud N. Hypogonadotropic hypogonadism and gonadotropin therapy. In de Groot L, McLachlan R, eds. www. ENDOTEXT.org, Chapter 5. South Dartmouth, MA: MDTEXT.COM.Inc.

4. Knuth UA, Hönigl W, Bals-Pratsch M, Schleicher G, Nieschlag E. Treatment of severe oligospermia with human chorionic gonadotropin/human menopausal gonadotropin: a placebo-controlled, double blind trial. *J Clin Endocrinol Metab* 1987; **65**(6): 1081–7.

5. Evers JH, Collins J, Clarke J. Surgery or embolisation for varicoceles in subfertile men. *Cochrane Database Syst Rev* 2009; **21**(1): CD000479.

6. Zini A, Boman JM. Varicocele: red flag or red herring? *Semin Reprod Med* 2009; **27**(2): 171–8.

7. Kamischke A, Nieschlag E. Analysis of medical treatment of male infertility. *Hum Reprod* 1999; **14** Suppl 1: 1–23.

8. Jung A, Schuppe HC. Influence of genital heat stress on semen quality in humans. *Andrologia* 2007; **39**(6): 203–15 (Review).

9. Palermo G, Joris H, Devroey P, Van Steirteghem AC. Pregnancies after intracytoplasmic injection of single spermatozoon into an oocyte. *Lancet* 1992; **340**(8810): 17–8.

10. Bhattacharya S, Harrild K, Mollison J, *et al.* Clomifene citrate or unstimulated intrauterine insemination compared with expectant management for unexplained infertility: pragmatic randomised controlled trial. *BMJ* 2008; **337**: a716.

11. Andersson AM, Jørgensen N, Frydelund-Larsen L, Rajpert-De Meyts E, Skakkebaek NE. Impaired Leydig cell function in infertile men: a study of 357 idiopathic infertile men and 318 proven fertile controls. *J Clin Endocrinol Metab* 2004; **89**(7): 3161–7

12. Devroey P, Silber S, Nagy Z, *et al.* Ongoing pregnancies and birth after intracytoplasmic sperm injection with frozen-thawed epididymal spermatozoa. *Hum Reprod* 1995; **10**(4): 903–6.

13. Tsirigotis M, Pelekanos M, Yazdani N, *et al.* Simplified sperm retrieval and intracytoplasmic sperm injection in patients with azoospermia. *Br J Urol* 1995; **76**(6): 765–8.

14. Houwen J, Lundin K, Söderlund B, *et al.* Efficacy of percutaneous needle aspiration and open biopsy for sperm retrieval in men with non-obstructive azoospermia. *Acta Obstet Gynecol Scand* 2008; **87**(10): 1033–8.

15. McLachlan RI, Rajpert-De Meyts E, Hoei-Hansen CE, de Kretser DM, Skakkebaek NE. Histological evaluation of the human testis – approaches to optimizing the clinical value of the assessment: mini review. *Hum Reprod* 2007; **22**(1): 2–16.

16. Stahl PJ, Masson P, Mielnik A, *et al.* A decade of experience emphasizes that testing for Y microdeletions is essential in American men with azoospermia and severe oligozoospermia. *Fertil Steril* 2009 Nov 5 [Epub ahead of print].

17. Meseguer M, Garrido N, Remohí J, *et al.* Testicular sperm extraction (TESE) and ICSI in patients with permanent azoospermia after chemotherapy. *Hum Reprod* 2003; **18**(6): 1281–5.

18. Schiff JD, Palermo GD, Veeck LL, *et al.* Success of testicular sperm extraction [corrected] and intracytoplasmic sperm injection in men with Klinefelter syndrome. *J Clin Endocrinol Metab* 2005; **90**(11): 6263–7.

19. Fullerton G, Hamilton M, Maheshwari A. Should non-mosaic Klinefelter syndrome men be labelled as infertile in 2009? *Hum Reprod* 2010; **25**(3): 588–97.

20. Schlegel PN, Li PS. Microdissection TESE: sperm retrieval in non-obstructive azoospermia. *Hum Reprod Update*. 1998; **4**(4): 439.

21. Schlegel PN, Su LM. Physiological consequences of testicular sperm extraction. *Hum Reprod* 1997; **12**(8): 1688–92.

22. Dork T, Dworniczak B, Aulehla-Scholz C, *et al.* Distinct spectrum of CFTR gene mutations in congenital absence of vas deferens. *Hum Genet* 1997; **100**: 365–77.

23. McLachlan RI and O'Bryan MK. State of the art for genetic testing of infertile men. *J Clin Endocrinol Metab* 2010; **95**: 1013–1024.

The management of anovulation (including PCOS)

Anthony J. Rutherford

Introduction

Anovulation is defined as a failure to release a mature oocyte on a regular monthly basis. Chronic anovulation is an important cause of infertility, accounting for approximately 20% of all causes. Establishing the correct diagnosis is essential so that the most effective therapy can be employed, as appropriate treatment can usually restore fertility. In general other common causes of infertility should be excluded before starting treatment, as more than one factor may be involved. Men should have had a semen analysis and women should have had the basic infertility work-up including an assessment of tubal patency. Lifestyle issues that could have a bearing on fertility need to be addressed before considering pharmacological or surgical intervention.

Basic physiology

In order to appreciate the various causes of anovulation and the potential treatment options, it is important to revisit an outline of ovarian physiology and follicular development.

Primordial follicles start to grow under influences yet unknown, totally independent of the pituitary hormones FSH and LH, until they reach around 0.25 mm in diameter. Further development to form an antral follicle requires FSH. After puberty, under the influence of FSH the follicles enlarge with proliferation of the granulosa cells to form a multilayered structure with a fluid-filled space known as an antrum, to which the oocyte is adherent, surrounded by follicular cells that form the cumulus oophorus. This process of development to a small antral follicle takes around three months.

The final development of one of these antral follicles through to a mature Graafian follicle is under the control of the hypothalamic-pituitary axis. Gonadotropin releasing hormone (GnRH), a decapeptide, is produced in neurons in the hypothalamus, and released into the hypophysial portal bloodstream at the median eminence. GnRH is released in a pulsatile manner, with the amplitude and rate of pulses determined by a number of factors which include a negative, and at times positive, feedback loop controlled by the steroid hormones estrogen and progesterone. In the follicular phase the pulse frequency varies between 60 and 90 minutes, and this decreases under the influence of progesterone in the luteal phase.

Towards the end of a non-conception ovulatory cycle the corpus luteum evolutes and progesterone and estradiol levels fall. This fall in estradiol removes the negative feedback on the hypothalamus, leading to an increase in gonadotropin secretion. The early cycle rise in

The Subfertility Handbook: A Clinician's Guide, Second Edition ed. Gab Kovacs. Published by Cambridge University Press. © Cambridge University Press 2011.

FSH further stimulates granulosa cell proliferation and differentiation, FSH receptor production, and an increase in the steroidogenic cytochrome P450 enzyme, aromatase. Aromatase is responsible for the conversion of androgens to the estrogens, estrone and estradiol. LH stimulates the production of androgens in the theca cells, which diffuse into the granulosa cells and form the substrate for estradiol production. Antral follicles have varying threshold requirements for FSH to progress and continue to develop. A small batch of antral follicles may start to grow but it is the follicle that has the lowest threshold for FSH that will develop and become the dominant follicle for that cycle. As the granulosa cells grow and aromatase is switched on, estradiol is produced, which facilitates further FSH receptor development in this dominant follicle. The rising estradiol also restores the negative feedback to the hypothalamus, leading to falling FSH levels. Falling FSH levels mean that the following cohort of antral follicles do not have sufficient FSH to survive and enter the process of atresia. This is the process of recruitment that leads to unifollicular development in humans. As the lead follicle grows, LH receptors also develop under the influence of FSH, allowing the follicle to respond to LH. By the mid-follicular phase the lead follicle can utilize both FSH and LH to continue growth and estradiol production. Although there are waves of small antral follicles developing throughout the cycle the low levels of FSH mean that no further recruitment takes place.

In the late follicular phase the rapidly increasing estradiol levels, essentially from the lead follicle, cause a change in the GnRH pulse generator, which results in the LH surge and ovulation. Following the LH surge, luteinization of the granulosa cells to form the corpus luteum leads to a shift to progesterone production with levels peaking in non-conception cycles at around 7 days post ovulation. In a conception cycle the hCG produced from the developing pregnancy maintains the corpus luteum until around 8 weeks gestation, when trophoblast takes over the endocrine function. In non-conception cycles the fall in estradiol and progesterone leads to the whole process starting again.

Classification of anovulation

In 1973 the World Health Organization published a simple classification of anovulation, which is still referred to today.

WHO I

These patients are characterized by a history of amenorrhea, a low estradiol, low or normal gonadotropins and a normal prolactin. They have a negative response to a progestogen challenge with no withdrawal bleeding. The most common examples include weight-related amenorrhea found in anorexic and bulimic patients, exercise-induced amenorrhea seen in athletes, and psychogenic amenorrhea. Rarer causes include genetic abnormalities of the hypothalamus (Kallmann's syndrome), pituitary (hypopituitarism), or physical disruption to the normal hypothalamic-pituitary axis, which may be either iatrogenic (surgery, cranial irradiation) or tumors such as a craniopharyngioma. In women recently delivered, catastrophic obstetric hemorrhage can lead to pituitary necrosis (Sheehan's syndrome) and secondary amenorrhea.

WHO II

This is by far the largest group and will form the predominant group presenting for treatment. They are characterized by a history of oligomenorrhea, although there may be some with amenorrhea. They are estrogenized and have a positive response to a progestogen challenge test, with a withdrawal bleed. FSH and prolactin levels are normal, but there may be a mildly elevated LH, with an altered LH/FSH ratio. The bulk of these women will have polycystic ovary syndrome (PCOS).

PCOS is probably the most common reproductive endocrinopathy, with a variable incidence depending on the populations studied, but thought to be between 5 and 10% of women of reproductive age. There is considerable heterogeneity in presentation, which underlines the diverse nature of the condition and why, to date, the complex genetic basis has not been identified. In 2003, a group of experts met in Rotterdam to establish diagnostic criteria, which it was hoped would enable appropriately defined clinical trials to be performed to further elucidate the condition [1]. The cardinal signs and symptoms of the condition are chronic anovulation, clinical or biochemical evidence of hyperandrogenism, and a polycystic appearance of the ovary on ultrasound. The Rotterdam consensus dictates that women with PCOS must have at least two out of these three criteria after exclusion of other potential underlying pathology.

The clinical manifestations of androgen excess include hirsutism and acne and less commonly alopecia. Biochemical evidence of hyperandrogenemia is seen in many but not all patients, with increased circulating levels of free testosterone, or a raised free androgen index (FAI). The morphological appearance of the polycystic ovary has been defined as the presence of 12 or more antral follicles between 2 and 9 mm in size on each ovary plus or minus an increase in ovarian volume. Preferably diagnostic scans should be performed on high-resolution ultrasound equipment. Only one ovary fitting this description is required to confirm the diagnosis. The majority of women with PCOS have higher levels of circulating LH and an elevated LH/FSH ratio.

Central obesity is a cardinal feature of women with PCOS with an increased waist–hip ratio. Insulin resistance and hyperinsulinemia are common features of obese and non-obese women with PCOS, with insulin sensitivity more pronounced in women with oligoamenorrhea. Furthermore, there is a 3–7-times increased risk of developing type II diabetes, particularly in obese women. There is also a higher incidence of a dyslipidemia, with increased serum triglycerides and lower levels of HDL cholesterol. Collectively, these abnormalities, along with hypertension, are features of the metabolic syndrome, which has been estimated to be double the incidence in women with PCOS compared to the general population. Those with the metabolic syndrome are known to have an increased risk of cardiovascular disease, although there are limited epidemiological data in women with PCOS to confirm the absolute risk.

WHO III

This group are characterized by oligoamenorrhea, and may present with menopausal symptoms, such as hot flushes, night sweats, and vaginal dryness. They will have raised gonadotropins and in amenorrheic women a low estradiol. Their serum anti-Müllerian hormone levels will be low or undetectable. These women essentially have ovarian failure. There may be an underlying genetic cause, such as Turner's mosaic (XO) or Fragile X syndrome, auto-immune, or it could be due to iatrogenic damage following surgery, radio- and/or chemo-therapy. In the majority a clear cause is not identified.

Hyperprolactinemia

These patients do not fit into the conventional WHO classification. They generally present with oligoamenorrhea and the majority will have galactorrhea. They will have a raised prolactin, and normal or low levels of gonadotropins. There may be sufficient estrogen to have a positive progestogen challenge test. Thyroid stimulating hormone (TSH) levels may be low.

A mildly raised prolactin can occur with anxiety. A significantly raised prolactin, particularly values above a 1000 mU/l, is likely to be associated with pathology. Pituitary prolactinomas are classified according to their size, with those under 10 mm known as a microadenoma, and those above as a macroadenoma. Approximately 7% of microadenomas left untreated will enlarge. Prolactin levels are generally proportional to tumor size. Most women of childbearing age with a microadenoma or macroademona will present with oligoamenorrhea and approximately 85% will report galactorrhea. Some will experience reduced libido, and symptoms of estrogen deficiency, while less common symptoms include headaches and visual field defects (due to suprasellar extension and compression of the optic chiasma). Non-secretory pituitary adenomas or tumors in the region of the hypothalamus may also cause hyperprolactinemia by compression or disruption of the pituitary stalk removing the inhibitory effect of dopamine on prolactin secretion. Other causes of hyperprolactinemia include associated endocrinopathies such as hypothyroidism, in adrenal insufficiency, and in some women with PCOS. It also occurs in renal disease and end-stage liver disease with cirrhosis. Moderate elevation of prolactin also occurs in women on various medications, alpha methyl dopa for hypertension, pyschotropic drugs such as phenothiazines and butyrophenones, and selective serotonin reuptake inhibitors. Chronic opiate abuse is another cause. Finally, all women presenting with amenorrhea and galactorrhea should be tested to exclude pregnancy.

Treatment

WHO I

Lifestyle modification

Changes in body weight have a profound influence on reproductive function. Those women with weight-related amenorrhea need to increase their calorific intake to restore their BMI to within the normal range. A certain proportion of body fat, thought to be about 22%, is required for normal ovulation. In women with weight-related amenorrhea, GnRH pulsatility reverts to a pattern similar to that seen in puberty, which in turn results in a typical multicystic ovary on pelvic ultrasound, and diminished LH. While ovulation can be restored by pulsatile administration of exogenous GnRH or gonadotropins (hMG or FSH/LH), this would be inappropriate until weight is restored. Nutrition plays an essential role in fetal development, and poor nutrition has a profound impact on the incidence of disease in adult life. Addressing the underlying psychological illness with appropriate support is the key to a successful outcome.

Athletes in training may have a BMI within the normal range but still develop amenorrhea because of increased muscle bulk. Interestingly athletes with a high body fat rarely have reproductive dysfunction. Those who exercise hard but do not have an adequate calorific intake are more likely to develop amenorrhea. Reduction of exercise or an increase in calorific intake is required to restore function.

Once weight is restored to normal it can take some time for normal cycles to resume. In these women, and others with a hypothalamic cause, the treatment options are to consider the use of synthetic GnRH to induce normal pituitary release of FSH and LH or consider exogenous gonadotropins. In pituitary causes, exogenous gonadotropins will be required.

Gonadotropin releasing hormone

Synthetic GnRH is commercially available as Gonadorelin. It is delivered via a small pump in a pulsatile manner either intravenously or subcutaneously. The route and site of administration make a difference to response, with lower doses of GnRH required with IV therapy. The upper arm results in higher peak serum concentrations as compared to injection into the abdomen. When both modes of delivery are considered, higher ovulation rates and pregnancy rates are obtained with IV therapy. In the first treatment cycle the pulse frequency and dose should be slightly longer (120 minutes) and the dose slightly lower (5 μg), to reduce the risk of multiple follicular development and multiple pregnancy. Treatment should be monitored carefully with ultrasound. In subsequent cycles the pulse frequency is reduced to between 60 and 90 minutes, and the dose increased to 10 μg. The GnRH therapy is continued throughout the cycle, although the pulse frequency may be reduced to up to 240 minutes in ovulatory cycles in the luteal phase to reduce costs. Another alternative to reduce costs is to give hCG once the follicle has reached a diameter of 17–18 mm, instead of continuing with the pump in the luteal phase. In addition to the factors outlined above, the success of treatment is determined by the careful selection of patients, with the best results obtained in women with hypothalamic amenorrhea, where ovulation rates can be up to 95% and pregnancy rates as high as 85% [2].

Gonadotropins

The first pregnancy using urinary-derived human menopausal gonadotropin (HMG), containing equal amounts of FSH and LH activity, was reported in 1962, in women with hypogonadotrophic hypogonadism [3]. HMG (Pergonal, Serono) was first licensed for clinical use in Israel in 1963, and Italy in 1965. The original preparation contained a high proportion of extraneous proteins with only 5% FSH and LH, and consequently needed to be administered by deep intramuscular injection. In some countries human pituitary gonadotropins (HPG), FSH of pituitary origin was used [4]. Unfortunately this led to the infection of some women with Creutzfeldt–Jakob disease [5].

The use of monoclonal antibody technology allowed development of a highly purified urinary FSH preparation, which could be administered by subcutaneous injection and had less batch-to-batch variation. It was clear that with a huge demand for gonadotropins driven by the explosion of assisted conception technology in the late 1980s there was a need for a more reliable source of base product than post-menopausal urine. Identification of the FSH alpha and beta subunit amino acid sequence, and the subsequent cloning of the gene which codes for FSH, led to the production of human FSH using DNA recombinant technology. The DNA for human FSH was incorporated into the host cell DNA of an immortalized cell line, CHO cells (CHO stands for Chinese hamster ovary). These cells then secrete human FSH. FSH is a glycosylated protein held in a specific active configuration by disulfide bridges. The enzymes needed for glycosylation are only found in mammalian cell lines. By selecting the CHO cells that produce the correct isoform of FSH and using these to form a master cell bank, which can be used in industrial quantities to manufacture a highly purified and potent FSH preparation, a potentially unlimited supply of gonadotropin is available. Gonal F (Serono) was launched in 1995, and Puregon (Organon laboratories) was released in 1996. Recombinant technology has now been used to make recombinant LH, hCG and more recently a longer-acting FSH by combining the active component of the FSH molecule to the carboxyterminal extension of the β-hCG molecule to develop a long-acting FSH. The latter may be of more value in patients having controlled ovarian stimulation for IVF. All of these preparations can be administered by subcutaneous injection using pen injection devices. Highly purified urinary gonadotropins containing FSH alone (Fostimon, IBSA; Brevelle, Ferring) or both FSH and LH activity (Menopur, Ferring; Merional, IBSA) are still manufactured and widely used.

In patients with hypogonadotropic hypogonadism, a combination of FSH and LH activity appears to be better than FSH alone, as LH stimulates androgen precursors for estrogen production.

The aim of ovulation induction treatment is to achieve unifollicular development to limit the risk of multiple pregnancy and ovarian hyperstimulation syndrome. The dose of gonadotropin required to achieve adequate stimulation is variable, and it is essential that all treatment is monitored with ultrasound. There are two principal methods known as the step up and step down regimens. The step up regimen involves starting with a low dose of gonadotropins, between 37.5 and 75 IU per day and kept at this level for up to 14 days, before increasing the dose in relatively small increments every 7 days until evidence of follicular growth; then the same dose is maintained until ovulation is achieved. The same dose is then used in subsequent cycles. The second method is known as the step down regimen, which consists of a higher loading dose of FSH which is subsequently reduced once follicular development is observed. The largest study so far comparing the two regimens was in patients with PCOS and found that the step up regimen is safer in terms of unifollicular development [6]. Once ovulation is restored, repeat treatment cycles allow a near normal cumulative conception rate, assuming other causes of infertility have been excluded.

WHO II

Lifestyle modification

In contrast, those with significantly increased weight, and in particular a raised waist–hip ratio commonly seen in women with PCOS, have an increased rate of anovulation, a poor response to ovulation induction treatment, and an increased risk of early pregnancy loss, increased risk of congenital abnormalities, for example spina bifida, and a myriad of late pregnancy complications including preeclampsia and gestational diabetes. A managed weight-loss program is far more likely to be successful in achieving weight loss, and losing a relatively modest amount of weight, as little as 5%, can restore normal ovulatory cycles and an excellent chance of conception. Combining diet and exercise is associated with a better chance of maintaining weight loss in the longer term. If simple measures alone do not achieve sufficient weight loss, the addition of pharmacological agents such as Orlistat (120 mg taken with each main meal), which inhibits fat absorption from the intestine, has been shown to be effective [6]. In those women with a BMI of greater than 44 kg/m² bariatric surgery could be considered, but only after careful counseling and assessment [2]. Whatever method is employed to lose weight it is important that medication is stopped, and a steady weight reached before the introduction of any ovulation induction treatment, to ensure a balanced nutritional intake at the time of conception.

Medical management

If weight reduction alone is unsuccessful there are a number of differing approaches for medical management. First-line treatment is oral medication with either an antiestrogen or more recently an aromatase inhibitor.

Clomiphene citrate

Clomiphene has now been used in clinical practice for over 50 years. It is a triphenylethylene derivative, a nonsteriodal structure first synthesized in 1956 [7]. The first clinical trials were published in 1961, and the drug was approved by the FDA for clinical use in 1967. It consists of a racemic mixture of two stereoisomers, zuclomiphene (38%) and euclomiphene (62%). The main mode of excretion is through the gut, with just over 50% lost 5 days after administration. Peak concentrations of zuclomiphene occur 6 hours after oral administration, and a steady state is reached after 48 hours, which then remains constant for about 14 days. Interestingly 10% of peak levels are still present after 28 days. Repeated doses at 28 day intervals lead to an accumulative effect, with basal levels increasing by 50% per month [7]. Therefore, from a practical perspective clomiphene may be more effective in subsequent months despite the dose remaining the same. This is important to consider when timing ovulation monitoring if multiple follicular development and the risk of multiple pregnancy are to be avoided. In contrast, euclomiphene, which is the principal cause of the antiestrogenic side effects, levels fall much more rapidly.

The mode of action is to act as a competitive antagonist of 17β-estradiol at its cytoplasmic nuclear receptor. Specifically, clomiphene binds to the estrogen receptors in the arcuate nucleus in the hypothalamus and the pituitary gland, leading to both an increased release of GnRH and heightening of the sensitivity of the pituitary gland to GnRH respectively. In women with normal menstrual cycles the GnRH pulse frequency is increased, whereas in those with PCOS who already have a higher pulse frequency the pulse amplitude is increased.

In clinical use clomiphene results in the lead follicle being significantly larger than a follicle in a natural cycle in the late follicular phase although the rate of growth is similar. The endometrium is significantly thinner four days prior to ovulation. Other hypoestrogenic side effects, which include hot flushes, and changes to the cervical mucus, are usually limited to the days of administration and up to five days later. For this reason clomiphene is administered for five days at the beginning of the menstrual cycle. The antiestrogenic effects can be counteracted by administration of exogenous estrogens, without having an impact on ovulation, but this is seldom required in clinical practice. Levels of estradiol and progesterone are generally higher in the luteal phase.

Although the dose of clomiphene used has varied between 25 mg and 250 mg, the majority of women who respond will do so to doses of 100 mg or less. Women who weigh more may require an increased dose, with 40% of women weighing over 90 kg needing a dose of greater than 100 mg. However, pregnancies occur rarely if greater than 150 mg is required, and so this is often the maximum dose prescribed [7].

The prospect for ovulation depends on the diagnosis. Ovulation rates are much higher in those who respond positively to a progestogen challenge. Clomiphene is of little value in those with classical WHO I anovulation. The degree of menstrual irregularity is also important as approximately 75% of women with oligoamenorrhea of up to 6 months will ovulate, in contrast to only 53% who have amenorrhea of greater than 6 months. In MacGregor's early series monthly fecundity rates varied between 19.7% and 21.3% in cycles 1 to 5, falling to 13.5% to 16.3% in cycles 6 to 10 [7]. The risk of multiple pregnancy is significant, with a 10% twin and a 1% triplet rate. Indeed, a survey of neonatal pediatricians in the UK in 1989 confirmed that, at that time, ovulation induction accounted for 34% of all higher multiple births, of which 27% arose after treatment with clomiphene [8]. To try to reduce this risk NICE recommended monitoring cycles with ultrasound [2]. This is far more accurate than measuring luteal progesterone, which on the whole tends to be higher after clomiphene treatment, and could arise from one or more follicles. Not every cycle needs to be monitored in detail, and once ovulation has been established, it would be reasonable to consider a single scan in the late follicular phase to confirm unifollicular ovulation.

The duration of clomiphene treatment is restricted to between 6 and 9 cycles. Epidemiological studies have raised a concern that the prolonged use of clomiphene (more than 12 cycles) is associated with an increased risk of ovarian malignancy [9]. The ASRM recommend limiting use to 6 cycles of treatment, which coincides with the time of maximum benefit. Rarely in someone who is ovulating, but has not conceived, a further three cycles may be beneficial. In those trying for a second pregnancy, clomiphene can be used following similar guidelines. Conception tends to occur in the same or an earlier cycle in 93% of women [7], and parity is known to reduce the risk of ovarian neoplasia.

Tamoxifen

Tamoxifen citrate is a trans-isomer of a triphenylethylene derivative. Peak plasma levels occur five hours after oral administration and it is principally excreted in the gut with a terminal elimination half-life of between 5 and 7 days. In the body it is extensively metabolized with its major metabolite, N-desmethyl tamoxifen, having similar actions to the native tamoxifen molecule. It is a selective estrogen receptor modulator, which has antagonistic actions on the estrogen receptor in some tissues such as breast and the hypothalamus, whereas weakly agonistic action occurs in others such as bone, the vaginal mucosa, and endometrium. The most common side effect is hot flushes, found in up to 30% of women. It is used in a similar fashion to clomiphene, at the beginning of the menstrual cycle between days 2 and 5 at a dose of between 20 and 80 mg, dependent on response. A meta-analysis of randomized controlled trials comparing clomiphene and tamoxifen has shown that there is no difference between the two agents in terms of ovulation induction, clinical pregnancy, or live birth [10].

Aromatase inhibitors

Aromatase is the cytochrome P450 enzyme responsible for the conversion of C19 androgens to C18 estrogens, androstenedione to estrone, and testosterone to estradiol, respectively. Aromatase is found in numerous tissues, which include the breast, adipose tissue, brain, placenta, and the ovaries of premenopausal women. Two third-generation aromatase inhibitors, anastrozole and letrozole, have been developed principally for use on postmenopausal women with estrogen-receptor-positive breast cancer as adjunct therapy to lower estrogen levels. These are nonsteroidal compounds that are selective aromatase inhibitors that are potent but reversible. They work by lowering estradiol, removing the negative feedback on the hypothalamus and pituitary gland to encourage increased FSH secretion. They also cause a transient build-up in the substrate androgens, which in turn appears to increase follicular sensitivity to FSH. The theoretical advantage of aromatase inhibitors over clomiphene is that they leave the estrogen-sensitive negative feedback on the hypothalamic pituitary access intact, which means as a follicle grows and secretes estradiol the negative feedback lowers FSH production, simulating a natural cycle, and allowing unifollicular development. Letrozole is the most commonly used medication and has been more extensively studied.

Letrozole is used off-license for ovulation induction. The usual dose of letrozole is between 2.5 and 5 mg taken orally between days 3 and 7 of the cycle. Maximum plasma levels are reached in approximately 60 minutes, with a terminal elimination half-life of

2 days. It is largely metabolized in the liver and then the inactive metabolite is excreted by the kidneys. The side-effect profile is kinder than that seen with clomiphene, and rarely limits use, but includes mild gastrointestinal side effects, headaches, musculoskeletal pains, and hot flushes. Although early studies suggested that there may be an increase in cardiac and skeletal abnormalities when used for ovulation induction, a later larger series appears to indicate that the risk of fetal abnormality is no greater than with other forms of treatment and similar to the normal population [11]. In clinical use a meta-analysis of randomized controlled trials have confirmed that the fecundity rate in WHO II patients is not significantly different to that associated with the use of clomiphene [12].

Insulin-sensitizing drugs

The majority of women with WHO II oligo-anovulation will have PCOS, which is a heterogeneous disorder characterized by hyperandrogenism, anovulation (leading to menstrual disturbance), and/or polycystic ovaries on ultrasound. There is now a significant body of evidence that implicates increased insulin resistance and compensatory hyperinsulinemia as a key factor in the pathogenesis of PCOS. The potential effect of insulin-sensitizing agents on ovulation was first noted in 1994 in studies primarily addressing metabolic and endocrine parameters [13]. The main insulin-sensitizing agent investigated in anovulation is Metformin, a biguanide antihyperglycemic drug. Metformin works by lowering gluconeogenesis in the liver, increasing insulin sensitivity in peripheral tissues, enhancing most of the actions of insulin, including increasing glucose transport, glycogen and lipid synthesis, decreasing fatty acid oxidation reducing free fatty acid levels. Hyperinsulinemia is found commonly in both lean and obese patients with PCOS, and this contributes to an increase in total and free circulating testosterone by directly increasing ovarian testosterone production and decreasing hepatic synthesis of sex hormone binding globulin. Metformin, by reducing hyperinsulinemia, leads to reduced total and free testosterone and a concomitant increase in estradiol levels.

Metformin has minimal protein binding, and as such has a widespread distribution. After oral administration peak plasma levels are reached between 1 and 3 hours. It is not metabolized and is cleared through the kidneys, with an elimination half-life of 6.2 hours. The most significant side effects of Metformin are gastrointestinal, and they are often significant enough to limit compliance. Diarrhea, abdominal discomfort, nausea and vomiting, and increased flatulence are common. Lactic acidosis is a rare but serious complication, but it is unlikely to be seen in patients of reproductive age without underlying medical pathology.

The role of insulin-sensitizing drugs in the treatment of PCOS is controversial. The latest Cochrane review of 27 RCTs found that although Metformin improves ovulation and pregnancy rates (more so when combined with clomiphene), it is not associated with any significant increase in live birth rates [14]. The exact dose of Metformin has not been established, but most clinical trials have used between 1500 mg and 2000 mg per day.

Gonadotropins

Gonadotropin therapy is indicated for those patients who are clomiphene resistant. This field has been extensively studied and subject to numerous Cochrane reviews. Recombinant FSH and the various urinary preparations give similar results in terms of ovulation induction rates (72–92%), pregnancy rates (11–16% per cycle), the risk of miscarriage and complications such as multiple pregnancy (4–18%) and OHSS (1–2%). The dose of medication and the regimens employed are the same as discussed earlier [6].

Surgical treatment of PCOS

Stein and Leventhal in 1935 were the first to demonstrate the potential impact of ovarian surgery in women with PCOS. Removing a wedge of ovarian tissue resulted in the return of regular menstrual cycles. Unfortunately such surgery often resulted in significant intrapelvic adhesion formation. Far less invasive laparoscopic surgery, using either diathermy or a variety of lasers, can produce similar results, restoring ovulation in the majority of women [15]. When compared to conventional medical ovulation induction therapy for patients with clomiphene-resistant PCOS, surgery is equally as effective as gonadotropins, while having the advantage of no ovarian hyper-stimulation, significantly fewer multiple pregnancies, and a lower cost per live birth [15].

The precise reason why ovarian tissue destruction leads to the resumption of ovulation is not understood. However, there are significant endocrine changes that occur immediately after and in the weeks following surgery. The ovarian androgens, testosterone and androstenedione, fall from day 1 after surgery, reaching a nadir by day 3 to 4 and then remain at this lower level. LH levels rise initially then gradually fall, with a more pronounced change seen in those who have an ovulatory response to surgery. The LH pulse amplitude is lower although the pulse frequency remains the same. Inhibin levels decrease rapidly initially, but then rise to normal after three to five weeks. FSH levels rise on the day of surgery and remain elevated for a few days before returning to a baseline value [16].

At laparoscopy one or both ovaries are punctured with a needle-point diathermy in 4 to 10 sites, and coagulated for 4 seconds at a strength of 40 watts. Caution is required as excessive diathermy can result in ovarian failure, and adhesions may still develop in approximately 10 to 20% of women. Our practice is to only make four puncture sites on both ovaries, and to liberally use a liquid adhesion barrier, Adept (to both cool ovaries and keep adjacent structures apart).

As laparoscopic surgery is invasive it is not considered first-line treatment for the majority of women with PCOS. It is best reserved for women who require a laparoscopy to assess tubal patency, those with persistently high baseline LH levels, those in whom it is difficult to produce a unifollicular response with gonadotropins, and finally those who are resistant to clomiphene and would have difficulty attending for the intensive monitoring required with gonadotropin therapy.

WHO III

Treatment of these women is to relieve their hypoestrogenic symptoms using the oral contraceptive pill or conventional combined hormone replacement therapy. Rarely, pregnancies occur spontaneously. The use of medication to increase endogenous FSH or the administration of exogenous gonadotropins is not effective. Oocyte donation is the only realistic way for these women to carry a pregnancy.

Hyperprolactinemia

In all patients with hyperprolactinemia presenting with oligoamenorrhea and infertility, treatment is required. Prior to treatment, pituitary imaging either with an MRI or CT scan will determine the presence of any tumor, its size and the extent of any suprasellar extension. Dopamine agonists are the primary treatment option for both micro- and macroadenomas as they rapidly reduce prolactin levels, followed by tumor shrinkage, and an improvement in pressure effects such as visual field defects in the majority of patients.

The most commonly used medications are bromocriptine and cabergoline, which are both ergot derivatives. Bromocriptine is a potent dopamine receptor agonist, which also has a direct effect on the pituitary lactotroph cells. Approximately 28% of an oral dose is absorbed and it is excreted principally in the feces with a half-life of 12 to 14 hours. Common side effects include nausea, constipation, headaches, nasal congestion, and dizziness caused by postural hypotension. Symptoms can be severe enough to limit compliance. To limit the side-effect profile bromocriptine is administered with a gradually increasing dose, starting at between 0.625 and 1.25 mg at night and building up to the usual maintenance dose of up to 10 mg daily in divided doses. Prolactin levels are monitored on a monthly basis and when they have fallen back to normal a lower maintenance dose can be employed. Cabergoline has a similar mode of action to bromocriptine, but has a much longer elimination half-life of around 80 hours, so it needs to be taken less frequently. It is extensively metabolized in the liver and excreted in both feces and urine. The side-effect profile is much kinder, which improves tolerance and compliance. The dose of carbergoline is increased gradually every four weeks from 0.25–0.5 mg, administered once per week, to the therapeutic range of 0.5–2 mg per week. In randomized controlled trials cabergoline has been shown to be more effective in normalizing prolactin levels than bromocriptine (83% compared to 59% respectively) [17]. Quinagolide is an alternative dopamine receptor agonist that can be used in place of bromocriptine or cabergoline, with the same dosing principles applied, gradual increase at 3 day intervals until the therapeutic dose is reached (75–150 µg).

Concerns have been raised for the use of cabergoline in women trying to conceive because of the absence of safety data in pregnancy. The manufacturers recommend discontinuing one month before pregnancy. Safety data for the use of bromocriptine are more encouraging, and for this reason it has been recommended as the preferred option by NICE for the use in infertility [2]. Another option is to use cabergoline to normalize prolactin while a patient uses barrier contraception then switch to bromocriptine for maintenance. Once pregnancy is achieved bromocriptine is stopped. Prolactin levels will rise in pregnancy but significant tumor enlargement occurs in less than 3% of women with a microadenoma. For those with a macroadenoma there is up to a 30% risk of tumor enlargement [17]. During pregnancy women should be monitored for signs and symptoms of an enlarging tumor at least during each trimester, and more commonly in those known to have tumor extension prior to pregnancy. Visual field assessment will usually suffice, and MRI is rarely indicated. Where there is significant tumor enlargement bromocriptine should be recommenced. Most women will need to start after completion of breast feeding.

In those who do not respond to medication, transsphenoidal surgery may be required. Success depends on surgical skill, and cure rates are high with a microadenoma (80 to 90%), but less so with macroadenomas (50%) with a high risk of recurrence [17].

References

1. The Rotterdam ESHRE/ASRM-sponsored PCOS consensus workshop group. Revised 2003 consensus on diagnostic criteria and long term health risks related to polycystic ovary syndrome (PCOS). *Hum Reprod* 2004; **19** (1): 41–7.

2. *NICE Assessment and Treatment for People with Fertility Problems.*

NICE Clinical Guideline, February 2004.

3. Lunenfeld B. Historical perspectives in gonadotrophin therapy. *Hum Reprod Update* 2004; **10**(6): 453–67.

4. Kovacs GT, Pepperell RJ, Evans JH. Induction of ovulation with human pituitary gonadotrophin (HPG):

the Australian experience. *Aust NZ J Med* 1989; **29**: 315–18.

5. Ludwig M, Felberbaum RE, Diedrich K, Lunenfeld B. Ovarian stimulation: from basic science to clinical application. *Reprod Biomed Online* 2002; 5 Suppl **1**(3): 73–86.

6. The Thessaloniki ESHRE/ASRM-Sponsored PCOS Consensus Workshop Group March 2–3, 2007, Thessaloniki, Greece. Consensus on infertility treatment related to polycystic ovary syndrome. *Fertil Steril* 2008; **89** (3): 505–22.

7. Dickey RP Holtkamp DE. Development, pharmacology and clinical experience with clomiphene citrate. *Hum Reprod Update* 1996; **2**(6); 483–506.

8. Levene MI, Wild J, Steer P. Higher multiple births and the modern management of infertility in Britain. The British Association of Perinatal Medicine. *Br J Obstet Gynaecol* 1992; **99**(7): 607–13.

9. Rossing MA, Daling JR, Weiss NS, *et al.* Ovarian tumors in a cohort of infertile women. *N Engl J Med* 1994; **331**: 771–6.

10. Steiner AZ, Terplan M, Paulson RJ. Comparison of tamoxifen and clomiphene citrate for ovulation induction: a meta-analysis. *Hum Reprod* 2005; **20**(6): 1511–15.

11. Tulandi T, Martin J, Al-Fadhli R, *et al.* Congenital malformations among 911 newborns conceived after infertility treatment with letrozole or clomiphene citrate. *Fertil Steril* 2006; **85**(6): 1761–5.

12. Requena A, Herrero J, Landeras J, *et al.*, Reproductive Endocrinology Interest Group of the Spanish Society of Fertility. Use of letrozole in assisted reproduction: a systematic review and meta-analysis. *Hum Reprod Update* 2008; **14**(6): 571–82.

13. Velazquez EM, Mendoza S, Hamer T, Sosa F, Glueck CJ. Metformin therapy in polycystic ovary syndrome reduces hyperinsulinemia, insulin resistance, hyperandrogenemia, and systolic blood pressure, while facilitating normal menses and pregnancy. *Metabolism* 1994; **43**: 647–54.

14. Tang T, Lord JM, Norman RJ, Yasmin E, Balen AH. Insulin-sensitising drugs (metformin, rosiglitazone, pioglitazone, D-chiro-inositol) for women with polycystic ovary syndrome, oligo amenorrhoea and subfertility. *Cochrane Database Syst Rev* 2010; **1**: CD003053. doi: 10.1002/14651858. CD003053.pub4.

15. Farquhar C, Lilford R, Marjoribanks J, Vanderkerchove P. Laparoscopic 'drilling' by diathermy or laser for ovulation induction in anovulatory polycystic ovary syndrome. *Cochrane Database Syst Rev* 2007; **3**: CD001122. doi: 10.1002/14651858. CD001122.pub3.

16. Hendriks ML, Ket JCF, Hompes PGA, Homburg R, Lambalk CB. Why does ovarian surgery in PCOS help? Insight into the endocrine implications of ovarian surgery for ovulation induction in polycystic ovary syndrome. *Hum Reprod Update* 2007; **13**(3): 249–64.

17. Klibanski A. Prolactinomas. *N Engl J Med* 2010; **362**: 1219–26.

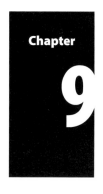

Chapter 9

The role of artificial insemination with partner semen in an ART program

W. Ombelet

Introduction

The first documented application of artificial insemination (AI) was done in London in the 1770s by John Hunter. A cloth merchant with severe hypospadias was advised to collect the semen in a warmed syringe and inject the sample into the vagina. JM Sims reported his findings of post-coital tests and 55 inseminations in 1873. Only one pregnancy occurred but this could be explained by the fact that he believed that ovulation occurred during menstruation.

The rationale behind intrauterine insemination (IUI) with partner sperm is bypassing the cervical-mucus barrier and increasing the number of motile spermatozoa with a high proportion of normal forms at the site of fertilization.

A few decades ago, homologous artificial insemination was only performed in cases of physiological and psychological dysfunction, such as retrograde ejaculation, vaginismus, hypospadias, and impotence. With the routine use of post-coital tests, other indications were added such as hostile cervical mucus and immunological causes with the presence of antispermatozoal antibodies.

However, the main reason for the renewed interest in IUI is the refinement of techniques for the preparation of washed motile spermatozoa which was associated with the introduction of in vitro fertilization (IVF) in 1978. These washing procedures are necessary to remove prostaglandins, infectious agents, and antigenic proteins. Another substantial advantage of these techniques is the removal of nonmotile spermatozoa, leukocytes, or immature germ cells. This may enhance sperm quality by decreasing the release of lympho-kines and/or cytokines, and also a reduction in the formation of free oxygen radicals has been observed. The final result is an improved fertilizing capacity of the sperm sample in vitro and in vivo.

Despite the extensive literature on the subject of artificial homologous insemination, controversy remains about the effectiveness of this very popular treatment procedure [1,2]. Contradictory results are observed because most studies are retrospective and vary in (1) the comparison of the study group (different groups of male subfertility), (2) the use or non-use of different ovarian hyperstimulation regimens, (3) the number of inseminations per treatment cycle, (4) timing of ovulation, (5) sites of insemination, (6) methods of sperm preparation, and (7) the use of additives such as kallicreine, pentoxyphylline, antioxidants etc. (Figure 9.1).

The Subfertility Handbook: A Clinician's Guide, Second Edition ed. Gab Kovacs. Published by Cambridge University Press. © Cambridge University Press 2011.

To be convinced of the exact value of IUI in the treatment of involuntary male sub-fertility, IUI has to be weighed against expectant management, timed coitus, IVF, and ICSI. This comparison should not only involve success rates but should also include a cost-benefit analysis, an analysis of the complication rate of the different treatment options, the invasiveness of the techniques, and patient compliancy.

In this chapter an attempt is made to examine the value and position of homologous intrauterine insemination in an ART program.

Effectiveness of IUI

According to the literature, the effectiveness of artificial insemination with partner semen seems to depend, at least partly, on the indication for which this treatment has been chosen.

Cervical factor subfertility

In the case of cervical factor subfertility, it seems logical to perform IUI. Bypassing the hostile cervix should increase the probability of conception. The results of a meta-analysis of randomized controlled trials comparing IUI with timed intercourse for couples with cervical factor infertility showed an improved probability of conception for IUI (odds ratio 3.6) [2]. However, cervical hostility is not frequently found. When the post-coital test is timed and performed adequately, and a male factor is excluded, only few couples will suffer from cervical hostility.

Unexplained subfertility

If an infertility work-up is unable to detect a plausible explanation for couples with a history of subfertility of at least one year, we use the term "unexplained infertility". Because a good explanation for the subfertility is lacking, the treatment is often empiric. A meta-analysis comparing IUI and timed intercourse in natural cycles showed no difference in results, therefore IUI in natural cycles seems ineffective in cases of unexplained infertility [2]. When controlled ovarian hyperstimulation (COH) is used, IUI becomes effective compared to timed intercourse. In two different studies it was shown that three cycles of COH-IUI in couples with unexplained infertility was just as effective as one IVF cycle in achieving pregnancy, but IVF was more expensive, not only for the couples but also for society [3,4].

Male factor subfertility

When a male factor is found in couples with long-standing infertility, expectant treatment seems to be disappointing, with a spontaneous conception rate of only 2% per cycle [5]. For IUI, with or without COH, a pregnancy rate of 10 to 18% per cycle is reported [6,7]. In a Cochrane review, Cohlen et al. [8] concluded that IUI is superior to timed intercourse (TI), both in natural cycles and in cycles with COH (natural cycles-IUI versus TI: OR 2.43; COH-IUI versus TI: OR 2.14). According to this review, IUI in natural cycles should be the treatment of choice in cases of moderate to severe male subfertility providing an inseminating motile count (IMC) of more than 1 million can be obtained after sperm preparation and in the absence of a triple sperm defect (according to WHO criteria).

Immunological male factor subfertility

The clinical significance of antisperm antibodies (ASA) in male subfertility remains unclear and the importance of circulating antisperm antibodies is probably low. However, most studies demonstrate a clear association between sperm surface antibodies and the fertility potential of the male. In 1997 we published a prospective study comparing the effectiviness of the first-line IUI approach versus IVF for male immunological subfertility [9]. The objective of this prospective study was to compare success rates after two different treatment protocols, COH-IUI versus IVF. Both IUI and IVF yielded unexpected high pregnancy rates in this selected group of patients with long-standing subfertility due to sperm surface antibodies. Since cost-benefit analysis comparing COH-IUI with IVF may favor a course of four IUI cycles, we concluded that IUI can be used as the first-line therapy in male immunological subfertility.

Although most fertility centers use IVF/ICSI in cases of immunological male subfertility [10] a well-organized prospective study is mandatory to examine the real value of IUI for this specific indication.

Risks and complications of IUI

Severe ovarian hyperstimulation syndrome (OHSS) may complicate all methods of treatment in which gonadotropins or recombinant FSH are used; however, OHSS seems to be rare after COH-IUI compared to IVF. The incidence of pelvic inflammatory disease after intra-uterine catheterization and/or transvaginal oocyte aspiration has been estimated to be 0.2% for IVF and 0.01–0.2% for IUI [11]. The major complication of assisted reproductive technologies remains, however, the high incidence of multiple pregnancies, responsible for considerable mortality, morbidity, and costs [12]. Careful monitoring remains essential and cancellation of the insemination procedure, escape IVF, and follicular aspiration before IUI are reasonable options. Transvaginal ultrasound-guided aspiration of supernumerary ovarian follicles increases both the efficacy and the safety of COH-IUI with gonadotropins. This method represents an alternative for conversion of overstimulated cycles to in vitro fertilization (escape IVF). Natural cycle IUI, clomiphene citrate and a minimal dose regimen with gonadotropins are valuable options to prevent the unacceptable high multiple gestation rate described after ovarian hyperstimulation.

Couple compliancy

Since IUI is a simple and non-invasive technique it can be performed without expensive infrastructure with a good success rate within three or four cycles. It is a safe and easy treatment procedure with minimal risks and monitoring. All these factors are responsible for a high couple compliancy for IUI compared to IVF. Table 9.1 gives an overview of the pros and cons of IUI compared to IVF/ICSI.

Cost of ART-related services

A number of studies have been performed on the cost-effectiveness of IUI when compared to IVF [3,13–15].

In a randomized prospective study, Goverde *et al.* [3] concluded that three cycles of IUI offer the same likelihood of a successful pregnancy as IVF. Their data clearly showed that IUI

Table 9.1 Overview of the pros and cons of IUI compared to IVF and ICSI

	Pros	Cons
IUI	Minimal equipment necessary Easy method Less invasive Less expensive Good couple compliancy ⇒ low drop-out rate Low risk for OHSS, PID	⇊ Success-rate per cycle ⇊ Success if IMC < 1 million ⇊ Success if morphology < 5% ⇑ Risk for LBW, prematurity (risk for antisperm antibodies)
IVF +/− ICSI	Minimal transmission of infection (IVF) Higher success-rate per cycle	More invasive ⇑ Risk for LBW, prematurity High risk of OHSS, PID ⇑ Multiple pregnancy rate ⇑ Risk of genetic disorders Lower couple compliancy ⇒ high drop-out rate

IMC, inseminating motile count; OHSS, ovarian hyperstimulation syndrome; PID, pelvic inflammatory disease; LBW, low birth weight (< 2500 g).

is a more cost-effective approach, not only for unexplained subfertility, but also for moderate male factor subfertility. This important message was confirmed in another study performed in the UK [13]. In this study the authors complemented existing clinical guidelines by including cost-effectiveness of different treatment options for infertility in the UK. A series of decision-analytical models were developed to reflect current diagnostic and treatment pathways for the different causes of infertility. According to this study, stimulated intra-uterine insemination for unexplained and moderate male factor infertility is a cost-effective approach. In a systematic review, Garceau *et al.* [14] also showed that initiating treatment with intrauterine insemination appears to be more cost-effective than IVF in most cases of unexplained and moderate male subfertility. In 1997 Van Voorhis and colleagues published the results of retrospective cohort studies in which they compared the cost-effectiveness of (stimulated) IUI with IVF or IVF-ICSI [15]. In couples with unexplained or mild male subfertility they concluded stimulated IUI to be more cost-effective than IVF and they recommended that IUI should be applied before starting IVF. The direct costs per delivery after (stimulated) IUI varied between $7800 and $10 300 whereas after IVF it was $37 000. In couples with an average total motile sperm count below 10 million IVF/ICSI seemed more cost-effective than IUI [15].

Factors influencing IUI success

Site of insemination

Artificial inseminations can be done intravaginally, intracervically (ICI), pericervically using a cap, intrauterine (IUI), transcervical intrafallopian (IFI) or directly intraperitoneal (IPI). Most studies refer to IUI, which seems to be an easy and better way of treatment. Studies comparing pregnancy outcome after IUI versus cervical cap insemination and transuter-otubal insemination favored the intrauterine method. In a large randomized controlled trial it was shown that among infertile couples, treatment with induction of superovulation and intrauterine insemination is three times as likely to result in pregnancy as is intracervical insemination and twice as likely to result in pregnancy as is treatment with either super-ovulation and intracervical insemination or intrauterine insemination alone [16].

Number of inseminations

Theoretically, improved chances of conception may be expected when two consecutive inseminations are performed since ovulation of oocytes does not occur in a synchronized pattern but rather in waves of release after hCG administration. Another appeal of double IUI is the attrition phenomenon by which IUI bypasses the cervical mucus. In the natural cycle the cervical mucus acts as a reservoir for sperm at midcycle and a single IUI might miss later-released cohorts of oocytes. In a Cochrane review, based on the results of two trials, double IUI showed no significant benefit over single IUI in the treatment of subfertile couples with partner semen [17]. The authors admitted that there are no meaningful data to offer advice on the basis of this review. According to this report, a large randomized controlled trial of single IUI versus double IUI is mandatory.

Natural cycle versus controlled ovarian hyperstimulation (COH)

The rationale behind the use of ovarian hyperstimulation in artificial insemination is the increase of the number of oocytes available for fertilization and to correct subtle unpredictable ovulatory dysfunction. Other advantages of superovulation with human menopausal gonado-tropins are the enhanced opportunity for oocyte capture, fertilization and implantation.

On the other hand, in a controlled study Cohlen *et al.* [18] concluded that in male subfertility cases ovarian stimulation only improved the success rate in moderate cases (IMC > 10 million). Comparing the effect of COH on pregnancy rates (PR) after IUI, hMG stimulation results in a significantly higher monthly fecundability compared to clomiphene citrate (CC) treatment. A retrospective study of 1100 IUIs in 412 couples showed a pregnancy rate of 17.7% per cycle after hMG stimulation compared to 10% per cycle after CC stim-ulation, but at the expense of a higher multiple pregnancy rate. This statistical difference was not influenced by the indication for IUI [19]. Considering the risk for multiple pregnancies and ovarian hyperstimulation syndrome (OHSS), a mild COH regimen should be used. Cohlen *et al.* [18] recommend IUI in natural cycles as the treatment of first choice in severe semen defects (IMC > 1 million, no triple semen defect). In couples with unexplained subfertility IUI in natural cycles should not be applied. Compared with intercourse, IUI does not increase the probability of conception. The combination of IUI with mild ovarian hyperstimulation does improves live birth rates and this combination can be used as a first-line treatment option in couples with unexplained subfertility. The choice between enhan-cing the probability of conception by increasing the number of available oocytes and minimizing the risk of achieving a multiple pregnancy should be taken with great care. Adjusting the individual dosage of FSH to strive after two oocytes seems to be the optimal strategy. Close ultrasound monitoring of all follicles larger than 10 mm in combination with strict cancellation criteria has been proven to minimize the risk of multiple pregnancy.

Exact timing of IUI

Exact timing is probably crucial in IUI treatment cycles. This can be explained by the fact that in IUI programs GnRH agonists and antagonists are seldom used. On the other hand, conflicting data are reported in the literature on which methodology has to be used. Ultrasound and hormonal monitoring with hCG induction probably allows the most exact timing but is relatively expensive and time-consuming. Urinary LH-timed IUI is commonly used but has the disadvantage that the LH surge can last for up to 2 days before ovulation in some patients.

Being aware of the importance of exact timing is essential in IUI, independent of the method being used.

Perifollicular vascularity of the follicles

Bhal *et al.* use Doppler imaging to identify those IUI cycles with high-grade perifollicular vascularity, and hence good oxygenation of the follicle with the maturing oocyte. The results again showed a significant correlation between perifollicular blood flow and pregnancy rate (57%) occurring in the group where all follicles had good blood flow, and significantly lower pregnancy rates where there was poor blood flow (11%). Significantly more multiple pregnancies developed when all the follicles exhibited good blood flow at the time of insemination. Monofollicular IUI cycles with poor blood flow are excluded by Bhal since they resulted in no pregnancies in his study.

Endometrial thickness/polyps

A trilaminar image rather than the exact endometrial thickness and/or Doppler measurement of the spiral and uterine arteries provides a favorable prediction of pregnancy in IUI [20]. Treatment should not be cancelled because of inadequate endometrial thickness. The use of ethinyl estradiol in clomiphene-stimulated cycles looks promising but requires confirmation in prospective randomized studies. If polyps are present, hysteroscopic polypectomy before IUI can be an effective measure to enhance pregnancy results, but robust data are still lacking.

Sperm preparation methods

The ejaculate is a composition of spermatozoa of different qualities and maturities suspended in the secretions of the epididymis, the testis, prostate, seminal vesicles, and bulbouretral glands. Cells from the urinary tract and prostate, leucocytes, and reactive oxygen species (ROS) are also present in the raw semen sample. Preparation and washing will remove ROS and also prostaglandins. These prostaglandins have to be removed since they will cause severe uterine cramps when a raw semen sample is used for IUI. The preparation will concentrate morphologically normal and motile spermatozoa, essential for good results in IUI. Most popular are the swim-up procedures, density gradient centrifugation and the use of Sephadex columns. Density gradient centrifugation results in concentrating significantly more spermatozoa that have normal chromatin packaging, reduced levels of chromatin and nuclear DNA anomalies as well as enhanced rates of nuclear maturity. Conflicting data are found on the superiority of any one prepartion technique in terms of fecundity. This can be explained by the fact that almost all methods of sperm washing and preparation surpass the low threshold number of motile spermatozoa ($> 1 \times 10^6$) needed for conception in vivo with no added benefit of additional sperm. According to a Cochrane review [21] there is insufficient evidence to recommend any specific preparation technique. Large high-quality randomized controlled trials, comparing the effectiveness of a gradient and/or a swim-up and/or wash and centrifugation technique on clinical outcome are lacking. Results from studies comparing semen parameters may suggest a preference for the gradient technique, but firm conclusions cannot be drawn and the limitations should be taken into consideration.

Addition of substances in sperm preparation

Whether the addition of substances such as pentoxyfylline, kallicreine, follicular fluid etc. may improve the results remains unclear and certainly unproven. On the other hand, it is important to recognize that sperm preparation methods may induce damage to spermatozoa by increasing ROS generation by spermatozoa and by removing the scavengers from the seminal plasma. Pentoxifylline, a motility stimulator, can also act as a ROS scavenger by reducing the generation of superoxide anion by spermatozoa, and may have a clinical role in the treatment of patients susceptible to ROS-induced damage (genital infections, smokers). More studies that investigate whether treating spermatozoa with solutions containing anti-oxidants during sperm preparation can improve pregnancy rates with IUI in selected cases are needed. Roudebush et al. [22] evaluated the effect of PAF (platelet-activating factor) exposure on sperm during semen processing for intrauterine insemination (IUI). They demonstrate a significantly higher pregnancy rate for the PAF-treated group in a subpopulation of couples without male factor subfertility. According to Roudebush, PAF clearly plays a significant role in reproductive physiology. It seems to influence ovulation, fertilization, preimplantation embryo development, implantation, and parturition. Exogenous PAF has been used to promote sperm motility, sperm capacitation and the acrosome reaction.

Which catheter to use

Lavie et al. [23] compared the results after IUI using two different catheters. Although one catheter was significantly less traumatic (objectified by ultrasound), only a trend towards increase in the chance of conception was found. According to the results of a structured review and meta-analysis, catheter choice during IUI does not seem to be a detrimental factor for success and the catheter type does not affect the outcome [24].

Fallopian tube sperm perfusion

Fallopian tube sperm perfusion (FSP) consists of mild ovarian stimulation with the aim of maturing two follicles, ovulation induction and insemination using a large volume (4 ml) of inseminate. Perfusion studies demonstrated that with this large volume, the inseminate will fill the uterine cavity, flow through the fallopian tubes and some of it will end up in the peritoneal space, the rationale being that this maximizes the chances the gametes will meet and fertilization will occur. Excellent results have been described in cases of unexplained infertility and in a donor insemination program [25]. Cantineau et al. [26] performed a systematic review based on a Cochrane review. They found that for non-tubal subfertility the results indicate no clear benefit for FSP over IUI. It has to be admitted that most studies examining the use of FSP versus routine IUI are rather small. A complicating factor is that in these studies, different protocols, different utensils, and different catheters for performing FSP have been used. This may well have influenced the outcome of the studies and contributed to the fact that currently there is no consensus on whether FSP or IUI is to be advocated.

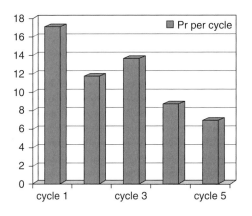

Figure 9.1 Retrospective analysis of 5000 IUI treatment cycles in the Genk program. A significant drop in success rate can be observed after the third cycle (Pr = clinical pregnancy rate per cycle).

The effect of the abstinence period

Prolonged abstinence time increases ejaculate volume, sperm count, sperm concentration, and the total number of motile spermatozoa, although the effect on sperm concentration is only small for oligozoospermic men. A prospective study performed in our unit in Genk showed the following results: abstinence did not influence pH, viability, morphology, total or grade A motility, or sperm DNA fragmentation. A short (24 hours) abstinence period negatively influenced chromatin quality [27]. It seems that looking for the optimal time of abstinence is not very important in IUI programs and is probably only valuable in selected male subfertility cases.

AI cycle number

It seems that a significant decline in cycle fecundity can be observed after the third or fourth IUI cycle, as reported in many studies. On the occasion of a retrospective analysis of more than 5000 IUI cycles in Genk we also found a significant decline after the third IUI cycle (Figure 9.1). The remaining couples do not seem to benefit from this method of treatment when compared to other methods of assisted reproduction such as IVF and ICSI.

Perinatal outcome following IUI

To our knowledge only four papers have been published reporting the obstetric and perinatal outcome after IUI. According to Nuojua-Huttunen *et al.* [28] and using the data obtained from the Finnish Medical Birth Register (MBR), IUI treatment did not increase obstetric or perinatal risks compared with matched spontaneous or IVF pregnancies. Wang *et al.* [29] examined preterm birth in 1015 IUI/AID singleton births compared to 1019 IVF/ICSI and 1019 naturally conceived births. They found that singleton IUI/AID births were about 1.5 times more likely to be born preterm than naturally conceived singletons, whereas the IVF/ICSI group were 2.4 times more likely to be born preterm than the naturally conceived group. In a retrospective cohort study, Gaudoin *et al.* [30] described a poorer perinatal outcome of singletons born to subfertile mothers conceived through COH-IUI compared to matched natural conceptions within the Scottish national cohort. This was caused by a higher incidence of prematurity and low-birth-weight infants. They suggest that intrinsic factors in subfertile couples predispose them to having smaller infants. We also performed a study to investigate differences in perinatal outcome of singleton and twin pregnancies after controlled ovarian hyperstimulation (COH), with or without artificial insemination (AI), compared to pregnancies after natural conception [31]. We used the data from the regional registry of 661 065 births in Flanders (Belgium) during the period 1993–2003. A total of 11 938 singleton and 3108 twin births could be selected. Control subjects were matched for maternal age, parity, fetal sex, and place and year of birth. We found a significantly higher incidence of extreme prematurity (< 32 weeks), very low birth weight (< 1500 g), stillbirths and perinatal death for COH/AI singletons. Twin pregnancies resulting from COH/AI showed a higher rate of neonatal mortality, assisted ventilation and respiratory distress syndrome. According to our results, COH/IUI singleton and twin pregnancies are significantly disadvantaged compared to naturally conceived children, with a higher mortality rate and a higher incidence of low birth weight and prematurity. We also believe that infertility itself predisposes to a worse perinatal outcome compared to naturally conceived babies.

Artificial insemination as a first-line treatment: a strategy proposal

In the selection of couples to be treated with IUI or IVF/ICSI, it would be interesting to establish cut-off values of semen parameters above which IUI is a real alternative for IVF/ICSI in male subfertility. According to the literature, IMC and sperm morphology are the most valuable sperm parameters to predict IUI outcome. A trend towards increasing conception rates with increasing IMC was reported, but the cut-off value above which IUI seems to be successful varies between 0.3 and 20 million [6]. In a large number of studies, 5% normal forms and 1 million motile spermatozoa after sperm preparation are believed to be potential cut-off values to select couples for IUI treatment.

A large retrospective analysis in Genk in a selected group of patients with normal ovarian response to clomiphene (CC) stimulation showed no significant difference in cumulative ongoing pregnancy rate after three IUI cycles between all patients providing the IMC was more than 1 million [32]. Furthermore, in cases with less than 1 million motile spermatozoa, IUI remains successful as a first-line option provided the sperm morphology score is 4% or more (cumulative ongoing pregnancy rate of 21.9% after three IUI cycles).

Figure 9.2 shows the treatment strategy used at the Genk Institute for Fertility Technology. Although the cumulative ongoing pregnancy rate after three IUI cycles is comparable with only one IVF cycle (25%), more than 90% of our couples agree to follow our protocol, being aware of the better success rate per cycle after IVF. Excellent counseling is mandatory and crucial.

But clinical practice can be very contradictory to common scientific knowledge. Data from Australia and New Zealand clearly show that almost 80% of fertility centers in the early 2000s were convinced of the cost-effectiveness of IUI, but nearly one-third of these centers still promoted IVF as a first-line treatment even with patent tubes and normal semen [33]. In their conclusion the authors stated that:

> Although it may take relatively more treatment cycles to achieve pregnancy, there are considerable advantages to the patient in terms of risk/benefit ratio and financial cost associated with IUI compared with IVF. In the current climate of evidence-based medicine, as clinicians we are obliged to translate this into our practice. It appears from our survey that in many units this is not happening. [33]

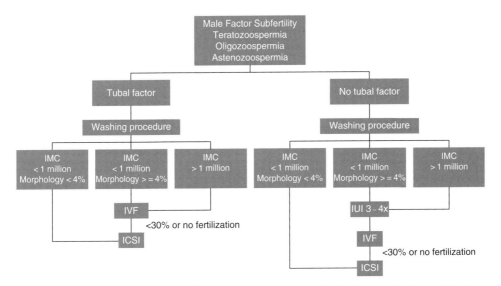

Figure 9.2 Opinion: proposed algorithm of male subfertility treatment at the Genk Institute for Fertility Technology.

Conclusion

IUI should be promoted as the best first-line treatment in most cases of subfertility provided at least one tube is patent and an IMC after sperm preparation of more than 1 million can be obtained. In this selected group of patients it is unwise to start with assisted reproductive techniques such as IVF and ICSI since these techniques are more invasive and less cost-effective, although the success rates per cycle are significantly better compared to IUI.

The future of IUI will depend on our ability to maintain the multiple pregnancy rate at an acceptable level and this will undoubtedly be the most important challenge in the near future. If the multiple pregnancy rate after artificial insemination is comparable to or lower than the multiple pregnancy rate after IVF, IUI with or without ovarian hyperstimulation should be used for most subfertile couples and not only for couples on a waiting list for IVF. Promoting IVF and ICSI to result in pregnancy "as quickly as possible" ignores the advantages of artificial insemination completely.

Acknowledgements

I gratefully acknowledge Ingrid Jossa for the technical support in preparing this chapter.

References

1. ESHRE Capri Workshop Group. Intrauterine insemination. *Hum Reprod Update* 2009; **15**: 265–77.

2. Cohlen BJ. Should we continue performing intrauterine inseminations in the year 2004? *Gynecol Obstet Invest* 2005; **59**: 3–13.

3. Goverde AJ, McDonnell J, Vermeiden JP, *et al.* Intrauterine insemination or in-vitro-fertilisation in idiopathic subfertility and male subfertility: a randomised trial and cost-effectiveness analysis. *Lancet* 2000; **355**: 13–18.

4. Peterson CM, Hatasaka HH, Jones KP, *et al.* Ovulation induction with gonadotropins and intrauterine insemination compared with in vitro fertilization and no therapy: a

prospective, nonrandomized, cohort study and meta-analysis. *Fertil Steril* 1994; **62**: 535–44.

5. Collins JA, Burrows EA, Wilan AR. The prognosis for live birth among untreated infertile couples. *Fertil Steril* 1995; **64**: 22–8.

6. Ombelet W, Deblaere K, Bosmans E, *et al.* Semen quality and intrauterine insemination. *Reprod Biomed* 2003; **7**: 485–92.

7. Stone BA, Vargyas JM, Ringler GE, *et al.* Determinants of the outcome of intrauterine insemination: analysis of outcomes of 9963 consecutive cycles. *Am J Obstet Gynecol* 1999; **180**: 1522–34.

8. Cohlen BJ, Vandekerckhove P, te Velde ER, *et al.* Timed intercourse versus intra-uterine insemination with or without ovarian hyperstimulation for subfertility in men. *Cochrane Database Syst Rev* 2000; **2**: CD000360.

9. Ombelet W, Vandeput H, Janssen M, *et al.* Treatment of male infertility due to sperm surface antibodies: IUI or IVF? *Hum Reprod* 1997; **12**: 1165–70.

10. Lombardo F, Gandini L, Lenzi A, *et al.* Antisperm immunity in assisted reproduction. *J Reprod Immunol* 2004; **62**: 101–9.

11. Bergh T, Lundkvist O. Clinical complications during in-vitro fertilization treatment. *Hum Reprod* 1992; **7**, 625–6.

12. Ombelet W, De Sutter P, Van der Elst J, *et al.* Multiple gestation and infertility treatment: registration, reflection and reaction: the Belgian project. *Hum Reprod Update* 2005; **11**: 3–14.

13. Philips Z, Barraza-Llorens M, Posnett J. Evaluation of the relative cost-effectiveness of treatments for infertility in the UK. *Hum Reprod* 2000; **15**: 95–106.

14. Garceau L, Henderson J, Davis LJ, *et al.* Economic implications of assisted reproductive techniques: a systematic review. *Hum Reprod* 2002; **17**: 3090–3109.

15. Van Voorhis BJ, Sparks AE, Allen BD, *et al.* Cost-effectiveness of infertility treatments: a cohort study. *Fertil Steril* 1997; **67**: 830–6.

16. Guzick DS, Carson SA, Coutifaris C, *et al.* Efficacy of superovulation and intrauterine insemination in the treatment of infertility. National Cooperative Reproductive Medicine Network. *N Engl J Med* 1999; **340**: 177–83.

17. Cantineau AE, Heineman MJ, Cohlen BJ. Single versus double intrauterine insemination in stimulated cycles for subfertile couples: a systematic review based on a Cochrane review. *Hum Reprod* 2003; **18**: 941–6.

18. Cohlen BJ, te Velde ER, van Kooij RJ, *et al.* Controlled ovarian hyperstimulation and intrauterine insemination for treating male subfertility: a controlled study. *Hum Reprod* 1998; **13**: 1553–8.

19. Ombelet W, Cox A, Janssen M, *et al.* Artificial insemination (AIH). Artificial insemination 2: using the husband's sperm. In Acosta AA, Kruger TF, eds. *Diagnosis and Therapy of Male Factor in Assisted Reproduction.* Nashville, TN: Parthenon Publishing, 1996; 397–410.

20. Tsai HD, Chang CC, Hsieh YY, *et al.* Artificial insemination; role of endometrial thickness and pattern, of vascular impedance of the spiral and uterine arteries, and of the dominant follicle. *J Reprod Med* 2000; **45**: 195–200.

21. Boomsma CM, Heineman MJ, Cohlen BJ, *et al.* Semen preparation techniques for intrauterine insemination. *Cochrane Database Syst Rev* 2007; **17**: CD004507.

22. Roudebush WE, Toledo AA, Kort HI, *et al.* Platelet-activating factor significantly enhances intrauterine insemination pregnancy rates in non-male factor infertility. *Fertil Steril* 2004; **82**: 52–6.

23. Lavie O, Margalioth EJ, Geva-Eldar T, *et al.* Ultrasonographic endometrial changes after intrauterine insemination: a comparison of two catheters. *Fertil Steril* 1997; **68**: 731–4.

24. Abou-Setta AM, Mansour RT, Al-Inany HG, *et al.* Intrauterine insemination catheters for assisted reproduction: a systematic review and meta-analysis. *Hum Reprod* 2006; **21**: 1961–7.

25. Kahn JA, Sunde A, Koskemies A, *et al.* Fallopian tube sperm perfusion (FSP) versus intra-uterine insemination (IUI) in

the treatment of unexplained infertility: a prospective randomized study. *Hum Reprod* 1993; **8**: 890–4.

26. Cantineau AE, Cohlen BJ, Heineman MJ. Intra-uterine insemination versus fallopian tube sperm perfusion for non-tubal infertility. *Cochrane Database Syst Rev* 2009; **15**: CD001502.

27. De Jonge C, LaFromboise M, Bosmans E, *et al.* Influence of the abstinence period on human sperm quality. *Fertil Steril* 2004; **82**: 57–65.

28. Nuojua-Huttunen S, Gissler M, Martikainen H, Tuomivaara L. Obstetric and perinatal outcome of pregnancies after intrauterine insemination. *Hum Reprod* 1999; **14**: 2110–15.

29. Wang JX, Norman RJ, Kristiansson P. The effect of various infertility treatments on the risk of preterm birth. *Hum Reprod* 2002; **17**; 945–9.

30. Gaudoin M, Dobbie R, Finlayson A, *et al.* Ovulation induction/intrauterine insemination in infertile couples is associated with low-birth-weight infants. *Am J Obstet Gynecol* 2003; **188**: 611–16.

31. Ombelet W, Martens G, De Sutter P, *et al.* Perinatal outcome of 12,021 singleton and 3108 twin births after non-IVF-assisted reproduction: a cohort study. *Hum Reprod* 2006; **21**: 1025–32.

32. Ombelet W, Vandeput H, Van de Putte G, *et al.* Intrauterine insemination after ovarian stimulation with clomiphene citrate: predictive potential of inseminating motile count and sperm morphology? *Hum Reprod* 1997; **12**: 1458–63.

33. Miskry T, Chapman M. The use of intrauterine insemination in Australia and New Zealand. *Hum Reprod* 2002; **17**: 956–9.

Chapter 10

Early pregnancy loss

Joe Leigh Simpson

Introduction

Reproduction is extraordinarily inefficient in humans. Only a distinct minority of conceptions result in liveborns. High pregnancy loss begins before implantation and continues with decreasing frequency throughout gestation. Among married women in the USA, 4% have experienced two clinical pregnancy losses and 3% three [1]. This high frequency of early pregnancy loss has a corollary – subfertility. Couples may experience repeated early losses and never realize pregnancy had been achieved. Instead, their problem is considered to be "infertility". Yet, the etiologies of early loss and "infertility" are similar and should be considered a clinical continuum. Here we shall focus on the most common causes. More details are available elsewhere where additional references are provided [2].

Frequency and timing of pregnancy losses

Embryos implant 6 days after conception. Physical signs are not generally appreciated until 5–6 weeks after the last menstrual period. Fewer than half of preimplantation embryos persist, as witnessed by ART success rates that rarely exceed 30–40% of cycles. Even after implantation, judged preclinically by the biochemical presence of β-hCG, approximately 30% of pregnancies are lost. Following clinical recognition, 10–12% are lost. Most clinical pregnancy losses occur prior to 8 weeks. Before widespread availability of ultrasound, embryonic demise was often not appreciated until 9–12 weeks' gestation, at which time there was bleeding and passage of tissue (products of conception). With widespread availability of ultrasound, it was shown that fetal demise actually occurs weeks before the time overt clinical signs are manifested. This conclusion was reached on the basis of cohort studies showing that only 3% of viable pregnancies are lost after 8 weeks' gestation [3]; studies involving obstetric registrants reached similar conclusions. Fetal viability thus ceases weeks before maternal symptoms appear. That almost all losses are retained in utero for an interval before clinical recognition means most losses could be termed "missed abortions". Actually this term is probably archaic.

After the first trimester, pregnancy losses occur but at a slower rate. Loss rates are only 1% in women confirmed by ultrasound to have viable pregnancies at 16 weeks. Two confounding factors influencing clinical pregnancy loss rates are clinically relevant. (1) Maternal age is positively correlated with pregnancy loss rates, a 40-year-old woman having twice the risk of a 20-year-old woman. This increase occurs in euploid as well as aneuploid pregnancies, as will be discussed below. (2) Prior pregnancy loss also increases loss rates but far less than

The Subfertility Handbook: A Clinician's Guide, Second Edition ed. Gab Kovacs. Published by Cambridge University Press. © Cambridge University Press 2011.

Table 10.1 Approximate recurrence risk figures useful for counseling women with repeated spontaneous abortions

	Number of prior abortions	Risk (%) of pregnancy loss
Women with liveborn infants only	0	5–10
Women with prior abortions and liveborns	1	20–25
	2	25
	3	30
	4	30
Women with prior abortuses and liveborns	3	30–40

Prepared by Simpson and Jauniaux [2] from multiple sources.

once believed. Among nulliparous women who have never experienced a loss, the likelihood of pregnancy loss is low: 5% in primiparas and 4% in multiparas (Table 10-1). Following one loss, risk of another is increased but does not exceed 30–40% even for women with three or more losses [4]. These risks apply not only to women whose losses were recognized at 9–12 weeks' gestation but also to those whose pregnancies were ascertained in the fifth week of gestation [5]. Of clinical relevance, there is no scientific evidence that women with three losses are etiologically distinct from those with two or even one loss.

The clinical consequence of the above information is that in order to be judged efficacious in preventing recurrent spontaneous abortions, therapeutic regimens must show success rates substantially greater than 70%. Essentially no therapeutic regimen can make this claim. The situation may be different if, rarely, four or more losses have occurred.

Chromosomal abnormalities in pregnancy losses

Preimplantation embryos

The frequency of losses in human preimplantation embryos is very high. Of morphologically normal embryos, approximately 25–50% show chromosomal abnormalities (aneuploidy or polyploidy) [6], depending on maternal age. The frequency of chromosomal abnormalities in morphologically normal embryos is at least 75%, principally aneuploidy and polyploidy. These data are based on studies using fluorescence *in situ* hybridization (FISH) with chromosome-specific probes for only seven to nine chromosomes; rates would be higher if based on 24 chromosome FISH (now possible) or array comparative genome hybridization (CGH). The 25–50% aneuploidy rate in morphologically normal embryos is consistent with 5–10% aneuploidy in sperm of ostensibly normal males and in 20% oocytes of women undergoing ART. Aneuploidy rates in oocytes and embryos predictably increase as maternal age increases.

Clinically recognized pregnancies

Approximately 50–60% pregnancy losses show chromosomal abnormalities, given 10–15% of clinical pregnancies ending in miscarriage; thus, 5–8% of all clinical pregnancies have chromosomal abnormalities. Several different categories of chromosomal abnormalities make up this total [2].

Autosomal trisomies constitute approximately 50% of cytogenetically abnormal spontaneous abortions. Trisomy for every chromosome has now been observed. The most common trisomies in abortuses are 16, 22, 21, 15, 13 and 14 (in descending order). The most common aberration in abortuses – trisomy 16 – is rarely, if ever, observed in liveborns in non-mosaic form. These six chromosomes in aggregate account for 60–70% of trisomies – an important consideration in selecting chromosome-specific probes in preimplantation genetic diagnosis (PGD) aneuploidy testing.

Most trisomies show a maternal age effect, but the effect varies among chromosomes. Increasing maternal age correlates positively with errors at meiosis I, the most common cytological explanation (95%) for trisomies. The proportion of trisomies that arise at meiosis I versus meiosis II varies among aneuploidies. Virtually all trisomy 16 cases are maternal in origin and arise at meiosis I. Errors in paternal meiosis account for 10% of acrocentric trisomies. In the rare nonacrocentric trisomies, paternal meiotic errors are equally likely to arise at meiosis I or II.

Double trisomy occurs, most often involving the X and an autosome. Maternal age is higher than found in single trisomy. The rarer trisomies also frequently coexist with more common trisomies (double trisomy). Thus distinguishing most (90%) normal embryos from most abnormal embryos may not necessarily require analysis of all 24 chromosomes.

Triploidy accounts for 25% of chromosomally abnormal abortuses and is typically 69, XXY or 69,XXX. The origin is usually dispermy. Triploidy may follow either fertilization by two haploid sperm or fertilization by a single diploid sperm. Tetraploidy ($4n = 92$) is uncommon, rarely progressing beyond 2–3 weeks of embryonic life.

Monosomy X accounts for 15–20% of chromosomally abnormal abortuses. Autosomal monosomy appears to be lethal prior to or just beyond implantation, and seems not to persist to clinical recognition. Early monosomy X abortuses usually consist of only an umbilical cord stump. If survival persists until later in gestation, anomalies characteristic of Turner syndrome may be seen; cystic hygroma, generalized edema, cardiac defects.

Relationship between recurrent losses and numerical chromosomal abnormalities

In both preimplantation and first-trimester abortions, recurrent aneuploidy occurs more often than expected by chance. Recurrent aneuploidy is a frequent explanation, at least until the number of losses reaches or exceeds four. In a given family successive abortuses are likely to be either recurrently normal or recurrently abnormal. Table 10.2 [7] shows that if the complement of the first abortus is abnormal, the likelihood is increased that the complement of the second abortus will also be abnormal [4]. Recurrence usually involves aneuploidy, although not necessarily the same chromosome. Rubio et al. [8] also have shown increased aneuploid embryos in couples undergoing repeated PGD for monogenic indications.

Expectations of the karyotype in recurrent abortion

The concept of recurrent aneuploidy has certain corollaries. Given that 50% of all abortuses are abnormal cytogenetically, aneuploidy should be detected in both recurrent abortuses as well as sporadic abortuses. When analyzing early pregnancy losses, Stern et al. [9] indeed

Table 10.2 Recurrent aneuploidy: relationship between karyotypes of successive abortuses

Complement of first abortus	Complement of second abortuses [7]					
	Normal	Trisomy	Monosomy	Triploidy	Tetraploidy	De novo rearrangement
Normal	142	18	5	7	3	2
Trisomy	31	30	1	4	3	1
Monosomy	7	5	3	3	0	0
Triploidy	7	4	1	4	0	0
Tetraploidy	3	1	0	2	0	0
De novo rearrangement	1	3	0	0	0	0

Data from Warburton et al. [7].

found a 57% prevalence of chromosomal abnormalities among abortuses of repetitively aborting women; the frequency was coincidentally identical among abortuses of sporadically aborting women. Among 420 abortuses obtained from women with repeated losses, Stephenson et al. [10] found 46% chromosomal abnormalities; 31% of the original sample was trisomic. In their comparison to unselected pooled data, 48% of abortuses were abnormal; 27% of that sample was trisomic. Higher-order losses (four or more) seem more likely to be cytogenetically normal, presumably because maternal factors are more often explanations in this group.

Recurrent losses and chromosomal rearrangement

A balanced translocation is found in 3–5% of couples experiencing repeated losses. These individuals are themselves phenotypically normal, but their offspring (abortuses or abnormal liveborns) may show chromosomal duplications or deficiencies as a result of normal meiotic segregation. The frequency of balanced translocations is higher in females than males, and there may be a family history of a stillborn or abnormal liveborn.

Detecting a translocation heterozygote does not correlate with maternal age, nor does the likelihood of detecting a balanced translocation substantively differ after one, two, or three miscarriages. In a study by Simpson at al. [11], detection rates in females after one, two, three, and four losses were 0.8%, 1.7%, 2.3%, and 2.9%, respectively. For males, the respective rates were 1.2%, 1.9%, 2.4%, and 0 (0/39). Other studies have shown similar results.

There are two general types of translocations: Robertsonian and reciprocal. Robertsonian translocations involve centric fusion of an acrocentric chromosome (13, 14, 15, 21, 22). The theoretical risk of a parent with translocation involving Nos. 14 and 21 t(14q;21q) having a liveborn child with Down syndrome is 33%. However, empirical risks are considerably less. Risks are only 2% if the father carries a translocation involving chromosome 21 and 10% if the mother carries such a translocation. Robertsonian (centric fusion) translocations involving chromosomes other than chromosome 21 show lower empirical risk. In t(13q:14q), the risk for liveborn trisomy 13 is 1% or less. Empiric risks are very much lower than theoretical risks because of the lethality of many segregant products (trisomies and monosomies).

In reciprocal translocations, interchanges occur between two or more metacentric chromosomes. Empirical data for specific translocations are usually not available, and generalizations are typically made on the basis of pooled data derived from many different translocations. As in Robertsonian translocations, theoretical risks for abnormal offspring (unbalanced reciprocal translocations) are much greater than empirical risks. Sex differences are less apparent. Empiric risks are 12% for offspring of either female heterozygotes or male heterozygotes. See Simpson and Jauniaux [2].

Distinct from the likelihood of unbalanced segregants is the quantitative likelihood of subsequent abortion. The likelihood of a live birth in couples who have rearrangement is 65–70%, not different in the general population of couples with recurrent pregnancy loss (RPL) – 65–70% (Table 10.1). However, there is an important caveat – time to achieve pregnancy. The mean time to achieve pregnancy is 5–10 years. This interval is not likely to be tolerable for older women, for which reason a translocation is considered in an individual for preimplantation genetic diagnosis (PGD) by authorative bodies [12].

Luteal phase defects

Implantation in an inhospitable endometrium is a plausible explanation for pregnancy loss. Progesterone deficiency in particular could result in the estrogen-primed endometrium being unable to sustain implantation. Luteal phase deficiency (LPD) has long been hypothesized, specifically due to inadequate progesterone secreted by the corpus luteum.

Once almost universally accepted as a common cause of fetal wastage, LPD is now generally considered an uncommon explanation. One difficulty is that endometrial histology identical to that observed with luteal phase "defects" exists also in fertile women. Efficacy of treatment is likewise unproved, principally because there are no randomized studies validating LPD as a genuine entity. Meta-analysis has shown [13] no beneficial effect of progesterone treatment. The current consensus is that LPD is either an arguable entity or cannot be proved to be treated successfully with progesterone or progestational therapy.

Luteal phase abnormalities arising during ovulation stimulation necessitated during assisted reproduction are a different phenomenon and considered appropriate to treat by administration of progesterone.

Thyroid abnormalities

Decreased conception rates and increased fetal losses are logically associated with overt hypothyroidism or hyperthyroidism. The role of subclinical thyroid dysfunction is less clear, and not generally considered an explanation for repeated losses. However, thyroid antibodies have been observed in several series, and some consider autoimmune thyroid disease a significant cause.

Elevations of maternal thyroid hormone per se are, however, clearly deleterious. This effect was shown by a family from the Azores in which a gene conferring resistance to thyroid hormone was segregating [14]. Those with an autosomal dominant mutation in the thyroid receptor β (TRβ) gene (Arg243Gln) secreted large amounts of thyroid-stimulating hormone (TSH) to compensate for end-organ resistance. During pregnancy, the fetus becomes unavoidably exposed to high levels of maternal TSH because TSH and T4 readily cross the placenta.

Loss rates were 22.8% in pregnancies of mothers who had the Arg243Gln mutation, 2.0% in those of normal mothers whose male partner had the mutation, and 4.4% in couples in which neither partner had the mutation.

Diabetes mellitus

Only women with poorly controlled diabetes mellitus have increased risk for fetal loss. Women whose glycosylated hemoglobin level was greater than four standard deviations above the mean showed higher pregnancy loss rates than either diabetic women showing lower glycosylated hemoglobin levels or euglycemic controls [15]. The vast majority of insulin-controlled diabetic women, who are better controlled, show no increase compared to a control population. In our study, pregnancy loss rates in diabetic women were 16.1% (62/386), compared with 16.2% (70/432) in controls. Almost all losses occurred early in pregnancy (< 8 weeks).

It follows also that neither subclinical nor gestational diabetes is a major etiological factor in pregnancy loss.

Intrauterine adhesions (synechiae)

Intrauterine adhesions could logically interfere with implantation or with early embryonic development. Adhesions most often arise after overzealous uterine curettage during the puerperium. Intrauterine surgery (e.g. myomectomy) is another explanation. Women with uterine synechiae usually manifest hypomenorrhea or amenorrhea, but 25–30% show repeated abortions. Adhesions doubtless cause early pregnancy failure on rare occasions, but the overall contribution to pregnancy loss is small.

Incomplete Müllerian fusion

Müllerian (uterine) fusion defects are well-accepted causes of second-trimester losses and pregnancy complications. Septate uteri are considered more likely to be associated with pregnancy loss than bicornuate, arcuate, or unicornuate uteri. Low birthweight, breech presentation, and uterine bleeding are commonly accepted correlates. However, the role incomplete Müllerian fusion plays in early (first-trimester) losses is probably overstated. Most studies lack controls or inappropriately pool early and later pregnancy losses. A pitfall in attributing second-trimester losses to uterine anomalies is that both phenomena occur so frequently that concurrent presence could well be coincidental. For example, bicornuate uteri or septate uteri are unexpectedly found in 1–3% of women undergoing laparoscopic sterilization.

With respect to clinical management, only losses occurring after the first trimester can confidently be considered to be attributed to uterine anomalies. Losses occurring in the first trimester, especially before 8 weeks, are much more likely to be the result of chromosomal abnormalities.

Leiomyomas

Leiomyomas are frequent and can produce clinical problems familiar to gynecologists. Leiomyomas plausibly could cause early pregnancy loss, but analogous to Müllerian fusion anomalies the coexistence of uterine leiomyomas and reproductive losses need not necessarily imply a causal relationship.

Location of leiomyomas is probably more important than size. Submucous leiomyomas are most likely to cause abortion. A plausible mechanism producing pregnancy loss is thinning of the endometrium over the surface of a submucous leiomyoma, predisposing to implantation in a poorly decidualized site. Rapid growth of leiomyomas could also occur secondary to the hormonal milieu of pregnancy, compromising blood supply and resulting in necrosis ("red degeneration") that subsequently leads to uterine contractions or infections.

With respect to clinical management, one should assume that leiomyomas have no etiological relationship to pregnancy loss. Surgery for this indication should be undertaken with great reluctance.

Incompetent internal cervical os

Characterized by painless dilatation and effacement, cervical incompetence usually occurs during the middle of the second trimester or the early part of the third trimester. This condition frequently follows traumatic events such as cervical amputation, cervical laceration, forceful cervical dilatation, or conization. No relationship to first-trimester losses should be expected given the small size of first-trimester embryos or fetuses.

Infections

Infections are known causes of late fetal losses and logical causes of early fetal losses. Microorganisms associated with spontaneous abortion include variola, vaccinia, *Salmonella typhi*, *Vibrio fetus*, malaria, cytomegalovirus, *Brucella*, toxoplasmosis, *Mycoplasma hominis*, *Chlamydia trachomatis*, and *Ureaplasma urealyticum*. Transplacental infection occurs with each of these microorganisms, and sporadic losses could logically result. However, infections as a cause of repetitive losses are less proven and actually unlikely.

Of the many organisms implicated in repetitive abortion, *U. urealyticum* and *M. hominis* seem most plausibly related to repetitive spontaneous abortions because they fulfill two important prerequisites. (1) The putative organism can exist in an asymptomatic state. (2) Virulence is not always so severe as to cause infertility due to fallopian tube occlusion and, hence, preclude the opportunity for pregnancy. Studies have also suggested a relationship between bacterial vaginosis, presumed due to *Gardnerella vaginalis*, and abortion. However, the latter is more typically if not exclusively associated with complications (premature delivery) in the second and third trimesters.

Given the lack of evidence for causality for recurrent losses, one may ask whether the infectious agents discussed above actually cause fetal losses or merely arise after fetal demise from other causes. Cohort surveillance for infections beginning in early pregnancy can help shed light on the true role of infections in pregnancy loss. The frequency of clinical infections was assessed prospectively in 386 diabetic subjects and 432 control subjects seen weekly or every other week during the first trimester [16]. Infection occurred no more often in 112 subjects experiencing pregnancy loss than in the 706 experiencing successful pregnancies. This held true both for the 2-week interval in which a given loss was recognized clinically as well as in the prior 2-week interval. Similar findings were observed in both control and diabetic subjects and further were substantiated when data were stratified into ascending genital infection only versus systemic infection only.

In conclusion, infections probably explain some pregnancy losses, but in the first trimester attributable risk is low even in sporadic cases. In recurrent losses, infections are much less likely.

Acquired thrombophilias (antiphospholipid and anticardiolipin antibodies)

An association between second- and third-trimester pregnancy loss and acquired thrombophilias is accepted, but the role thrombophilias play in first-trimester losses is less certain. Antibodies detected in women with pregnancy loss are diverse, encompassing nonspecific antinuclear antibodies (ANA) as well as antibodies against such specific cellular components as phospholipids, histones, and double- or single-stranded DNA. Antiphospholipid antibodies (aPL) have been most often implicated, specifically lupus anticoagulant (LAC) antibodies and anticardiolipin antibodies (aCL).

In the 1980s many descriptive studies initially seemed to show increased aCL levels in women with first-trimester pregnancy losses. However, frequencies of various antiphospholipid antibodies (LAC, aCL, aPL) were later shown to be similar in women who experienced and who did not experience first-trimester abortions. Given the still uncertain relationship, treatment regimens should be embarked upon with caution. Aspirin and heparin are not unreasonable but uncertain first-trimester results contrast with the generally accepted beneficial effect observed in women having a previous second-trimester loss [17]. Intravenous immunoglobulin is not recommended.

Inherited thrombophilias

Inherited maternal hypercoagulable states have been associated with increased fetal losses unequivocally in the second trimester and less so in the first trimester. Postulated associations include factor V Leiden (Q1691G→A), prothrombin 20210G→A, and homozygosity for the 677C→T polymorphism in the methylene tetrahydrofolate reductase gene (MTHFR). Meta-analysis of 31 studies published as of 2003 revealed associations between recurrent (two or more) fetal loss, less than 13 weeks and these thrombophilias: factor V Leiden (G1691A), activated protein C resistance, prothrombin (20210A) gene, and protein S deficiency [18]. Conversely, MTHFR, protein C, and antithrombin deficiencies were not associated with recurrent pregnancy loss. A second meta-analysis of 16 studies published by Kovalevsky *et al.* [19] reported an association between recurrent pregnancy loss, defined as two or more losses in the first two trimesters, and maternal heterozygosity for either factor V Leiden or prothrombin 20210G7→A.

There is less evidence for an association between inherited thrombophilias and recurrent early (< 10 weeks' gestation) pregnancy loss. However, some have recommended testing for factor V Leiden, activated protein C resistance, fasting homocysteine, antiphospholipid antibodies, and the prothrombin gene. Pending salutary results in randomized clinical trials, treatment for recurrent first-trimester losses with heparin and/or other antithrombotic or anticoagulant therapies must be initiated with caution.

Psychological factors

Impaired psychological well-being has long been claimed to predispose to early fetal losses. An older but still illustrative investigation ostensibly showing a benefit of psychological well-being was that of Stray-Pedersen and Stray-Pedersen [20]. One group consisted of

16 pregnant women previously experiencing repetitive abortions who received increased attention but no specific medical therapy. This group was more likely (85%) to complete their pregnancies than 42 women in a second group not given such close attention (36% successful outcome). A major experimental pitfall was that only women living "close" to the university were eligible to be placed in the increased-attention group. Women living further away served as "controls" by default, and could have differed from the experimental group in ways other than mere geographic proximity. However, in an expanded study conducted later by the same group, the same high success rate was observed in women given "tender loving care". Still, no genuine control group existed. Multiple potential confounding factors were not taken into account, making it difficult to determine whether the outcome was truly salutary with respect to the background rate of 60–70% (Table 10.1). In our study of 132 pregnancy losses involving both control and diabetic women none were associated with physical or psychological (e.g. bereavement) trauma [15].

Does PGD have a role in managing recurrent pregnancy losses?

Chromosomal aneuploidy is a very common explanation for preimplantation and early pregnancy loss. We have further noted that non-random distribution occurs in successive miscarriages (recurrent aneuploidy); abortuses tend to be either successively aneuploid or euploid [4,7]. Thus, a strong rationale exists for performing PGD aneuploidy testing and transferring only euploid embryos. RCTs have not been performed, but PGD seems beneficial, especially with respect to avoiding further abortions [21]. One good surrogate involves comparison to objective criteria like the Brigham formula, which takes into account maternal age and the number of prior abortions to derive the likelihood of a pregnancy loss. Munné *at al.* observed losses in only 13% of couples who used PGD, compared to an expected rate (Brigham) of 33% [21]. Benefit was greatest for women over age 35 years (39% vs. expected 13%; $P < .001$). However, no RCTs have been performed.

This author believes that PGD for aneuploidy testing should probably be undertaken only if there are 6–8 embryos, allowing reasonable likelihood of finding euploid embryos to transfer [22]. Ideally at least one loss should have documented aneuploidy. If no information is available, one can verify prior aneuploidy by performing FISH on archived specimens embedded in paraffin.

Finally, the approach to a couple with recurrent pregnancy losses is summarized in Table 10.3.

Table 10.3 Recommended management of recurrent pregnancy losses

First-trimester losses only
 Counseling concerning frequency at various stages of pregnancy
 Counseling concerning known etiologies, specifically cytogenetic (50–60%)
 Counseling concerning empiric recurrence risk (30–40% at most)
 Parental karyotypes to exclude balanced translocation
 Thyroid function tests (TSH, T4, prolactin)
 Karyotype on prior abortus
 Discussion on benefits and risks of PGD aneuploidy testing

First- plus second-trimester losses
 Evaluation of uterine anomalies (hysterosalpingogram or 3D ultrasound)
 Acquired thrombophilias (anticardiolipin and antiphospholipid)
 Hereditary thrombophilias (factor V Leiden, prothrombin 20210G→A, MTHFR 677C→T)

References

1. U.S. Department of Health and Human Services: Reproductive impairments among married couples., U.S. Vital and Health Statistics Series 23, No. 11, Hyattsville, MD, 1982, p. 12.

2. Simpson JL, Jauniaux ERM. Pregnancy loss In Gabbe, SA, Niebyl, JF, Simpson, JL eds. *Obstetrics: Normal and Problem Pregnancies*, 5th edn. New York: Churchill-Livingstone, 2007; 628–49.

3. Simpson JL, Mills JL, Holmes LB, *et al*. Low fetal loss rate after ultrasound-proven viability in early pregnancy. *JAMA* 1987; **258**: 2555–7.

4. Warburton D, Dallaire L, Thangavelu M. *et al*. Trisomy recurrence: a reconsideration based on North American data. *Am J Hum Genet* 2004; **75**: 376–85.

5. Simpson JL, Gray RH, Queenan JT, *et al*. Risk of recurrent spontaneous abortion for pregnancies discovered in the fifth week of gestation. *Lancet* 1994; **344**: 964.

6. Munné S, Alikani M, Tomkin G, Grifo J, Cohen J. Embryo morphology, development rates, and maternal age are correlated with chromosome abnormalities. *Fertil Steril* 1995; **64**: 382–91.

7. Warburton D, Kliner JH, Stein Z, *et al*. Does the karyotype of a spontaneous abortion predict the karyotype of a subsequent abortion? Evidence from 273 women with two karyotyped spontaneous abortions. *Am J Hum Genet* 1987; **41**: 465–83.

8. Rubio C, Simon C, Vidal F, *et al*. Chromosomal abnormalities and embryo development in recurrent miscarriage couples. *Hum Reprod* 2003; **18**: 182–8.

9. Stern JJ, Dorfmann AD, Gutierrez-Najar AJ, Cerrillo M, Coulam CB. Frequency of abnormal karyotypes among abortuses from women with and without a history of recurrent spontaneous abortion, *Fertil Steril* 1996; **65**: 250–3.

10. Stephenson MD, Awartani KA, Robinson WP. Cytogenetic analysis of miscarriages from couples with recurrent miscarriage: a case-control study. *Hum Reprod* 2002; **17**: 446–51.

11. Simpson JL, Meyers CM, Martin AO, *et al*. Translocations are infrequent among couples having repeated spontaneous abortions but no other abnormal pregnancies. *Fertil Steril* 1989; **51**: 811–14.

12. Fritz MA, Schattman G. Reply of the Committee: parental translocations and need for preimplantation genetic diagnosis? Distorting effects of ascertainment bias and the need for information-rich families. *Fertil Steril* 2008; **90**: 892–3.

13. Karamardian LM, Grimes DA. Luteal phase deficiency: effect of treatment on pregnancy rates. *Am J Obstet Gynecol* 1992; **167**: 1391–8.

14. Anselmo J, Cao D, Karrison T, *et al*. Fetal loss associated with excess thyroid hormone exposure. *JAMA* 2004; **292**: 691–5.

15. Mills JL, Simpson JL, Driscoll SG, *et al*. NICHD-DIEP Study: incidence of spontaneous abortion among normal women with insulin-dependent diabetic women whose pregnancies were identified within 21 days of conception. *N Engl J Med* 1988; **319**: 1617–23.

16. Simpson JL, Mills JL, Kim H, *et al*. Infectious processes: an infrequent cause of first trimester spontaneous abortions. *Hum Reprod* 1996; **11**: 668–72.

17. Rai R, Backos M, Rushworth F, *et al*. Polycystic ovaries and recurrent miscarriage: A reappraisal. *Hum Reprod* 2000; **15**: 612–15.

18. Rey E, Kahn SR, David M, *et al*. Thrombophilic disorders and fetal loss: a meta-analysis. *Lancet* 2003; **361**: 901–8.

19. Kovalevsky G, Gracia CR, Berlin JA, *et al*. Evaluation of the association between hereditary thrombophilias and recurrent pregnancy loss. *Arch Intern Med* 2004; **164**: 558–63.

20. Stray-Pedersen B, Stray-Pedersen S. Etiologic factors and subsequent reproductive performance in 195 couples

with a prior history of habitual abortion. *Am J Obstet Gynecol* 1984; **148**: 140–6.

21. Munné S, Chen S, Fischer J, *et al.* 2005. Preimplantation genetic diagnosis reduces pregnancy loss in women aged 35 years and older with a history of recurrent miscarriages. *Fertil Steril* 2005; **84**: 331–5.

22. Simpson, JL. Preimplantation genetic diagnosis at twenty years. *Prenat Diag* 2010; **30**: 682–95.

In vitro fertilization: indications, stimulation and clinical techniques

Cheng Toh Yeong and P. C. Wong

Introduction

In vitro fertilization (IVF) and other assisted reproductive techniques are now fully accepted modalities of treatment for subfertility in our modern world. Current IVF practice has its roots in the pioneering research carried out in the twentieth century into ovarian physiology; the isolation, purification, and production of gonadotropins; as well as the ground-breaking work by Edwards and others which led to the birth of Louise Brown on July 25, 1978, in Oldham, England.

It has been shown that 84% of couples not using contraception and having regular sexual intercourse will conceive within one year; another 8% will conceive in their second year of trying. Hence, infertility can be defined as the failure to achieve a pregnancy within one year of regular unprotected intercourse. The infertility rate is 4.5% in married women aged 16–20, 31.8% in married women aged 35–40, and 70% in married women over the age of 40. Of all cases of infertility, 35% may be attributed to the male, and 55% to the female; the remaining 10% is undetermined [1].

The International Committee for Monitoring Assisted Reproductive Technology's (ICMART) Eighth World Report analyzes assisted reproductive technology (ART) practice and results for the year 2002 from 53 countries by type of ART, women's age, number of embryos transferred, and multiple births. Over 601 243 initiated cycles resulted in a delivery rate (DR) per aspiration of 22.4% for conventional IVF, 21.2% for ICSI and a DR per transfer of 15.3% for frozen embryo transfer. For conventional IVF and ICSI, there was an overall twin rate of 25.7% per delivery and a triplet rate of 2.5%. The number of babies born worldwide through ART in 2002 was estimated to range between 219 000 and 246 000. [2]. All these statistics remind us how tremendous improvements have been made since the first IVF birth in 1978.

The indications for IVF have increased with the development of newer techniques such as ICSI, surgical sperm retrieval, embryo biopsy, and cryopreservation techniques, and IVF has become the cumulative step for the diagnosis and treatment for unexplained infertility. The procedure has few side effects and the acceptance of this treatment by the general public has opened up newer areas of social and legal concerns, e.g. egg donation, surrogacy, sex balancing, and egg or ovarian tissue freezing. Nevertheless, with ovarian hyperstimulation syndrome (OHSS) and multiple pregnancies still being the main concerns, the paradigm should shift to proper assessment of ovarian reserve, refining stimulation protocols using newer and safer or fewer drugs to minimize OHSS, and development of international guidelines

The Subfertility Handbook: A Clinician's Guide, Second Edition ed. Gab Kovacs. Published by Cambridge University Press. © Cambridge University Press 2011.

on the optimal number of embryos to be transferred so that the aim of a single healthy offspring can be achieved.

The role of IVF in the management of subfertile couples is not in question; its development and progress over the last couple of decades is staggering but it is imperative that we remind ourselves that this is an expensive treatment and its stressful impact on the mental and physical health of the patient should not be underestimated.

Indications

Tubal infertility

Accounting for about 20% of the causes for subfertility, the definition of tubal infertility is the presence of persistent tubal obstruction, absence of Fallopian tubes or tubal damage which has led to the inability to conceive for more than 12 months. The various ways in which the female patient can be evaluated for tubal infertility include hysterosalpingogram, hysterosalpingo-contrast sonography (HyCoSy), chromatography at the time of laparoscopy, selective transcervical tubal cannulation, and falloposcopy, which are discussed in detail in Chapter 4.

Endometriosis

This is a disease characterized by the presence of endometrial tissue (endometrial glands and stroma) outside the uterine cavity. It affects approximately 10% of reproductive-age women and is a leading cause of pelvic pain and infertility. Diagnosis is based on morphological aspects of the lesions and an accompanying histological confirmation of endometriotic tissue [3,4].

Many possible mechanisms may explain the association between endometriosis and infertility in women. In severe endometriosis, distortion of pelvic anatomy and pelvic adhesions may account for the infertility [4]. However, severe endometriotic lesions are not present in all women suffering from endometriosis-related infertility. In patients with minimal endometriosis, peritoneal endometrial lesions may lead to alterations in peritoneal cell populations and peritoneal fluid, resulting in infertility [5,6]. With respect to therapeutic options for endometriosis-related infertility, surgical removal of superficial and deep lesions and adhesiolysis may result in spontaneous pregnancy.

In the literature, it is not well documented whether temporary or repetitive exposure to high estrogen levels such as those encountered during ovarian stimulation for IVF contributes to endometrial recurrences. In 2006, a retrospective study analyzed the risk of recurrences in patients with moderate to severe endometriosis undergoing ovarian stimulation for insemination or IVF [7]. The conclusion of this research was that IVF treatment is less associated with endometriosis recurrence than insemination. Ovarian stimulation protocols for IVF seem to have no unwanted effects in terms of endometriosis recurrence.

Apart from the risk of an ovarian abscess, endometriomas raise the problem of whether or not they should be treated prior to starting an ovarian stimulation cycle. A large endometrioma may hamper follicular development as well as the monitoring of ovulation induction, resulting in an inadequate response [8]. For smaller endometriomas and for the cases where surgery is not considered, the long-term down-regulation protocol may be indicated, but it should be taken into account that its effects on the cyst volume are highly uncertain. It is

Table 11.1 Age-related infertility

Age	Subfertile (%)
Less than 30 years old	25
30 to 35 years old	33
35 to 40 years old	50
Greater than 40 years old	> 90

proposed that if the cyst is > 6 cm, it should be drained/removed [9]. Cystectomy is associated with a lengthening of stimulation duration and an increase in gonadotropin doses required, while the number of collected oocytes is significantly reduced [10]. Moreover, it has also been associated with premature menopause by a risk factor of 2.4 times (95 CI; 0.5–6.8) [11].

Age-related infertility

Many women experience age-related infertility owing to social trends that lead to deferred childbearing and to the current age of the "baby boom" generation. Age-related infertility (Table 11.1) is due to oocyte abnormalities and reduced ovarian reserve [11].

Likewise, paternal aging has been implicated in higher risk for infertility. A recent review of studies on the effects of male age on semen quality and fertility concluded that increasing age is associated with decreased semen volume and motility and poorer sperm morphology, but not with decreased sperm concentration [12]. Male fertility declines somewhat with age, particularly in men older than 50 years of age, but the results of many of these studies are confounded by female partner age. There is no absolute age at which men cannot father a child [13].

Ovarian dysfunction

Currently, IVF is considered only as a third-line option in patients with polycystic ovarian syndrome and anovulation. The first line of treatment is ovulation induction in these women with agents such as clomiphene citrate or HMG alone, or combined with intra-uterine inseminations is generally preferred, as once restoration of ovulation is achieved the chances of pregnancy will return. The second line of treatment is laparoscopic ovarian cautery. If COH is used for PCOS patients, they are particularly liable to develop ovarian hyperstimulation syndrome (OHSS). IVF together with in vitro maturation has been used to manage PCOS patients to eliminate the side effects of OHSS (discussed in Chapter 12).

Unexplained infertility

Couples with unexplained infertility are those with

- normal luteal phase progesterone
- tubal patency assessed by hysterosalpingography and/or laparoscopy
- normal semen sample according to WHO guidelines.

IVF is becoming popular when there is no specific explanation for infertility as it may be able to overcome a variety of problems. Ten randomized controlled trials were identified

[14] to determine, in the context of unexplained infertility, whether IVF improves the probability of live birth compared with (i) expectant management, (ii) clomiphene citrate (CC), (iii) intrauterine insemination (IUI) alone, (iv) IUI with controlled ovarian stimulation, and (v) gamete intrafallopian transfer (GIFT).

The authors [14] concluded that there was a trend towards higher live birth rates per woman/couple associated with IVF compared with intrauterine insemination with or without ovarian stimulation and GIFT. The beneficial effect of IVF on this outcome over these treatments was not statistically significant. There was also a trend towards higher multiple pregnancy rates with IUI and ovarian stimulation compared to IVF.

Therefore, IVF might result in more pregnancies than other options for unexplained infertility, but this is still uncertain and more research is needed on birth rates, adverse outcomes and costs in order to prescribe this modality of treatment as a first option.

Egg donation

The initial indication for egg donation was originally for women with premature ovarian failure (POF), defined as menopause occurring before the age of 40 years. POF affects approximately 1% of the female population. The next indication was for women carrying transmittable genetic abnormalities which could affect their offspring.

In recent years, it is being used for women with diminished ovarian reserve. It has long been known that women over 40 years old have reduced fertility in general and a poorer chance of success after IVF.

Other potential candidates for egg donation include women who have previously failed multiple IVF attempts, particularly when poor egg quality is suspected, and women carrying a genetic abnormality, e.g. Huntington's disease.

In many countries where the availability of egg donors remains low or paid donation is illegal, the practice of egg sharing with clear counseling and protocols has managed not to compromise the chance of achieving a pregnancy or live birth for the egg-sharer or the recipient compared with standard IVF/ICSI patients[15].

Surrogacy

The two separate methods of surrogacy offering a full or partial genetic link are gestational and genetic.

Gestational surrogacy takes place when both the intended mother and father use their own gametes (usually) and the genetically related embryo is transferred into the surrogate mother via IVF. The indications for gestational surrogate include disorders confined to the uterus and tubes. These include previous hysterectomy, surgeries for fibroids (myomectomy) which may affect the uterus's ability to grow with a pregnancy, damage from infection, congenital abnormalities of the uterus (as seen in DES exposure), or severe adhesions which distort the uterine cavity (Ashermann's syndrome).

In genetic surrogacy the woman donates the oocyte as well as carrying the fetus and thus the baby is genetically related to the surrogate mother (i.e. the surrogate mothers are inseminated with the intended fathers' sperm). Conditions such as menopause or advanced maternal age, premature ovarian failure, genetic disorders of the woman, severe ovulatory disorders (refractory polycystic ovaries, fertility drug insensitivity, etc.), previous chemotherapy which has destroyed the ovaries, surgically absent ovaries, or severe endometriosis which has damaged the ovaries are all possible indications for a surrogate.

Preimplantation genetic diagnosis

Preimplantation genetic diagnosis (PGD) in which embryos created in vitro are analyzed for specific inheritable genetic defects by FISH technology or PCR techniques so that only those that are free of these defects are transferred into the patient. PGD was originally developed as an alternative to prenatal diagnosis and selective abortion for couples at high risk of having a child with a severe Mendelian genetic disorder, e.g. muscular dystrophy. However, over the last 10 years, the indications for PGD have broadened to include inherited and sporadic chromosomal abnormalities (e.g. translocation disorders causing recurrent miscarriages), genetic abnormalities associated with adult-onset disorders (e.g. Huntington's disease), blood group incompatibilities and HLA tissue typing, and even to screen for cancer genes (e.g. familial polyposis) [16].

Male factor

A male factor is solely responsible in at least 20% of subfertile couples and contributory in another possibly 20%. The main causes of male factor infertility are divided into four main groups, i.e. idiopathic, testicular, posttesticular and pretesticular, with the former two accounting for more than 80% of cases.

The goal is to identify conditions where sperm can be obtained for subsequent ICSI. Even in some men with azoospermia, sperm cells can be surgically obtained from the epididymis (PESA) or by testicular biopsy. The establishment of ICSI for couples means that most causes of male infertility can now be treated. In conditions where no sperm can be obtained and therefore they are not amenable to ART, these couples can be offered adoption or donor insemination.

The typical IVF cycle

1. Stimulation for multiple follicular development
2. Monitoring follicular growth and development
3. Trigger of follicular maturation
4. Oocyte recovery and identification
5. Insemination/ICSI
6. Embryo culture
7. Embryo replacement
8. Luteal phase support
9. Confirmation of pregnancy

Controlled ovarian hyperstimulation (COH), monitoring and trigger of follicular maturation (steps 1, 2 and 3) will be considered together.

Superovulation is the term for stimulating the growth of multiple follicles with the release of eggs from each follicle. This is an integral part of IVF treatment. Trounson and colleagues at the Monash group had shown elegantly [17] that the increased number of eggs at the time of oocyte retrieval was directly correlated to the pregnancy rate.

The ideal stimulation protocol should be simple, allowing patient self-administration at home, requiring minimal monitoring, and avoiding premature luteinization, spontaneous ovulation, optimizing endometrial development and reducing risks for hyperstimulation.

Ovulation stimulation must be individualized according to the ovarian reserve status of the patient and if applicable from a previous treatment cycle's response.

Ovulation induction agents

Clomiphene citrate

Whilst used in the first stimulated cycles to achieve IVF pregnancies [19] it is now seldom used for contemporary IVF.

Gonadotropins

These are the principal agents used in controlled ovarian stimulation in IVF.

In the early twentieth century FSH-containing hormones were isolated from post-mortem pituitaries (HPG) or from the urine of postmenopausal women – human menopausal gonadotropin (hMG). Through further advances in DNA technology and the transference of human genes encoding for the common α and hormone-specific β subunit of the glycoprotein hormone into Chinese hamster ovary cell lines, pharmaceutical companies are able to produce human recombinant FSH (recFSH).

Human menopausal gonadotropins have been, for over two decades, used extensively for ovulation induction with the aim of increasing the number of oocytes available for fertilization. The initial preparations were not very pure which led to great batch-to-batch inconsistency, with only less than 5% of the proteins present being bioactive. Improvements in protein purification led to purified urinary FSH (uFSH) and later, with recombinant DNA technology, the production of recFSH. These products have greatly improved purity and consistency and can be administered by protein weight rather than by bioactivity.

GnRH agonist

GnRH agonists have been in use for more than 20 years and, due to the intrinsic agonist activity, there is an initial flare effect rendering the ovaries quiescent two weeks later only for the stimulation proper to begin. They are then maintained to prevent LH release and premature ovulation.

GnRH antagonist

GnRH antagonists allow for immediate suppression and recovery of pituitary function and can be used any time in the early or mid follicular phase of a treatment cycle to prevent a premature LH surge.

Stimulation regimes

We will describe four basic stimulation regimes below but stress that any proposed stimulation protocol should be individualized according to the maternal age, her ovarian reserve, body mass index, past medical, endocrine and fertility history, indication for treatment and also in accordance with the specific fertility and ethical regulations in the country without compromising the safety of the patient in terms of OHSS.

Luteal gonadotropin-releasing hormone agonist stimulation protocol

1. Start GnRH-a on day 21 of a regular menstrual cycle. The luteal start is confirmed by a serum progesterone level > 4 ng/ml or by a transvaginal scan showing the presence of a corpus luteum. By starting GnRH-a in the luteal phase the risk of ovarian cyst formation is decreased.
2. Spontaneous menses expected 10–12 days after the administration of GnRH-a.

3. Transvaginal scan to evaluate the lining of the endometrium after menses started and serum estradiol to confirmed down-regulation before starting stimulation using gonadotropins (rec-FSH , or urinary FSH or combination) daily.
4. Serial ultrasound and E_2 levels monitor follicular development; measuring the number and size of follicles and also the development of the endometrium and its morphology.
5. Once follicular size reaches 18–22 mm, administer rec-hCG, typically 5000–10 000 IU SC or IM.
6. Oocyte retrieval 34–36 hours after hCG.

Alternatively, a variation of this protocol is to overlap with the usage of the oral contraceptive pill (PDR) with the intention to program treatment and also preventing ovarian cyst formation and inadvertent pregnancy when the GnRH-a is given. With this method the oral contraceptive is usually administered for 21 days (although can be shorter), and GnRH-a is commenced 3–5 days before the completion of the oral contraceptive and FSH is commenced in the usual fashion as described above.

Fixed, multi-dose GnRH antagonist protocol

1. Transvaginal ultrasound and serum E_2 are arranged on day 2/3 of the period after oral contraceptive pretreatment.
2. After confirmation of quiescent ovaries and low E_2 level, SC recFSH is commenced daily for ovarian stimulation. GnRH antagonist 0.25 mg daily is then given as a fixed protocol starting on day 6 of the stimulation until the day of hCG administration. Alternatively, for the flexible multi-dose protocol, the GnRH antagonist is started when the leading follicle is 14 mm and /or serum LH levels > 10 IU/l and continued till day of trigger.
3. Ovulation triggering is achieved by subcutaneous injection of 10 000 IU of hCG when leading follicles reach 18–20 mm together with at least three mature follicles 16 mm detected on ultrasound scan. This is followed by transvaginal ultrasound-guided oocyte retrieval ≈34–36 h later.

Flare-up or BOOST GnRH agonist protocol

1. Daily 0.05 mg/day GnRH-a from day 2 of the cycle.
2. recFSH started from day 3.
3. GnRH agonist is administered subcutaneously and continued daily until and including the day of human chorionic gonadotropin (hCG) administration.
4. A total of 10 000 units of rec-hCG 250 mcg is administered SC when the leading follicle reaches 17–18 mm in diameter followed 34–36 h later by an ultrasound-guided transvaginal oocyte retrieval.

Natural cycle

Although Louise Brown was conceived in a natural cycle, this is rarely used in 2010.

1. All the patients have a vaginal ultrasound scan of the pelvis on day 2 of the cycle. Patients with an ovarian cystic structure > 14 mm in diameter are cancelled.
2. All the patients undergo vaginal ultrasound monitoring beginning on day 9 of the cycle, followed by daily scans once the leading follicle reaches 15 mm in diameter.
3. Serum estradiol and LH concentrations are measured after each ultrasound examination.
4. Once the follicle reaches 17 mm in diameter, each patient is given a series of five test bands for urinary detection of the LH surge.
5. The patient is then asked to perform a test every 6 hours until hCG administration. rec-hCG 250 mcg is administered to all patients when the largest diameter of the follicles

reaches 18 mm and in the presence of estradiol concentrations 100 pg/ml with the absence of any LH surge.

6. Transvaginal ultrasound-directed oocyte retrieval is performed 35 hours later. In the case of a spontaneous LH surge, oocyte retrieval is scheduled 33 hours after the observation of a positive coloration with urinary testing.

7. Treatment is abandoned if inadequate follicular growth is observed (defined as the absence of increase in follicular diameter after two ultrasound scans), if the serum estradiol concentration is falling or < 100 pg/ml or if there is evidence of a premature LH surge (defined as an LH value three times the basal LH value determined on day 2 and with a follicle < 17 mm in diameter).

There is a high likelihood of premature ovulation and missed ovulation in the natural cycle and hence intensive monitoring is necessitated. Even so, the rate of cycle cancellation is deemed too high by most clinicians for this method to be used routinely in practice.

Complications of ovulation stimulation and IVF techniques

Complications can occur during the ovulation induction, the oocyte collection procedure, and postoperatively.

Ovarian hyperstimulation syndrome (OHSS) is considered the most serious complication of ovulation induction. It can vary from being a mild illness to a severe, life-threatening disease requiring hospitalization. OHSS can occur as soon as a few days after receiving hCG ("early OHSS") or later ("late OHSS"). Multiple pregnancy has been shown to be associated with a higher risk of late OHSS.

The frequency of IVF complications other than OHSS has been only sporadically reported. For oocyte collection, bleeding has been reported in 0.03–0.5% and infections in 0.02–0.3% of embryo transfers [20].

Oocyte recovery and identification

Oocyte recovery in day surgery theater is now usually performed under general anesthesia or intravenous sedation as oocyte retrieval is carried out under ultrasound guidance.

The patient is first placed in a lithotomy position, cleaned and draped. The transvaginal probe with a needle guide attached is then inserted into the vagina to visualize both ovaries and their follicles. Meanwhile the aspiration system is readied and vacuum pressures are checked (100 mmHg) by aspirating culture media with the specially designed disposable needles. The lower more accessible ovary is targeted first and the needle is inserted under ultrasound guidance into the first follicle. The follicular fluid is then aspirated into a test tube placed in a warmer block and the test tube is handed over to the waiting embryologist located in the adjoining IVF laboratory. All the follicles on one side are systematically aspirated without flushing , with care at all times to avoid the nearby pelvic side-wall vessels. Once all the follicles on one side have been aspirated, the needle is withdrawn and used to aspirate warm culture media in a test tube to flush the system through.

The surgeon then moves over to the opposite ovary and the needle is again inserted under ultrasound guidance to target the remaining follicles. Once again, the follicles are systematically punctured and aspirated (without flushing) until all the follicles are tapped. Once completed, the needle is withdrawn and the system flushed again with warm culture media to ensure no egg is left behind in the needle system.

The uterus is scanned and the endometrial thickness measured before the ultrasound probe is removed.

The vagina is cleaned with sterile gauze swabs and hemostasis is confirmed before the procedure is deemed completed.

Postoperatively, the patient is monitored in the recovery ward and reviewed 2–6 hours later before discharge.

When the embryologist receives the test tube containing the follicular fluid, she/he pours the contents into a Petri dish and examines the contents under a binocular dissecting microscope for the oocyte cumulus complex (OCC). Once the OCC is identified, it is quickly transferred into a buffered medium. It is washed thrice in the medium to remove red blood cells before it is transferred into a culture dish containing culture medium. The dish containing all the OCCs is placed in the incubator. This dish remains in the incubator until the time of insemination, which is about 4 hours post oocyte retrieval.

Oocytes are graded based on the expansion of the cumulus complex and the tightness of the corona cells:

Grade 1 oocytes are immature oocytes which have few cumulus cells and tightly packed corona cells. On removing the cumulus cells, the presence of a germinal vesicle (GV) is clearly seen.

Grade 2 oocytes have tightly packed cumulus and corona cells. On removing the cumulus cells no GV is seen and there is no polar body present and they are referred to as metaphase I oocytes.

Grade 3 oocytes have very expanded cumulus; corona cells are loosely packed with a visible polar body and they are referred to as metaphase II oocytes.

Post-mature oocytes are Grade 4 oocytes which have clumpy cumulus cells, incomplete or irregular corona cells and the ooplasm of these oocytes is dark or very granular.

Atretic oocytes are Grade 5 oocytes which have no cumulus or very few cumulus cells, irregular corona cells, and dark and misshapen ooplasm.

Insemination

The man's semen sample is processed in the morning of the oocyte retrieval. The density gradient technique followed by washing in culture medium is the most common method used for recovery of motile sperm with normal morphology. The processed sperm sample is placed in the incubator until the time of insemination or intracytoplasmic spermatozoa injection (ICSI).

Fertilization is achieved by either insemination or ICSI. This is performed 4 hours post oocyte retrieval.

Insemination is done for patients with high sperm count and normal morphology sperm. Each OCC is placed in a droplet containing 150 000 motile sperm/ml.

ICSI is done for patients who have poor sperm quality or antisperm antibodies and also for patients who had fertilization failure in a prior cycle. Each mature oocyte is injected with one sperm each.

Embryo culture

After insemination or ICSI the oocytes are placed in the incubator until the next day.

A fertilization check is done 18 hours post insemination or ICSI. The oocytes are checked for the presence of two pronuclei. The fertilized oocytes are placed in the incubator until the next day, which is referred to as day 2. Embryos are scored daily from day 2 until day 6. On day 2 the embryos should be at the four-cell stage. Day 3 embryos should be at the eight-cell stage, day 4 embryos should be at the compacted stage and day 5 and 6 embryos should be at the blastocyst stage. Embryos are graded based on the regularity of the blastomeres and presence of fragments. Good-quality embryos have regular blastomeres with no fragmentation. Average-quality embryos have regular blastomeres with moderate fragments. Poor-quality embryos have irregular blastomeres with a lot of fragments.

Embryo transfer

Embryo transfer (ET) is done on either day 2, day 3, day 4, or day 5. Prior to embryo transfer, the embryologist selects the best embryo(s) for transfer. The number of embryos transferred depends on the patient's eligibility. There is no need for dietary restrictions on the day of ET. It is suggested that patients should have a moderately full but not overfull bladder at the time of embryo transfer so they should not routinely empty their bladder on arrival. However, this can be left to the discretion of the treating doctor.

The patient is put in the lithotomy position and the cervix is then cleansed with sterile culture medium to remove mucus. All embryo transfers for patients are to be performed with soft catheters (if possible). The embryos are loaded for transfer in a 18 cm Wallace embryo transfer catheter. Embryos are deposited at 5.5 cm from external cervical or 1–2 cm from the fundus unless the uterus is abnormally small or large. If it is not possible to smoothly pass a soft catheter, a stiffer catheter or an introducer may be used. If transfer is still not possible at this point a single-tooth tenaculum may be used. After the embryos have been deposited in the uterus the doctor should keep the pressure on the syringe plunger the whole time while withdrawing the catheter to reduce the chance of the embryos being aspirated back into the catheter at this stage. Following transfer the catheter is handed back to the embryologist to ensure that the embryos are no longer present in the catheter. If one or more embryos do return in the catheter the embryologist will reload them into another catheter and they should be replaced back into the uterus approximately 1 cm below the level at which the embryos had been previously deposited. After use the empty transfer catheter is disposed of in the clinical waste bag in the laboratory.

The use of a transabdominal ultrasound may be preferred to help visualize the entry of the catheter or in difficult transfers. Rarely it may be necessary to pass other catheters with metal obturators or to pass a metal sound or Hegar dilator to allow embryo transfer to be performed. In extreme circumstances, the transfer may need to be delayed to allow IV sedation to be administered or the embryos may even need to be frozen and subsequent frozen embryo transfer performed after cervical dilatation.

The patient's remaining good-quality embryos are cryopreserved for future use. Embryos can be cryopreserved by either slow freezing or vitrification. Slow freezing is a procedure where the embryos are loaded into freezing straws and placed in a freezing machine that is capable of achieving low temperatures very gradually. Vitrification is a rapid method of cryopreservation. In this method the loaded straws are plunged directly into liquid nitrogen. During cryopreservation, embryos are protected from cryodamage due to the presence of cryoprotectants in the freezing solution.

Luteal phase support

Although the use of luteal support has been debated since the early days of IVF, the use of progesterone support in a long-acting GnRH-a-stimulated IVF cycle yields significantly better pregnancy rates compared to placebo or no treatment [21]. The route and type of luteal support has evolved from the early days where hCG injections were given three times on day 3, day 6 and day 9 post egg collection to the use of progesterone gel, pessaries, and injections. Recent meta-analysis [22] shows comparable pregnancy rates with the vaginal and intramuscular route for progesterone and suggests that with better patient tolerance, and being less time-consuming, less painful and with a better side-effect profile, the vaginal route is gaining popularity. There is still no consensus as to the duration for luteal supplementation although most units would stop at the first ultrasound scan at 6–7 weeks. However, a RCT comparing administration of vaginal progesterone for 14 days after oocyte pickup, with extended administration for 3 weeks after a positive test, revealed no difference in live birth rates [23].

There is no firm evidence suggesting the need for routine use of progesterone in ovulation induction cycles using clomiphene citrate or hMG.

Conclusion and pregnancy rates

The efficacy of IVF treatment and how to express success rates have been topics of debate but to the patient the key performance indicator remains whether a live birth is attained. Results vary according to geography, various regulations laid down by respective governing bodies and selection of patients. Traditionally, pregnancy rate per cycle has been used to compare results but gradually cumulative pregnancy outcome over the course of treatment may become more pertinent to the couple. A recent paper by Malizia *et al.* [24] demonstrated among 6164 patients undergoing 14 248 cycles that the cumulative live birth rate after six cycles was 72% (95% confidence interval [CI], 70–74%). Among patients who were younger than 35 years of age, the corresponding rate after six cycles was 65% (95% CI, 64–67%). Among patients who were 40 years of age or older, the live birth rate was 23% (95% CI, 21–25%). The cumulative live birth rate decreased with increasing age, and the age-stratified curves (< 35 vs. ≥40 years) were significantly different from one another ($P < 0.001$).

We see that IVF is an effective treatment option in the younger age groups but it cannot reverse age-related infertility.

References

1. Zegers-Hochschild F, Nygren KG, Adamson GD, *et al.* The ICMART glossary on ART terminology. *Hum Reprod* 2006; 21: 1968–70.

2. World Collaborative Report on Assisted Reproductive Technology, 2002. *Hum Reprod* 2009; 24(9): 2310–20.

3. El Bishry G, Tselos V, Pathi A. Correlation between laparoscopic and histological diagnosis in patients with endometriosis. *J Obstet Gynaecol* 2008; 28: 511–15.

4. Walter AJ, Hentz JG, Magtibay PM, Cornella JL, Magrina JF. Endometriosis: correlation between histologic and visual findings at laparoscopy. *Am J Obstet Gynecol* 2001; 184: 1407–13.

5. American Fertility Society. Revised American Fertility Society classification of endometriosis: 1985. *Fertil Steril* 1985; 43: 351–2.

6. Practice Committee of the American Society for Reproductive Medicine.

Endometriosis and infertility. *Fertil Steril* 2004; **82**(Suppl 1): S40–5.

7. D'Hooghe TM, Denys B, Spiessens C, Meuleman C, Debrock S. Is the endometriosis recurrence rate increased after ovarian hyperstimulation? *Fertil Steril* 2006; **86**: 283–90.

8. Gupta S, Agarwal A, Agarwal R, Loret de Mola JR. Impact of ovarian endometrioma on assisted reproduction outcomes. *Reprod Biomed Online* 2006; **13**: 349–60.

9. Dechard, H, Dechanet C, Brunet C, *et al.* Endometriosis and in vitro fertilisation: a review. *Gynecol Endocrinol* 2009; **25**: 717–21.

10. Demirol A, Guven S, Baykal C, Gurgan T. Effect of endometrioma cystectomy on IVF outcome: a prospective randomized study. *Reprod Biomed Online* 2006; **12**: 639–43.

11. Busacca M, Riparini J, Somigliana E, *et al.* Postsurgical ovarian failure after laparoscopic excision of bilateral endometriomas. *Am J Obstet Gynecol* 2006; **195**: 421–5.

12. Lebovic D, Gordon JD, Taylor RN. Female infertility. In *Reproductive Endocrinology and Infertility – Handbook for Clinicians*, 1st edn. Arlington, VA: Scrub Hill Press, 2005; 194.

13. Kidd SA, Eskenazi B, Wyrobek AJ. Effects of male age on semen quality and fertility: a review of the literature. *Fertil Steril* 2001; **75**: 237–48.

14. Pandian Z, Bhattacharya S, Vale L, Templeton A. In vitro fertilisation for unexplained subfertility. *Cochrane Database Syst Rev* 2005; **2**: CD003357. doi: 10.1002/14651858.CD003357.pub2.

15. Thum MY, Gafar A, Wren M, *et al.* Does egg-sharing compromise the chance of donors or recipients achieving a live birth? *Hum Reprod* 2003; **18**: 2363–7.

16. Davis T, Song B, Cram DS. Preimplantation genetic diagnosis of familial adenomatous polyposis. *Reprod Biomed Online* 2006; **13**(5): 707–11.

17. Trounson AO, Wood EC. IVF and related technology. The present and the future. *Med J Aust* 1993, **58**: 853–7.

18. Trounson AO, Leeton JF, Wood C, Webb J, Wood J. Pregnancies in humans by fertilization in vitro and embryo transfer in the controlled ovulatory cycle. *Science* 1981; **212**: 681–2.

19. Adashi EY. Clomiphene citrate initiated ovulation: a clinical update. *Sem Reprod Endocrinol* 1986; **4**: 255–75.

20. Nyboe Andersen A, Gianaroli L, Felderbaum R, de Mouzon J, Nygren KG. Assisted reproductive technology in Europe, 2001. Results generated from European registers by ESHRE. *Hum Reprod* 2005; **20**: 1158–76.

21. The Practice Committee of the American Society of Reproductive Medicine. Progesterone supplementation during the luteal phase and in early pregnancy in the treatment of infertility: an educational bulletin. *Fertil Steril* 2008; **89**: 789–92.

22. Zarutskie PW, Phillips JA. A meta-analysis of the route of administration of luteal phase support in assisted reproductive technology: vaginal versus intramuscular progesterone. *Fertil Steril* 2009; **92**(1): 163–9.

23. Nyboe AA, Popovic-Todorovic B, Schmidt KT *et al.* Progesterone supplementation during early gestations after IVF or ICSI has no effect on delivery rates: a randomized controlled trial. *Hum Reprod* 2002; **17**: 357–61.

24. Malizia BA, Hacke MR, Penzias AS. Cumulative live birth rates after In vitro fertilisation. *NEJM* 2009; **30**: 236–43.

Chapter 2

In vitro maturation

Baris Ata, Shauna Reinblatt and Seang Lin Tan

Introduction

In vitro fertilization (IVF) treatment not only proved to be the most effective treatment of subfertility but also extended treatment opportunities with its complementary procedures such as intracytoplasmic sperm injection, testicular sperm retrieval, gamete and embryo cryopreservation, and preimplantation genetic diagnosis. IVF has completely changed the field of reproductive medicine.

Although the first IVF birth was achieved with "the reimplantation of a human embryo" derived from a single oocyte retrieved in a natural cycle, soon it was realized that pregnancy and birth rates per treatment cycle could be increased with simultaneous transfer of multiple embryos following retrieval of multiple mature oocytes with controlled ovarian stimulation (COS). Simultaneous transfer of multiple embryos substantially increased pregnancy rates and on average they reached 20–40% per started cycle. The results achieved by most treatment centers exceed spontaneous conception rates in healthy fertile couples [1].

Production of multiple embryos requires COS with exogenous gonadotropin administration combined with gonadotropin releasing hormone analogs. Unfortunately, COS is not without limitations. First, the cost of drugs poses a substantial financial burden and at times prevents a couple's access to treatment. The cost of medications can reach as high as 40% of overall treatment cost. Second, COS requires frequent monitoring scans and creates further direct and indirect costs, loss of working time and inconvenience. Furthermore, the most important medical problem associated with COS is the risk of ovarian hyperstimulation syndrome (OHSS). OHSS is a potentially lethal condition, most commonly occurring as an iatrogenic complication of COS. It is characterized by ovarian enlargement and increased capillary permeability, causing fluid shift to the third space. This results in ascites formation, hypovolemia, hemoconcentration and hypercoagulability. OHSS may be further complicated by acute renal failure, hypovolemic shock, thromboembolic episodes and adult respiratory distress syndrome, and in extreme cases it can be fatal. The risk of OHSS can be as high as 6% in young women with polycystic ovarian syndrome (PCOS) [2]. More recently, COS has been suggested to have detrimental effects on developing oocytes, embryos derived from these oocytes, and/or endometrial receptivity.

The ideal treatment, therefore, would combine the pregnancy rates of conventional IVF without the risks and costs associated with COS. The small antral follicles present in the human ovary harbor immature oocytes that are not amenable to fertilization by sperm before

The Subfertility Handbook: A Clinician's Guide, Second Edition ed. Gab Kovacs. Published by Cambridge University Press. © Cambridge University Press 2011.

they complete maturation and reach metaphase II (MII) stage. The immature oocytes resume meiosis upon removal from the follicle and they have the capacity to complete meiotic division and can be fertilized in vitro. More than 80% of oocytes were reported to resume meiosis independent of the menstrual cycle day and gonadotropin support in IVM medium. Collection and in vitro maturation (IVM) of these already existing immature oocytes provides multiple MII oocytes that can be fertilized in vitro.

Research on immature oocytes dates as far back as the 1930s although the first pregnancy and live birth from in vitro matured oocytes in humans was only reported by Lucinda Veeck and colleagues in 1983 in the context of a stimulated IVF cycle. They reported two pregnancies resulting from IVM of immature oocytes collected in gonadotropin-stimulated IVF cycles. However, IVF with COS had already become the norm and it was not until 1991 when Cha and colleagues first reported intentional collection of immature oocytes from women undergoing gynecological surgery that IVM began to gain momentum. The immature oocytes donated by these women were matured in vitro and the resulting embryos were transferred to a recipient with premature ovarian failure [3]. The recipient delivered healthy triplet girls.

Three years later, Trounson and colleagues reported the collection of immature oocytes from women with PCOS for their own use. The immature oocytes collected were matured in vitro with gonadotropin-enriched medium, then fertilized, and a healthy live birth following transfer of resultant embryos was reported. Unfortunately, the initial pregnancy rates were low, and it took another five years for breakthrough research to allow success rates to exceed 35% per cycle in appropriately selected patient groups[4,5].

Currently, IVM is not only a recognized treatment alternative for couples who need assisted reproductive technologies (ART), but also is considered as an innovative fertility preservation method which extends the options for patients with various diseases that preclude treatment with conventional methods. However, compared to widespread application of IVF, IVM is still practiced by relatively few clinics worldwide.

Indications for IVM

Young women with high antral-follicle counts achieve the highest pregnancy rates with IVM [6]. Therefore IVM is considered an established treatment option for women with polycystic ovaries (PCO) or PCOS who need treatment with ART. However, the application of IVM technology is not limited to these women alone, and can be extended to benefit other patient populations.

Over-responders to gonadotropin stimulation

Women who over-respond to gonadotropins during an IVF cycle face the risk of OHSS. Among the strategies available to decrease OHSS, the only method proven to absolutely prevent it is to withhold the injection of human chorionic gonadotropin (hCG) for final oocyte maturation, i.e. to cancel the cycle. Obviously, this strategy leads to frustration for both the patient and the physician. IVM combined with IVF can be a valid option for patients who demonstrate an over-response to COS and are considered to be at risk of OHSS during an already started IVF cycle. Giving the hCG injection when the leading follicle size is 12–14 mm, before the conventional hCG criteria for IVF are met, followed by oocyte collection 36–38 hours later may prove to be an effective strategy. Early oocyte collection prevents any further increase in the number of granulosa cells available for later luteinization. Given the fact that the vasoactive molecules leading to early OHSS are secreted from luteinized granulosa cells, a decrease in the incidence of early OHSS can be anticipated.

Collection of some mature oocytes alongside the immature oocytes is possible at this stage of follicle development. Lim and colleagues reported a 36.6% clinical pregnancy rate using a similar strategy in 123 women who had ≥ 20 follicles with a mean diameter ≥ 10 mm after ≥ 5 days of gonadotropin stimulation. None of the women in this cohort developed OHSS [7]. Moreover, 18.9% of the 1554 oocytes collected were in vivo matured.

Poor responders to gonadotropin stimulation

The sole aim of COS is the retrieval of several mature oocytes that can be fertilized in vitro and unfortunately women do not respond similarly to gonadotropin stimulation. Some women fail to develop a reasonable number of mature follicles despite COS. The most common cause of such poor response seems to be the age-related decline in ovarian reserve, which cannot be overcome by different stimulation strategies. The problem is not confined to older women and some younger women also respond poorly to COS.

Identification and prediction of poor responders remains a challenge for the clinicians and none of the several stimulation protocols available has unequivocally proven to provide a significant improvement in ovarian responsiveness. For women in whom poor ovarian response does not seem to be due to a rectifiable cause inherent to the particular treatment cycle, i.e., inappropriate choice of stimulation protocol, skipped medication, etc., justification of trying other stimulated cycles is questionable and IVM may provide a viable option in such cases.

Some women have multiple antral follicles that are unresponsive to gonadotropins in a stimulated cycle and lack an optimal ovarian response warranting further stimulation. Immature oocyte collection with or without hCG administration may be an alternative to cycle cancellation. Encouraging results have been reported with both strategies [8,9]. Women with a poor response during an IVF cycle underwent immature oocyte collection with or without hCG priming and pregnancy rates of 31.6% and 40.4% were achieved in 19 and 55 cycles, respectively.

On the other hand, there are the women with genuine decreased ovarian reserve. They have antral follicles that are capable of responding to gonadotropin stimulation with growth, but the number of antral follicles is decreased. Given the fact that gonadotropin stimulation fails to provide the desired number of in vivo matured oocytes in such women, IVM in an unstimulated cycle or combined with natural-cycle IVF may provide a reasonable option. In fact, in eight women with a poor response, defined as ≤ 4 follicles growing or oocytes collected in a previous stimulated IVF cycle, we achieved a similar number of embryos available for transfer in the subsequent IVM cycle [10]. Six women reached embryo transfer (75%), and one achieved a live birth, yielding a 16.7% live birth rate per transfer in this small group of genuine poor responders.

Oocyte donation

Today oocyte donation is a recognized treatment option for women with severely decreased ovarian reserve, women of advanced reproductive age, women affected by/carriers of certain genetic disorders, women who repeatedly have poor oocyte and/or embryo quality or multiple unexplained failed treatment cycles. An ideal oocyte donor is defined by a young age and high ovarian reserve among other characteristics. Donors routinely undergo COS in order to maximize the number of mature oocytes available for donation and eventually to increase pregnancy rates in recipients. However, COS puts these young donors with high ovarian reserve under a high risk of early OHSS. Besides the risk of OHSS, the inconvenience of the numerous injections required and the yet to be proven risk of cancer associated with repeated use of ovulation induction drugs cause reluctance on the part of potential oocyte donors. IVM can become the method of choice for oocyte donation cycles as young women with high antral follicle counts constitute the best candidates for IVM and yield good pregnancy rates. Avoiding ovarian stimulation may decrease the risks and inconvenience for oocyte donors. Such an approach may also serve to increase the availability of altruistic oocyte donors.

We collected on average 12.8 immature oocytes from 12 oocyte donors with a mean age of 29 years. Sixty-eight percent of the oocytes matured in vitro and 62 embryos were available for transfer to 12 recipients with a mean age of 37.7 years. On average, four embryos were transferred (range 2–6) and a clinical pregnancy rate of 50% was achieved. Two women had first-trimester miscarriages while four had healthy live births, yielding a live birth rate of 33% [11].

Fertility preservation

There have been substantial improvements in both diagnosis and treatment of cancer over the last decades. Improved treatment methods have resulted in a steady increase in the survival rates. Accordingly, a growing number of women who have survived cancer are faced with the risk of infertility resulting from gonadotoxic oncological treatment. Moreover, chemotherapy for non-oncological conditions such as systemic lupus erythematosus or other autoimmune disorders, surgery for endometriosis and non-malignant ovarian neoplasms, and genetic disorders such as Turner syndrome and Fragile X pre-mutation are among other factors that can cause irreversible gonadal damage and seriously decrease future fertility potential [12–14]. Many women with such conditions and whose current circumstance precludes a pregnancy find themselves facing potential childlessness.

IVF and embryo cryopreservation (EC) is the only method of female fertility preservation that is endorsed by the American Society of Clinical Oncology and American Society of Reproductive Medicine. However, conventional IVF and embryo cryopreservation requires 2–5 weeks to complete, produces relatively high estradiol levels, which may be deleterious in certain hormone-sensitive malignancies, and requires a male partner. IVM expands the fertility preservation options for women who are not candidates for IVF-EC for various reasons. Women with hormone-sensitive tumors may undergo immature oocyte collection and cryopreserve resultant embryos. In addition to eliminating the need for expensive drugs and the inconvenience of injections, IVM enables oocyte retrieval at any phase of the menstrual cycle and completion of the fertility preservation procedure in 2–10 days, preventing a delay in treatment of the primary disease [15,16].

We reported three women without male partners seeking fertility preservation prior to chemotherapy, who presented for the first time in the luteal phase of their menstrual cycle and were to undergo gonadotoxic treatment immediately [16]. Five to seven immature oocytes were recovered with luteal phase oocyte retrieval from these patients. Three to five MII oocytes were vitrified following IVM. Two of these three women later underwent one and two more collections, respectively, in the follicular phase of the next cycle(s) and additional immature oocytes were vitrified following IVM.

For patients without a male partner, oocyte cryopreservation represents the least invasive option compared to ovarian tissue cryopreservation. Recent advances in vitrification techniques have markedly improved the efficacy of oocyte cryopreservation [17,18]. In a clinical trial at the McGill Reproductive Centre (MRC) involving 38 infertile women, oocyte vitrification (OV) using the McGill Cryoleaf resulted in a mean cryosurvival rate of 81% post-thawing, a 76% fertilization rate, a clinical pregnancy rate per cycle of 45%, a live birth rate of 40% and 22 healthy babies [19]. We achieved 67.5% cryosurvival, 64.2% fertilization, 20% clinical pregnancy and 20% live birth rates following vitrification of in vitro matured oocytes in the same trial [19]. A novel fertility preservation strategy involves immature oocyte retrieval in an unstimulated menstrual cycle or from ovarian tissue biopsies, followed by IVM and OV or EC [15,20].

Immature oocytes can also be collected from ovarian biopsy specimens and can be vitrified following IVM [20]. This combination of ovarian-tissue cryobanking and IVM represents a new strategy for fertility preservation. We retrieved 11 immature oocytes from a wedge resection specimen in a 16-year-old patient with mosaic Turner syndrome (20% 45,XO and 80% 46,XX karyotype). Eight of these oocytes were vitrified following IVM. In four women with cancer, we harvested 11 immature and 8 mature oocytes from wedge biopsy specimens. Eight of the 11 immature oocytes reached MII stage following IVM and were vitrified [21].

In conclusion, IVM combined with embryo or oocyte vitrification provides previously unavailable options for some patients and improves the services provided by a fertility preservation program. To date, the MRC has provided fertility preservation to more than 180 patients with breast, hematological, brain, soft-tissue, colorectal and gynecological cancers. Primary-care physicians and oncologists should discuss the fertility preservation options early during treatment of their patients and, if desired, refer them to an ART center that offers the full range of fertility preservation options.

Monitoring and management of an IVM cycle

Monitoring starts with a baseline scan performed in the early follicular phase of the menstrual cycle, preferably between days 2 and 5 of a natural menstrual cycle or a withdrawal bleed, induced with progesterone administration in amenorrheic women. The number and size of the antral follicles and endometrial texture and thickness are recorded. The uterus and ovaries are examined for any abnormalities. In a retrospective analysis including the antral follicle count (AFC), ovarian volume and peak ovarian stromal blood flow velocity as independent variables, AFC was found to be the most important predictor of the number of retrievable oocytes [6]. A second scan is performed around cycle day 8 when it is anticipated that the largest follicle has reached 10–12 mm in diameter and the endometrial thickness is at least 6 mm. The presence of a dominant follicle does not require cancellation of the treatment cycle because smaller follicles are found to contain viable oocytes, even in the presence of a dominant follicle. In fact, we have reported that the implantation and clinical pregnancy rates were the highest in cycles where hCG was given when the leading follicle was 12 mm [22].

The role of gonadotropin administration before oocyte collection in IVM cycles is still controversial. Some authors have suggested that a short course of gonadotropin administration can improve the clinical outcome of IVM cycles through increasing developmental competence of immature oocytes and/or the number of in vivo matured oocytes collected in an IVM cycle [23]. However, randomized controlled trials comparing the outcome of gonadotropin-primed IVM cycles with that of IVM cycles without any priming have yielded conflicting results [23–26]. Based on our own experience and the favorable trend observed in trials of hCG priming, we administer hCG at a dose of 10 000 IU 38 hours before immature oocyte collection; however, stimulation with HMG is reserved for patients with an endometrial thickness of less than 6 mm on the day of the second scan [5].

We failed to observe any improvement in laboratory or clinical outcomes with a higher hCG dose of 20 000 IU in a randomized controlled trial [27]. The rationale behind injecting hCG 38 hours before immature oocyte collection is the observation of an increase in the number of in vivo matured oocytes collected, the rate of oocyte maturation in the first 24 hours after collection and the embryo implantation and clinical pregnancy rates when the interval between hCG administration and oocyte collection was extended to 38 hours rather than the traditional 35 hours [28]. Our results suggest that the presence of in vivo matured oocytes can be associated with higher pregnancy rates in hCG-primed IVM cycles [29]. A significantly higher proportion of embryos derived from in vivo matured oocytes attained good morphological characteristics compared with those derived from in vitro matured oocytes in these cycles [29]. Moreover, oocytes that complete in vitro maturation in the first 24 hours after collection seem to have a higher rate of cleavage, and embryos derived from such oocytes have a higher rate of blastocyst formation compared with their counterparts that complete maturation later [30]. Finally, in IVM cycles we observe a trend towards higher chromosomal abnormality rates in embryos derived from oocytes that complete maturation later than 24 hours after collection versus embryos derived from oocytes achieving maturation within the first 24 hours. The incidence of chromosomal abnormality seems to be similar in embryos derived from in vivo matured oocytes or immature oocytes that reach the MII stage within the first 24 hours after collection (unpublished data).

Studies assessing the effect of endometrial thickness on pregnancy rates in IVF cycles have yielded conflicting results, and the predictive value of endometrial thickness on treatment outcome is at best marginal, if there is any at all. However, some reports suggest a significant decrease in pregnancy rates when endometrial thickness is less than 7 mm. Owing to the fact that immature oocyte collection occurs relatively earlier in the menstrual cycle as compared to conventional IVF cycles, the applicability of findings from IVF studies to IVM practice is questionable. This notwithstanding, in a retrospective analysis of 155 unstimulated IVM cycles, we have found mean endometrial thickness to be significantly higher in conception cycles though the absolute difference was only 0.8 mm (10.2 mm versus 9.4 mm in conception and non-conception cycles respectively, $P = 0.04$). More interestingly, a trend analysis demonstrated a significant increase in pregnancy rates in parallel with endometrial thickness (clinical pregnancy rates were 9.4, 15.9, 27.6, and 28% for endometrial thickness of < 8, 8–9.9, 10–11.9, and ≥ 12 mm, respectively, chi-square test for trend, $P = 0.036$) [31].

Sequential exposure to estrogen and progesterone seems to be required for the endometrium to become receptive to embryo implantation. Studies on oocyte donation cycles and frozen thawed embryo transfer cycles have suggested an increase in delivery rates when endometrial exposure to estrogen before progesterone administration was between 11 days and 9 weeks. Given the shorter duration of the proliferative phase in IVM cycles, we initiate estrogen on the day of oocyte collection and postpone progesterone supplementation to the day of fertilization [32]. Initially, we adopted an individualized protocol with estrogen doses of 6 mg and 12 mg per day for women whose endometrial thickness is more or less than

6 mm, respectively. We later adopted an additional strategy of administering 150 IU/day of HMG to women whose endometrial thickness was less than 6 mm on the day of the second scan and whose follicles were still small. The rationale is to boost endogenous estrogen levels while supporting the growth of the follicles in the cohort.

A retrospective comparison of these two strategies in 48 cycles demonstrated a similar increase in mean endometrial thickness with both methods, from 4.5 mm to 7.7 mm and from 4.7 mm to 7.3 mm in HMG and estradiol cycles respectively [33]. However, compared with oral administration of 17β-estradiol, HMG injections were associated with an increase in the number of in vivo matured oocytes collected (cycles with more than one in vivo matured oocyte, 54.5% vs. 34.6%), implantation (15% vs. 8.2%) and pregnancy rates (36.4% vs. 23.1%). The differences were not statistically significant. However, this might be due to the limited sample size of the study as well as the absence of a genuine difference. We prefer HMG injections over oral estradiol for women with a thin endometrium, unless the leading follicle is 10–12 mm, in which case we will start oral estrogen in a dose of 6–12 mg/day instead of HMG so that the size of the leading follicle will not exceed 12 mm by the time the endometrium reaches adequate thickness. The medications are continued until endometrial thickness reaches 8 mm or the leading follicle reaches a mean diameter of 12 mm.

Immature oocyte collection

The basic principles of transvaginal ultrasound-guided oocyte retrieval for IVM are the same as those for IVF oocyte collection. Most patients tolerate the procedure under conscious sedation with intravenous midazolam and fentanyl.

Following vaginal preparation with sterile saline, 1% bupivacain is injected to achieve paracervical block. As the follicles are smaller than follicles aspirated in IVF cycles, we use a smaller-gauge needle (19–20G) with a shorter bevel. Multiple ovarian punctures are often required because the follicles are spread diffusely throughout the ovarian stroma and the collection is more technically demanding. The aspiration pressure is reduced to 75–80 mmHg, lower than the conventional IVF aspiration pressure. This is to avoid the denudation of surrounding granulosa cells, which has been shown to be important to the nuclear maturation process.

Because the fine-bore needle gets blocked frequently with bloodstained aspirate and ovarian stroma, we flush the needle lumen with heparinized saline between punctures.

Embryology laboratory procedures

The follicular aspirate is first examined under a stereomicroscope to identify cumulus-oocyte complexes (COC). Identification of small immature oocytes surrounded by fewer granulosa cells is more difficult compared to mature oocytes collected in an IVF cycle and they can be overlooked. Therefore, the follicular aspirate is filtered through a nylon mesh strainer with 70-μm pores after removal of initially identified COCs. The filtered aspirate can be reexamined after washing with HEPES buffered human serum albumin-containing medium. Maturation status of the oocytes is assessed immediately after collection. Oocytes reaching the MII stage on the day of collection are denuded and fertilized together with any in vivo matured oocytes, while immature oocytes are cultured in IVM medium and periodically assessed for maturation status. They are denuded and fertilized upon completion of nuclear maturation.

Although similar implantation and pregnancy rates have been reported following fertilization of in vitro matured oocytes with intracytoplasmic sperm injection (ICSI) or IVF, ICSI has been commonly practiced in IVM cycles due to a theoretical risk of zonal hardening during the in vitro culture period. In fact, fertilization rates with ICSI were shown to be higher than with IVF in the same study (84.1% vs. 56.3%) [34]. Another reason for preferring ICSI over IVF in IVM cycles is some immature oocytes having been denuded for assessment of polar-body extrusion. Oocytes devoid of cumulus cells may have decreased chemotactic potential for sperm in the medium. We routinely perform ICSI at 2–4 hours after polar-body extrusion. Culture conditions for fertilized oocytes and cleavage-stage embryos derived from in vitro matured oocytes are the same as those in IVF cycles.

Embryo transfer

The timing of embryo transfer and the number of embryos to be transferred are determined based upon the number and quality of available embryos. Growth and quality of available embryos are evaluated with respect to fertilization time of each embryo. Embryo transfer is commonly performed on the third day after oocyte collection. In general, embryo implantation rates in IVM cycles are lower than in IVF cycles. Therefore, on average, 1–2 more embryos are transferred in order to maintain similar pregnancy rates without increased multiple pregnancy rates [35].

High implantation and pregnancy rates have been achieved by performing blastocyst transfers in selected IVM patients [36]. A clinical pregnancy rate of 51.9% and an implantation rate of 26.8% have been reported with blastocyst transfer in patients with > 7 zygotes and > 3 good-quality embryos on the third day post-fertilization in IVM cycles [36]. Assisted hatching is routinely employed before embryo transfer in our IVM program due to the above-mentioned concerns about zonal hardening.

Luteal phase support

As mentioned previously, the luteal phase support protocol employed in our IVM program includes 50 mg/day i.m. progesterone injections and 6 mg/day estradiol valerate p.o. in three divided doses. Luteal phase support is continued until completion of the first trimester for pregnant patients.

IVM treatment outcome

Pregnancy rates

Age of the woman and the number of oocytes collected are the two most important determinants of pregnancy following an IVM cycle. Young women with PCO are the best candidates for IVM treatment. In 2009, we achieved an embryo implantation rate of 19.5% and a clinical pregnancy rate per embryo transfer (CPR) of 55.2% in women with PCO or PCOS with an average age of 32.6 ± 3.6 years. Successful results have been reported by other centers around the world. Pregnancy rates seem to be significantly higher when an in vivo matured oocyte has been collected.

Pregnancy loss

In a retrospective analysis of 1581 women who had a positive pregnancy test following ART with IVM, IVF or ICSI in our unit during a five-year period, we found biochemical pregnancy loss rates to be similar among these patients (17.5% for IVM pregnancies, 17% for IVF, and 18% for ICSI pregnancies, $P = 0.08$). However, the clinical miscarriage rate was significantly higher in IVM pregnancies (25.3%) than in IVF (15.7%) and ICSI (12.6%) pregnancies ($P < 0.01$) [37]. It is known that women with PCOS have higher miscarriage rates, regardless of the method of conception. Miscarriage rates reaching 25% after ovulation induction, and ranging from 25 to 37% following IVF, have been reported in such women. Therefore, the higher miscarriage rate observed in the IVM group can be explained by the higher incidence of PCOS in these patients. Indeed, while only 8% and < 1% of women in the IVF and ICSI groups had PCOS, respectively, the incidence of PCOS in the IVM group was 80%. Importantly, miscarriage rates were not different between IVM and IVF pregnancies among women with PCOS, 24.5% versus 22.8%, respectively [37].

Obstetric outcome

We further analyzed obstetric outcomes of pregnancies following ART and compared them with those of spontaneous conceptions [35]. The study population consisted of all pregnancies delivered at the McGill University Health Centre after ARTs (namely, IVM, IVF, or ICSI) with a birth weight of at least 500 g at the time of confinement, from January 1, 1998, to December 31, 2003. IVM pregnancies constituted 15.9% of 344 ART pregnancies during the study period. The reason for the relatively low number of ART deliveries is that many women who conceived with ART at the MRC delivered at other hospitals in Québec or outside the province. Therefore, inclusion of these externally delivered cases and reporting all conceptions was impossible.

The incidences of twin and high-order multiple pregnancies were not different among IVM (21% and 5%), IVF (20% and 3%), and ICSI (17% and 3%) pregnancies. The incidence of cesarean delivery was similar among singleton pregnancies conceived with different treatments (IVM 39%, IVF 36%, and ICSI 36%). Likewise, the mean birth weights of all infants conceived with ART were similar among all ART groups. The proportion of low birth weight and very low birth weight infants was similar across ART children. Apgar scores at 1 and 5 minutes, the proportion of infants with an Apgar score ≤ 6 at 1 and 5 minutes, and the incidence of acidosis were all similar among IVM, IVF, ICSI, and spontaneous-conception deliveries. Our figures compare favorably with results reported by other IVM programs, supporting our conclusions.

Congenital abnormalities, physical and neuromotor development

Currently available data suggest an increase in the prevalence of major congenital malformations, chromosomal anomalies, and imprinting disorders in children born following ART. However, whether infertility per se or treatment of it is the reason for higher incidence is controversial. In our series of 55 IVM newborns, there were only two major congenital abnormalities; one case of ventriculoseptal defect and one of omphalocele [35]. There were nine major congenital abnormalities (two hydronephroses, one Fallot's tetralogy, one single ventricle, two atrio-septal defects, one hydrocephaly and intraventricular hemorrhage, and two trisomies) and 14 minor abnormalities among 350 infants born to the 344 age- and parity-matched spontaneously conceived controls. Compared with spontaneous conceptions, the observed odds ratios (ORs) for any congenital abnormality were 1.42 (95% confidence interval [CI] 0.52–3.91) for IVM, 1.21 (95% CI 0.63–2.32) for IVF and 1.69 (95% CI 0.88–3.26) for ICSI, respectively. None of these was statistically significant [35]. Interestingly, the odds ratio was lower for IVM than for ICSI, even though ICSI was used for all IVM cases. This can be regarded as indirect evidence of the reported high congenital abnormality rate with ICSI being due to poor sperm per se, because ICSI with normal sperm did not increase the odds of congenital abnormality to the same extent.

In a study involving 21 children conceived through IVM, the chromosomal constitution and mental development of children were compared with those of spontaneously conceived children [38]. All of the IVM children were found to have normal karyotype and mean developmental index score, similar to controls in this small-sized study. Another study of 46 IVM babies reported similar findings [39]. In the latter study, the neuro-psychological development of children was assessed until 24 months and was found to be within population standards. The physical growth of IVM children also appears to be similar to that of spontaneously conceived children [38,39]. Currently available data seem reassuring and do not suggest an increased risk of congenital malformations, physical or neurological developmental delay in IVM children.

Conclusions

IVM is a relatively new technology and clinical experience with this technique is limited compared to conventional IVF. Despite the achievement of satisfactory results in selected patient groups, overall embryo implantation and pregnancy rates are still lower than those achieved with IVF. However, IVM should not be regarded as a competitor of IVF, but rather a complementary assisted reproductive technology that provides unique opportunities. Patients who are at high risk of OHSS, those with unexpectedly hyper- or poor responses during controlled ovarian hyperstimulation, those with recurrent unexplained IVF failures, as well as those who are facing imminent gonadotoxic chemotherapy can benefit from the advantages of IVM.

Essentially, all ART laboratory procedures can be performed with in vitro matured oocytes if the need arises. The first successful IVM cycles combined with preimplantation genetic screening and percutaneous testicular sperm aspiration have already been reported by our team [40,41]. IVM has enabled successful treatment of patients with empty follicle syndrome in previous stimulated IVF cycles [42]. Patients can undergo several IVM cycles and we previously reported a series of patients who achieved repeated live births with IVM treatment [43].

Currently, IVM represents the least invasive and the simplest option for ART patients, and with further improvement in success rates, it can become the "ultimate" patient-friendly protocol that has been sought for in this era of patient-friendly milder assisted reproductive treatments.

References

1. Tan SL, Royston P, Campbell S, *et al.* Cumulative conception and livebirth rates after in-vitro fertilisation. *Lancet* 1992; **339**: 1390–4.

2. MacDougall MJ, Tan SL, Balen A, Jacobs HS. A controlled study comparing patients with and without polycystic ovaries undergoing in-vitro fertilization. *Hum Reprod* 1993; **8**: 233–7.

3. Cha KY, Koo JJ, Ko JJ, *et al.* Pregnancy after in vitro fertilization of human follicular oocytes collected from nonstimulated cycles, their culture in vitro and their transfer in a donor oocyte program. *Fertil Steril* 1991; **55**: 109–13.

4. Chian RC, Gülekli B, Buckett WM, Tan SL. Priming with human chorionic

gonadotropin before retrieval of immature oocytes in women with infertility due to the polycystic ovary syndrome. *N Engl J Med* 1999: **18**: 1624–6.

5. Chian RC, Buckett WM, Tulandi T, Tan SL. Prospective randomized study of human chorionic gonadotrophin priming before immature oocyte retrieval from unstimulated women with polycystic ovarian syndrome. *Hum Reprod* 2000; **15**: 165–70.

6. Tan SL, Child TJ, Gulekli B. In vitro maturation and fertilization of oocytes from unstimulated ovaries: predicting the number of immature oocytes retrieved by early follicular phase ultrasonography. *Am J Obstet Gynecol* 2002; **186**: 684–9.

7. Lim KS, Yoon SH, Lim JH. IVM as an alternative for over-responders. In Tan SL, Chian RC, Buckett W, eds. *In-Vitro Maturation of Human Oocytes: Basic Science to Clinical Application*. London: Informa Healthcare, 2007.

8. Liu J, Lu G, Qian Y, Mao Y, Ding W. Pregnancies and births achieved from in vitro matured oocytes retrieved from poor responders undergoing stimulation in in vitro fertilization cycles. *Fertil Steril* 2003; **80**: 447–9.

9. Liu J, Lim JH, Chian RC. IVM as an alternative for poor responders. In Tan SL, Chian RC, Buckett W, eds. *In-Vitro Maturation of Human Oocytes: Basic Science to Clinical Application*. London: Informa Healthcare, 2007; 333–44.

10. Child TJ, Gulekli B, Chian RC, Abdul-Jalil AK, Tan SL. In-vitro maturation (IVM) of oocytes from unstimulated normal ovaries of women with a previous poor response to IVF. *Fertil Steril* 2000; **74**: S45.

11. Holzer H, Scharf E, Chian RC, *et al.* In vitro maturation of oocytes collected from unstimulated ovaries for oocyte donation. *Fertil Steril* 2007; **88**: 62–7.

12. Elizur SE, Chian RC, Holzer HE, *et al.* Cryopreservation of oocytes in a young woman with severe and symptomatic endometriosis: a new indication for fertility preservation. *Fertil Steril* 2009; **91**: 293 e1–3.

13. Huang JY, Buckett WM, Gilbert L, Tan SL, Chian RC. Retrieval of immature oocytes followed by in vitro maturation and vitrification: a case report on a new strategy of fertility preservation in women with borderline ovarian malignancy. *Gynecol Oncol* 2007; **105**: 542–4.

14. Lau NM, Huang JY, MacDonald S, *et al.* Feasibility of fertility preservation in young females with Turner syndrome. *Reprod Biomed Online* 2009; **18**: 290–5.

15. Rao GD, Chian RC, Son WS, Gilbert L, Tan SL. Fertility preservation in women undergoing cancer treatment. *Lancet* 2004; **363**: 1829–30.

16. Demirtas E, Elizur SE, Holzer H, *et al.* Immature oocyte retrieval in the luteal phase to preserve fertility in cancer patients. *Reprod Biomed Online* 2008; **17**: 520–3.

17. Huang JY, Chen HY, Tan SL, Chian RC. Effect of choline-supplemented sodium-depleted slow freezing versus vitrification on mouse oocyte meiotic spindles and chromosome abnormalities. *Fertil Steril* 2007; **88**: 1093–100.

18. Huang JY, Chen HY, Park JY, Tan SL, Chian RC. Comparison of spindle and chromosome configuration in in vitro- and in vivo-matured mouse oocytes after vitrification. *Fertil Steril* 2008; **90**: 1424–32.

19. Chian RC, Huang JY, Gilbert L, *et al.* Obstetric outcomes following vitrification of in vitro and in vivo matured oocytes. *Fertil Steril* 2009; **91**: 2391–8.

20. Huang JY, Tulandi T, Holzer H, Tan SL, Chian RC. Combining ovarian tissue cryobanking with retrieval of immature oocytes followed by in vitro maturation and vitrification: an additional strategy of fertility preservation. *Fertil Steril* 2008; **89**: 567–72.

21. Huang JY, Tulandi T, Holzer H, *et al.* Cryopreservation of ovarian tissue and in vitro matured oocytes in a female with mosaic Turner syndrome: case report. *Hum Reprod* 2008; **23**: 336–9.

22. Son WY, Chung JT, Herrero B, *et al.* Selection of the optimal day for oocyte retrieval based on the diameter of the

dominant follicle in hCG-primed in vitro maturation cycles. *Hum Reprod* 2008; **23**: 2680–5.

23. Son WY, Yoon SH, Lim JH. Effect of gonadotrophin priming on in-vitro maturation of oocytes collected from women at risk of OHSS. *Reprod Biomed Online* 2006; **13**: 340–8.

24. Fadini R, Dal Canto MB, Mignini Renzini M, *et al.* Effect of different gonadotrophin priming on IVM of oocytes from women with normal ovaries: a prospective randomized study. *Reprod Biomed Online* 2009; **19**: 343–51.

25. Mikkelsen AL, Smith SD, Lindenberg S. In-vitro maturation of human oocytes from regularly menstruating women may be successful without follicle stimulating hormone priming. *Hum Reprod* 1999; **14**: 1847–51.

26. Mikkelsen AL, Lindenberg S. Benefit of FSH priming of women with PCOS to the in vitro maturation procedure and the outcome: a randomized prospective study. *Reproduction* 2001; **122**: 587–92.

27. Gulekli B, Buckett WM, Chian RC, *et al.* Randomized, controlled trial of priming with 10,000 IU versus 20,000 IU of human chorionic gonadotropin in women with polycystic ovary syndrome who are undergoing in vitro maturation. *Fertil Steril* 2004; **82**: 1458–9.

28. Son WY, Chung JT, Chian RC, *et al.* A 38 h interval between hCG priming and oocyte retrieval increases in vivo and in vitro oocyte maturation rate in programmed IVM cycles. *Hum Reprod* 2008; **23**: 2010–6.

29. Son WY, Chung JT, Demirtas E, *et al.* Comparison of in-vitro maturation cycles with and without in-vivo matured oocytes retrieved. *Reprod Biomed Online* 2008; **17**: 59–67.

30. Son WY, Lee SY, Lim JH. Fertilization, cleavage and blastocyst development according to the maturation timing of oocytes in in vitro maturation cycles. *Hum Reprod* 2005; **20**: 3204–7.

31. Child TJ, Gulekli B, Sylvestre C, Tan SL. Ultrasonographic assessment of endometrial receptivity at embryo transfer in an in vitro maturation of oocyte program. *Fertil Steril* 2003; **79**: 656–8.

32. Child TJ, Abdul-Jalil AK, Gulekli B, Tan SL. In vitro maturation and fertilization of oocytes from unstimulated normal ovaries, polycystic ovaries, and women with polycystic ovary syndrome. *Fertil Steril* 2001; **76**: 936–42.

33. Elizur SE, Son WY, Yap R, *et al.* Comparison of low-dose human menopausal gonadotropin and micronized 17beta-estradiol supplementation in in vitro maturation cycles with thin endometrial lining. *Fertil Steril* 2009; **92**: 907–12.

34. Soderstrom-Anttila V, Makinen S, Tuuri T, Suikkari AM. Favourable pregnancy results with insemination of in vitro matured oocytes from unstimulated patients. *Hum Reprod* 2005; **20**: 1534–40.

35. Buckett WM, Chian RC, Holzer H, *et al.* Obstetric outcomes and congenital abnormalities after in vitro maturation, in vitro fertilization, and intracytoplasmic sperm injection. *Obstet Gynecol* 2007; **110**: 885–91.

36. Son WY, Lee SY, Yoon SH, Lim JH. Pregnancies and deliveries after transfer of human blastocysts derived from in vitro matured oocytes in in vitro maturation cycles. *Fertil Steril* 2007; **87**: 1491–3.

37. Buckett WM, Chian RC, Dean NL, *et al.* Pregnancy loss in pregnancies conceived after in vitro oocyte maturation, conventional in vitro fertilization, and intracytoplasmic sperm injection. *Fertil Steril* 2008; **90**: 546–50.

38. Shu-Chi M, Jiann-Loung H, Yu-Hung L, *et al.* Growth and development of children conceived by in-vitro maturation of human oocytes. *Early Hum Dev* 2006; **82**: 677–82.

39. Soderstrom-Anttila V, Salokorpi T, Pihlaja M, Serenius-Sirve S, Suikkari AM. Obstetric and perinatal outcome and preliminary results of development of children born after in vitro maturation of oocytes. *Hum Reprod* 2006; **21**: 1508–13.

40. Ao A, Jin S, Rao D, *et al.* First successful pregnancy outcome after preimplantation genetic diagnosis for aneuploidy screening in embryos generated from natural-cycle in vitro fertilization combined with an in vitro maturation procedure. *Fertil Steril* 2006; **85**: 1510 e9–11.

41. Abdul-Jalil AK, Child TJ, Phillips S, *et al.* Ongoing twin pregnancy after ICSI of PESA-retrieved spermatozoa into in-vitro matured oocytes: case report. *Hum Reprod* 2001; **16**: 1424–6.

42. Hourvitz A, Maman E, Brengauz M, Machtinger R, Dor J. In vitro maturation for patients with repeated in vitro fertilization failure due to "oocyte maturation abnormalities". *Fertil Steril* 2010; **94**: 496–501.

43. Al-Sunaidi M, Tulandi T, Holzer H, *et al.* Repeated pregnancies and live births after in vitro maturation treatment. *Fertil Steril* 2007; **87**: 1212 e9–12.

Chapter 3

The use of donor insemination

Vanessa J. Kay and Christopher L. R. Barratt

Introduction

Insemination using donated sperm is one of the oldest infertility treatments known, with pregnancies being recorded apparently as far back as the eighteenth century [1]. Advances in sperm storage and cryopreservation techniques resulted in the first human pregnancy from cryopreserved semen in 1953 [2]. Until the 1970s fresh semen was often used, producing superior pregnancy rates compared with cryopreserved semen. After it was shown that HIV could be transmitted via donor insemination (DI) [3], a mandatory quarantine with 6 months cryopreservation of semen was introduced in order to prevent the transmission of sexually transmitted diseases.

Over the last two decades there has been a substantial decline in the use of donor sperm [4]. This was mainly due to the introduction of an alternative treatment for male infertility in 1992, i.e. intracytoplasmic sperm injection (ICSI). Once ICSI was shown to be an effective treatment most couples preferred to use their own sperm, rather than undergo the less invasive treatment using donor sperm. This was motivated by the strong urge to be genetically related to offspring [5]. The dramatic rise in the use of ICSI is paralleled by a decline in DI in the UK (Figure 13.1), a trend seen throughout the world [6]. Significant changes in regulatory framework introduced in a number of countries, including removal of donor anonymity and changes in guidelines for re-imbursement of expenses for gamete donors, are also likely to have contributed to the decline in DI.

Against this background, DI remains a very important treatment option with acceptable pregnancy rates. In a large recent study of DI the delivery rate was 14% per treatment cycle with a cumulative delivery rate of 77% after 12 cycles [7]. In order to optimize pregnancy rates with DI, careful consideration should be given to various aspects of this service, including the recruitment and screening of sperm donors, cryopreservation of semen, and the screening and management of recipients. The purpose of this chapter is to examine these important aspects of treatment to enable the reader to consider how to optimize DI services in the future.

Clinical indications for DI

Treatment using DI was initially designed to treat male factor infertility. However, DI remains a therapeutic option for male factor infertility when either too few or no sperm are obtained at surgical sperm aspiration. But, DI can also be considered when ICSI treatment has failed or in couples who for various reasons decide against ICSI, e.g. cost

The Subfertility Handbook: A Clinician's Guide, Second Edition ed. Gab Kovacs. Published by Cambridge University Press. © Cambridge University Press 2011.

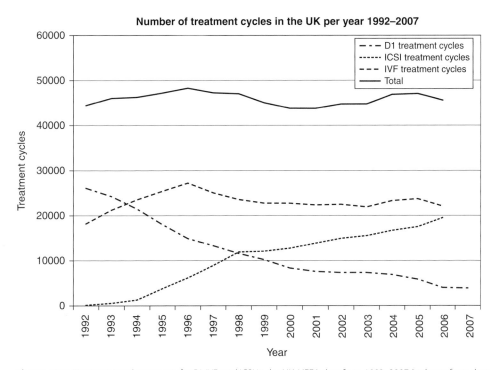

Figure 13.1 Treatment cycles per year for DI, IVF, and ICSI in the UK. HFEA data from 1992–2007 (redrawn from data available in reference 4 and www.hfea.gov.uk).

implications, ICSI treatment not available, ethical considerations regarding creation of embryos, and/or concerns regarding risks of ICSI treatment.

More recently, changes in social attitudes towards the use of donor sperm have resulted in more single and lesbian women being offered treatment. Whilst in 1979 only 9.5% of American physicians would have treated an unmarried woman with DI, by 1990 the figure had risen to 35% [8]. In the UK a similar trend is noted, with an increase in the proportion of lesbian and single women being offered DI treatment: from 18% in 1999 to 38% in 2006 [9]. Such is the degree of change in attitude that lesbian and single women are the commonest indication for DI treatment in some countries: e.g. in Belgian women undergoing DI 55% consist of lesbian couples, followed by single women (23%), with male infertility making up the remaining 22% [7]. Although there appears to be widespread acceptance by society of single parents and lesbian couples, there remains contention in many countries whether women without a male partner should have the same rights to treatment as couples. In the UK there has recently been a change in the regulation that no longer requires taking into account the need for a father when considering the welfare of the child. However, currently DI is not routinely available on the NHS for this indication, creating the possibility of being accused of discrimination and leading to potential court cases under rights laws if single or lesbian women are denied their right to motherhood.

There are a variety of other indications for DI, including infectious disease in the male partner, risk of genetic disorder transmission and severe rhesus isoimmunization. These conditions are now less frequent indications for DI due to modern advances, e.g. effective sperm washing for HIV in discordant couples, preimplantation genetic diagnosis for many genetic disorders, and improvements in perinatal medicine for severe rhesus disease. With the ongoing development and establishment of new techniques further changes in indication for DI are to be expected in the future.

Regulatory framework for recruitment of sperm donors

Due to a number of changes in regulatory framework, it has become increasingly difficult to recruit the ideal sperm donor due to a decreasing number of men being willing to donate. This is exemplified by the clear trend in removal of anonymity of semen donors – first initiated in Sweden in 1985. In Holland removal of anonymity initially reduced the number of sperm donors and hence restricted the possibility of DI treatment [10]. Certainly in the UK, in the lead-up period to the change in legislation a number of clinics reported a considerable shortage of sperm donors [11]. However, there are some reassuring data suggesting that with an appropriate donor recruitment strategy, this decline in sperm donors will be temporary [11]; data from the UK suggest a 6% increase in the number of men now registering as sperm donors [4]. Despite this, there are still considerable difficulties in obtaining donated sperm in many UK clinics [12] and this may be partly related to changes in the attitudes of sperm donors following the removal of anonymity, such as anecdotal evidence that more non-anonymous donors are only willing to donate to one recipient.

An important factor shown to strongly influence the recruitment of sperm donors is the use of financial incentives. Regulations vary across different countries, with an increasing number of countries restricting the financial incentive. For example in the UK, a nationwide report (the SEED review 2005 [13]) concluded that in addition to expenses, donors could be compensated for loss of earnings of up to £55.19 per day (maximum £250 for each course of sperm donation – although "course" was not rigorously defined). An inequality in financial incentives has resulted in an expanding market in commercial sperm banks in certain countries, with, in extreme cases, package holiday deals being available. In 2008 in the UK 15% of donor sperm used were imported [4].

Although the SEED review [13] concluded that financial reasons should not be the primary motivation for donation and thus financial benefits should be restricted, it can be argued that the removal of anonymity should be linked to an increased payment to compensate donors for having to provide this identifying information.

Another issue that influences the availability of donated semen is the limit on the number of families that a donor is allowed to father. The limit varies in different parts of the EU and appears to be set entirely arbitrarily; e.g. in France the limit is 5, whilst in Holland it is 25. There are persuasive arguments why this should be higher than the currently recommended UK limit of 10, including the low genetic risk of inadvertent consanguinity with the shift from anonymous to open-identity donation [14]. A review of these guidelines is planned by the Human Fertilization and Embryo Authority (HFEA) in 2010/2011 in light of recruitment difficulties.

Screening of sperm donors

The characteristics of the sperm donor are crucial to the success of a DI program. Therefore any recruitment program should aim to recruit the optimal donor. There is, however, difficulty in defining the characteristics of the best donor and this has to be balanced against the limited number of sperm donors currently available due to the above-mentioned recruitment difficulties within the current regulatory framework. National guidelines now exist for screening potential sperm donors, for medical, social, and genetic characteristics, and for blood-borne viruses and sexually transmitted disease [15]. However, there remains controversy over two key issues.

What should be the minimal quality of semen?

There is a plethora of data showing that semen quality is critical for success in DI, e.g. data from CECOS show that the mean fecundity is doubled if the number of motile sperm per straw (insemination) is increased from below 5 to over 10 million motile cells [16]. The process of cryopreservation of sperm and subsequent thawing for use is known to cause a significant loss of sperm motility and viability. In view of the reduced fertilizing potential of cryopreserved sperm, it is important to select only donors who have high-quality semen. Therefore as a minimum we should be within WHO guidelines for normal semen [17] but in order to improve DI success rates it may be reasonable to only utilize sperm from the top 20% of samples. Unfortunately, the use of additional sperm function tests has not resulted in the selection of higher-quality donors and thus we are still dependent on traditional semen parameters.

What should be the age limit?

Unlike women, the age threshold for infertility in men is less clear. There is evidence showing that older men have reduced semen quality [18] and some data showing an increased risk of abnormalities in offspring, such as autism [19]. Debate continues regarding the age limit for sperm donors. Current HFEA guidance recommends that the upper age limit for sperm donors should be 45 years [4]. By contrast a report from the British Fertility Society in 2008 [12] suggested that consideration be given to increasing the maximum age limit to 50 years. This report was released before the joint professional guidelines on screening were published, which recommend an upper sperm donor age limit of 40 [15]. In order to optimize success rates some sperm banks have an even lower age limit to below 35 years, similar to that suggested for oocyte donation.

Donor insemination service model

Whilst recruiting semen donors is challenging, time-consuming and difficult, it has always been so [20]. There is a very high attrition rate throughout the recruitment, screening, and selection process. Often, fewer than 5% of men who enquire about being a semen donor actually end up being accepted [21].

In order to provide an efficient donor recruitment service, a number of stages are required, which can be carried out in various ways. Attrition of donors has been shown to occur throughout this process, with rejection of semen analysis being the main culprit [11] (Table 13.1). This may be minimized by targeting specific groups who are likely to be fertile and may well consider donation, e.g. partners at antenatal clinics, students, sporting events, students, family planning clinics, pre-vasectomy clinics, and men already donating to sperm research projects. A significant proportion of donors are also lost between first contact and submission of semen sample. In order to minimize this high attrition rate the service should be centered on the donors' convenience, e.g. prompt answering of telephone enquiries, convenient location and opening times of the semen laboratory.

Table 13.1 Attrition of donors

	Number (% of potential donors)	Attrition (% of total applicants still in program)
Applicants	1101 (100.0)	
Rejected at initial phone call	87 (7.9)	92.1
Defaulted semen analysis	308 (28.0)	64.1
Rejected semen analysis	595 (54.5)	10.1
Released donors	40 (3.6)	3.6

Adapted from Paul *et al.*, [11].

Within the current regulatory framework donor recruitment can be encouraged by "payment in kind". This is when a donor is offered an incentive to donate, e.g. in exchange for becoming a sperm donor he is offered a reduced cost of pre-vasectomy sperm cryopreservation or IVF treatment (also known as sperm sharing).

The development of a national recruitment infrastructure has been recommended by the British Fertility Society in order to improve the current supply of sperm donors in the UK [12]. A hub-and-spoke model was proposed, in which a number of larger centers would take responsibility for the management and coordination of donated samples and the smaller units would only undertake some stages of the processing and handling of donated samples and providing treatment. A pilot scheme funded by the Department of Health has been approved at St Mary's Hospital, Manchester, UK, to explore this model of a national sperm donation program.

Cryopreservation of semen

Cryopreservation of semen undoubtedly reduces the success rates of DI. Historical controls provide ample evidence that, in comparable doses, cryopreserved semen produces fewer pregnancies (52% cumulative pregnancy rate vs. 83% cumulative pregnancy rate, cryopreserved vs. fresh semen respectively) [22]. However, as a result of the need to screen donors for HIV there is an absolute necessity to use cryopreserved semen. Since the original methods of vapor freezing with glycerol, there have been many improvements in cryopreservation regimes which significantly enhance the preservation of the functional ability of cryopreserved cells. However, in a number of national situations the success rates have not improved significantly above 10% per cycle. This is disappointing especially when such success rates were being achieved using intracervical insemination with cryopreserved semen in the 1970s. With our enhanced knowledge base, we should be able to routinely achieve >15% live birth rates per cycle.

Screening of recipients

Clearly, an important factor affecting the success of DI is the fertility of the female partner. Female fertility is influenced in many ways. It is well established that the age at which women decide to start a family is increasing, e.g. the mean age of childbearing has increased in England and Wales from 26.4 years in 1978 to 28.9 years by 1998 (see statistics from UK government) [23]. Female age is known to be an important prognostic factor in all fertility treatments. Pregnancy rates with DI are known to decrease with age, especially once a woman is over the age of 40 years (overall pregnancy rate < 35 years is 18.5% and > 40 years is 5.4%) [24]. More recently, De Brucker et al. (2009) confirmed that cumulative pregnancy rates after 12 cycles decreased with increasing age, from 87% at 20–29 years, to 52% at 40–45 years [7]. They concluded that women up to the age of 42 years had acceptable delivery rates and should be encouraged to pursue treatment.

Another issue that adversely affects female fertility is obesity, which has been increasing by 10–40% in Europe in the last 10 years (see data from International Obesity Taskforce) [25]. Women who are overweight are more likely to be infertile and have lower success rates with all fertility treatments, including assisted conception [26]. Whilst it is known that obesity causes infertility due to anovulation, there is increasing evidence that even when anovulation has been excluded, obesity affects the chance of spontaneous pregnancy, with a linear decrease in pregnancy once body mass index is over $29\,kg/m^2$ [27]. This is of particular relevance in DI, when ovulatory dysfunction should be excluded or corrected with appropriate treatment before commencing DI. There is little doubt that success with DI can be improved by rationing access to treatment by female age and weight. However, there remains contention as to the precise criteria at which these restrictions should apply.

The rate of pelvic infection with Chlamydia is known to be rising rapidly, with an increase of 61% in UK clinics from 1996 to 1999 and being highest in women under age of 20 years [28]. It is well established that C. trachomatis, even when asymptomatic, causes pelvic inflammatory disease leading to tubal infertility [29]. Tubal disease will decrease pregnancy rates from DI [30]. Moreover, with the advancing age of recipients, other pelvic pathologies that reduce fertility will become increasingly common, such as endometriosis and uterine fibroids.

Previous studies have reported that asymptomatic ovulatory women with no history of pelvic disease have only a low incidence of abnormal findings at hysterosalpingiography (HSG) (2.8%) [31]. Moreover, the probability of finding pelvic pathology was only 1.8% in a study of couples with severe male factor infertility willing to undergo ICSI [32]. It has been established in DI recipients that pelvic pathology is less common in women whose partners are azoospermic compared with those with oligoasthenoteratozoospermic parthers [33]. A likely explanation is that in men with poor semen quality there are more likely to be coexisting female factors, as the highly fertile women have already conceived spontaneously.

Given this low rate of pelvic disease, it has been advised that tubal assessment should only be performed in women with a history suggestive of tubal damage or after three unsuccessful treatment cycles [34]. However, in view of the increasing prevalence of chlamydia infection, the rising maternal age and the shortage of donor sperm, it may be reasonable to consider offering tubal assessment prior to DI treatment.

Another issue to consider is the optimal method to assess for pelvic pathology. Laparoscopy and HSG are currently the two most widely used methods. Laparoscopy is more invasive, but has been shown to detect more pelvic pathology and, if required, treatment can be performed during the procedure. In women undergoing intrauterine insemination (IUI) with a normal HSG, laparoscopy identified severe pelvic disease in 4% that resulted in change of treatment to IVF or open surgery. A further 21% had less severe pelvic disease (endometriosis and adhesions), which was treated laparoscopically followed by intrauterine insemination [35]. However, prospective studies are required to evaluate the cost-effectiveness, and whether the changes that result from laparoscopy improve pregnancy rates. In NICE Guidelines it has been recommended that HSG is used to screen for tubal disease and laparoscopy is reserved for women with a history or clinical findings suggestive of pelvic disease [34].

Management of recipients

Optimal timing and site of insemination – unresolved issues?

In spite of improvements in cryopreservation methods, spermatozoa survival in a functional state in the female reproductive tract will be reduced. As such, it is important to inseminate the spermatozoa in the preovulatory period to account for the limited (reduced) fertile window of the cryopreserved spermatozoon. A variety of papers have discussed the "best" methods to do this: basal body temperature, ultrasound follicle tracking, luteinising hormone dipsticks, etc.; but accurate timing of inseminations, taking into account the considerable variations between and within patients in ovulatory patterns, is absolutely necessary.

Perhaps because of the reduced fertilizing potential of cryopreserved sperm, a number of authors have suggested that two inseminations per treatment cycle are necessary. The evidence to support the use of two rather than one well-timed insemination remains inconsistent and thus, in view of the potential shortage of semen, one well-timed insemination with high-quality semen should be sufficient.

The main method of insemination of CECOS is intracervical [36] with intrauterine insemination (IUI) being used following unsuccessful intracervical insemination – for example after 12 failed cycles. However, the trend in the USA and now in the UK is for first-line treatment using IUI [37] often using IUI-ready preparations. It is difficult to assess whether IUI is really necessary as a first choice as often when studies have compared the use of IUI with intracervical inseminations the conception rates in the latter have been very poor compared to normal practice [38]. However, a recent Cochrane review of DI cycles where ovarian stimulation was used supported the use of IUI rather than cervical insemination [39].

How long should we treat?

Traditionally the approach has been to routinely treat for 6 or 12 cycles. Recently, however, perhaps with the trend to more individual patient management and increases in patients' expectations, the approach has been to treat for shorter periods in the belief that success rates would decline significantly as the number of cycles increased. However, a recent large study has shown that continual treatment is justifiable. In a group of 928 deliveries there was an overall expected cumulative delivery of 77% after 12 cycles [7]. This encourages the treatment (where appropriate) of patients for up to 12 months.

Future development and conclusions

With the advent of ICSI many assumed that DI would become a very limited treatment. Although the numbers of cycles have reduced considerably there has been an increasing trend for DI to be used for other groups of patients such as single women and lesbians. Unfortunately the changes in regulation etc. have restricted the availability of donor semen which has in a number of countries limited treatment. It is anticipated that with time this will be addressed and the number of DI cycles is likely to increase from its current low base.

Unfortunately there has not been the emphasis on clinical research with DI in the last 20 years so simple questions such as optimal timing of inseminations and number of insemination have yet to be fully resolved. Hopefully with the increased number of cycles and the limitations in supply of donor semen removed such simple questions can easily be addressed.

Acknowledgements

Work in the authors' laboratories is supported by Scottish Enterprise, TENOVUS, The Wellcome Trust and NHS Tayside. The authors are grateful to all members of the research group and IVF unit for their support and help in the production of this manuscript.

References

1. Magyar LA. History of artificial insemination. *Ther Hung* 1991; **39**: 151–3.

2. Bunge RG, Keettel WC, Sherman JK. Clinical use of frozen semen: report of four cases. *Fertil Steril* 1954; **5**: 520–9.

3. Stewart GJ, Tyler JP, Cunningham AL, *et al.* Transmission of human T-cell lymphotropic virus type III (HTLV-III) by artificial insemination by donor. *Lancet* 1985; **14**: 581–5.

4. www.hfea.gov.uk.

5. Schover LR, Thomas AJ, Miller KF, *et al.* Preferences for intracytoplasmic sperm injection versus donor insemination in severe male factor infertility: a preliminary report. *Hum Reprod* 1996; **11**: 2461–4.

6. Nyboe Andersen A, Carlsen E, Loft A. Trends in the use of intracytoplasmatic sperm injection marked variability between countries. *Hum Reprod Update* 2008; **14**: 593–604.

7. De Brucker M, Haentjens P, Evenepoel J, *et al.* Cumulative delivery rates in different age groups after artificial insemination with donor sperm. *Hum Reprod* 2009; **24**(8): 1891–9.

8. Shapiro S, Saphire DG, Stone WH. Changes in American AID practice during the past decade. *Int J Fertil* 1990; **35**: 284–91.

9. Human Fertilisation and Embryo Authority. A long term analysis of the HFEA Register data (1991–2006). Available at: www.hfea.gov.uk/docs/Latest_long_term_data_analysis_report_91–06.pdf.pdf.

10. Janssens PM, Simons AH, van Kooij RJ, Blokzijl E, Dunselman GA. A new Dutch Law regulating provision of identifying information of donors to offspring: background, content and impact. *Hum Reprod* 2006; **21**: 852–6.

11. Paul S, Harbottle S, Stewart JA. Recruitment of sperm donors: the Newcastle-upon-Tyne experience 1994–2003. *Hum Reprod* 2006; **10**(21): 150–8.

12. British Fertility Society. Working party on sperm donation service in the UK: report and recommendations. *Hum Fertil* 2008; **11**(3): 147–158.

13. Human Fertilisation and Embryology Authority. *SEED Report. A Report on the Human Fertilisation & Embryology Authority's Review of Sperm, Egg and Embryo Donation in the United Kingdom.* London, HFEA; 2005. Available at: www.hfea.gov.uk/docs/SEEDReport05.pdf.

14. Sawyer N. Sperm donor limits that control for the 'relative' risk associated with the use of open-identity donors. *Hum Reprod* Feb 2010. doi: 10.1093/humrep/deq038.

15. Association of Biomedical Andrologists; Association of Clinical Embryologists; British Andrology Society; British Fertility Society; Royal College of Obstetricians and Gynaecologists. UK guidelines for the medical and laboratory screening of sperm,

egg and embryo donors. *Hum Fertil* 2008; **11**: 201–10.

16. Le Lannou D, Lansac J, Federation CECOS. Artificial procreation with frozen donor sperm: the French experience of CECOS. In Barratt CLR, Cook ID, eds. *Donor Insemination*. Cambridge: CUP, 1993; 152–69.

17. Cooper TG, Noonan E, von Eckardstein S *et al.* World Health Organization reference values for human semen characteristics. *Hum Reprod Update* 2009; EPub ahead of print.

18. Sartorius GA, Nieschlag E. Paternal age and reproduction. *Hum Reprod Update* 2010; **16**: 65–79.

19. Anello A, Reichenberg A, Luo X, *et al.* Brief report: parental age and the sex ratio in autism. *J Autism Dev Disord* 2009; **39**: 10; 1487–92.

20. Barratt CLR, Cooke ID, eds. *Donor Insemination*. Cambridge: CUP, 1993.

21. David G, Czyglik F, Mayaux MJ, Martin-Boyce A, Schwartz D. Artificial insemination with frozen sperm: protocol, method of analysis and results for 1188 women. *Br J Obstet Gynaecol* 1980; **87**: 1022–8.

22. Keel BA, Webster BW. Semen cryopreservation methodology and results. In Barratt CLR, Cook ID, eds. *Donor Insemination*. Cambridge: CUP, 1993; 71–96.

23. www. statistics. gov.uk.

24. Ferrara I, Balet R, Grudzinskas JG. Intrauterine insemination with frozen donor sperm. Pregnancy outcome in relation to age and ovarian stimulation regime. *Hum Reprod* 2002; **17**: 2320–4.

25. www.iotf.org.

26. Wang JX, Davies M, Norman RJ. Body mass and probability of pregnancy during assisted reproduction treatment: retrospective study. *BMJ* 2000; **321**: 1320–1.

27. Van der Steeg JW, Steures P, Eijkemans MJC, *et al.* Obesity affects spontaneous pregnancy chances in subfertile, ovulatory women. *Hum Reprod* 2008; **23**(2): 324–8.

28. PHLS, DHSS and PS and the Scottish ISD (D) 5 Collaborative Group. *Sexually Transmitted Infections in the UK: New Episodes Seen at Genitourinary Medicine Clinics, 1995 to 2000*. London: Public Health Laboratory Service, 2001.

29. Paavonen J, Eggert-Kruse W. Chlamydia trachomatis: impact on human reproduction. *Hum Reprod Update* 1999; **5**: 433–47.

30. Bradshaw KD, Guzick DS, Grun B, Johnson N, Ackerman G. Cumulative pregnancy rates for donor insemination according to ovulatory function and tubal status. *Fertil Steril* 1987; **48**: 1051–4.

31. Stovall DW, Christman GM, Hammond MG, Talbert LM. Abnormal findings on hysterosalpingography: effects on fecundity in a donor insemination program using frozen semen. *Obstet Gynecol* 1992; **80**: 249–52.

32. Balasch B. Investigation of the infertile couple in the era of assisted reproductive technology: a time for reappraisal. *Hum Reprod* 2000; **15**: 2251–7.

33. Emperaire JC, Gauzere-Soumireu E, Audebert AJ. Female fertility and donor insemination. *Fertil Steril* 1982; **37**: 90–3.

34. NICE Guidelines. *Fertility: Assessment and Treatment for People with Fertility Problems, Clinical Guideline 11*. February 2004.

35. Tanahatoe S, Hompes PGA, Lambalk CB. Accuracy of diagnostic laparoscopy in the infertility work-up before intrauterine insemination. *Fertil Steril* 2003; **79**: 361–6.

36. Le Lannou D, Lansac J and Federation CECOS. Artificial procreation with frozen donor semen: the French experience of CECOS. In Barratt CLR, Cook ID, eds. *Donor Insemination*. Cambridge: CUP, 1993; 152–69.

37. Wolf DP, Patton PE, Burry KA, Kaplan PF. Intrauterine insemination-ready versus conventional semen cryopreservation for donor insemination: a comparison of retrospective results and a prospective, randomized trial. *Fertil Steril* 2001; **76**: 181–5.

38. Marshburn PB, McIntire D, Carr BR, Byrd W. Spermatozoal characteristics from fresh and frozen donor semen and their correlation with fertility outcome after intrauterine insemination. *Fertil Steril* 1992; **58**: 179–86.

39. Besselink DE, Farquhar C, Kremer JA, Marjoribanks J, O'Brien P. Cervical insemination versus intra-uterine insemination of donor sperm for subfertility. *Cochrane Database Syst Rev* 2008; **16**(2): CD000317.

Using donor oocytes

Pedro N. Barri and Elisabet Clua

Introduction

Since 1984, when Lutjen and collaborators published the first pregnancies following oocyte donation [1], its effectiveness and its applications have increased constantly. Women are delaying childbirth and trying to conceive when they are > 35 years old and at this age their chances of achieving a pregnancy with their own oocytes suffer a progressive and dramatic drop. It is currently estimated that oocyte-donation cycles represent approximately 10% of all IVF cycles that are carried out annually worldwide.

The efficacy of oocyte-donation programs has increased considerably in the last decade and we are now in a position to say that half of the donation cycles allow a clinical pregnancy to be achieved. The growing social demand for this technique involves the need for a greater number of donations and could raise difficulties of access to the technique and a number of ethical and/or legal problems that must be taken into consideration. In Spain oocyte donation must be anonymous, the donors must be between 18 and 35 years old, and they receive financial compensation of 1000 euros for each donation cycle. It is recommended that a donor should not do more than four donation cycles in a two-year period and the number of children born from one donor is limited to six. Moreover, legislation varies in different countries so that in Europe a social movement known as "cross-border reproductive care" has arisen, which reflects the ability of infertile couples to travel to another country where they can receive the treatment that is legally prohibited to them in their own.

It is estimated that in the USA more than 100 000 young women have donated oocytes, either altruistically or motivated by financial compensation [2]. Considering that the donors are young and may not yet have fulfilled their reproductive wishes, it is incumbent on the professionals who treat these women to minimize the risks of this technique and ensure that the treatment is comfortable for the donors.

Indications

Our oocyte-donation program started in 1986 and at that time most of the patients who were to be recipients had no ovarian activity. The first pregnancies were easily obtained after administration to the recipients of protocols that combined estrogens and gestagens to prepare the endometrium, making it receptive to the embryos that were to be received after the oocyte donation [3].

Since 1992 we have moved from 94% of recipients without ovarian activity, who needed a donation of oocytes as the only possibility of having children, to 52% in recent years.

The Subfertility Handbook: A Clinician's Guide, Second Edition ed. Gab Kovacs. Published by Cambridge University Press. © Cambridge University Press 2011.

Table 14.1 Indications for oocyte donation

	1992 (n = 92) Preg/cycle	%	2005 (n = 303) Preg/cycle	%
Agonadal women	22/87	25.3	93/158	58.8
Primary ovarian failure	4/16	25.0	22/34	64.7
Secondary ovarian failure	18/71	25.3	71/124	57.3
Gonadal women	1/5	20.0	81/145	55.8
Age+failure IVF cycles	0/3	–	65/116	56.0
Poor oocyte quality	1/2	50.0	16/29	55.0

Currently, half of the recipients conserve their gonadal function and undertake oocyte donation for other reasons [4]. The main indications for which a woman undergoes oocyte donation are usually occult ovarian failure, advanced age and repeated failure of IVF (Table 14.1). For this reason, the demand for donations has grown exponentially in the last decade and in most countries there is an evident scarcity of donors that is not solved by donor-capture campaigns. In our experience with a group of 468 potential donors we found that a high percentage of them did not pass through the preliminary screening, either for personal reasons or because of pathologies detected in this stage, and only 105 went on to make the donation (22.4%). Leaving aside those countries in which a significant financial compensation is permitted (in the USA the national average for standard donor compensation exceeds $4500), altruistic donation is unusual and it is becoming really difficult to have a sufficient number of oocyte donations to meet the growing demand.

Results

The women who donate oocytes are young, with no previous pathology and with a high reproductive potential. This explains the high clinical pregnancy rates that are usually achieved with this treatment. Recent figures from our program and from the registries of the Spanish Fertility Society clearly show that clinical pregnancy rates exceed 50%, and the implantation rates are above 30%, but despite transferring at most two embryos the multiple pregnancy rates are too high at above 30% (Table 14.2). The evolution of the pregnancies is usually favorable but with a cesarean section rate of over 50% and with rates of miscarriage below 20%. With regard to the risk of fetal malformations, in this population of 252 births we observed 8 major fetal malformations (3.2%), which is to say that the level of fetal malformations is within the range expected in our population (Table 14.3).

There is a series of variables that must be analyzed separately to find the influence that they have on clinical pregnancy rates.

Age

In Spain there is no upper limit on the age of the recipients although this technique is formally discouraged in women aged over 50 years. In this context, we have observed no significant differences between the ages of the recipients who became pregnant and of those who did not. Nor have we seen differences in the miscarriage rate.

Table 14.2 Oocyte donation pregnancy rates

	I. U. Dexeus	Spanish Fertility Society
Recipients (n)	462	4601
Embryos / ET ($\bar{X}$)	1.9	2
Pregnancies (n)	252	2190
Pregnancy rate / ET (%)	52.2	51
Implantation rate (%)	34.2	33
Miscarriage rate (%)	15.5	19
Multiple pregnancy rate (%)	26	36

Table 14.3 Oocyte donation fetal malformations

Pierre Robin syndrome
Abdominal wall defect
Fallot's tetralogia
Down's syndrome + cardiopathy
Down's syndrome (paternal origin)
Hydrocephalia
Skeletal displasia
8/252 (3.2%)

The age of the donors is limited in our country to the 18–35-year age range, and within this interval we have not observed that the donor's age has any significant repercussion on the possibility of obtaining a pregnancy. However, we have noticed that the risk of miscarriage increased significantly and progressively when the donor's age exceeded 29 years.

Screening of donors

Under current Spanish legislation and the Guidelines of the Spanish Fertility Society donor screening must fulfil the following criteria.

- Donors must be over 18 and under 35 years of age, in good psychological and physical condition, and be tested for phenotype characteristics and genetic, hereditary, and infectious diseases.
- Oocyte donation is anonymous and must be performed as a non-remunerative, formal, confidential, and mutual agreement between the donor and the center. Donation must never be regarded as lucrative and cannot be promoted for financial benefit.
- Karyotype and cystic fibrosis mutation analysis must be performed in donors and in partners of recipients.

Table 14.4 Egg donation guidelines: Spanish Fertility Society

Donors must be over 18 and under 35 years of age, in good psychological and physical conditions; law 14/2006 requires each donor to be tested for phenotype characteristics, and genetic, hereditary, and infectious disease, according to a fixed study protocol.
Must be performed as a non-remunerative, formal, confidential, and mutual agreement between donor and the center. Donation must never be regarded as lucrative and cannot be promoted by financial benefit. Anonymous.
Maximum six newborns allowed per donor
As donors may carry karyotype abnormalities or cystic fibrosis mutations, it is recommended that potential donors are tested and carriers counseled.
Specific genetic screening should be performed when the partner of the egg recipient is also the carrier of a genetic disease.
The use of the donor eggs creates the potencial for rhesus incompatibility. All donors should have their blood group and rhesus status recorded for matching purposes.
To minimize the risk of transmission of viruses and bacterial infections the prospective donors should screen negative for: hepatitis C (VHC), hepatitis B (HBsAg), human immunodeficiency virus (HIV) 1 and 2, syphilis (*Treponema pallidum*), gonorrhea (*Neisseria gonorrhoea*) and chlamydia (*Chlamydia trachomatis*).
The egg donor must be informed of the potential risks of controlled ovarian stimulation and egg collection. Consent form must be signed.
Maximum compensation per egg donation cycle is 600–1000€.
The age of the recipient should not influence the number of embryos transferred, although a maximum of one or two embryos is recommended.
Recipients > 45 years should be counseled about the risks of pregnancy at that age and have to undergo a complete medical check-up prior to the treatment.
Egg donation is discouraged after age 50.

Data from Matorras R. *The Infertile Couple. Recommendations from the Spanish Fertility Society.* Madrid: Adalia Farma, 2007.

- Egg donors will be informed about the potential risks of controlled ovarian stimulation and oocyte retrieval. An informed consent form will be signed.
- Maximum compensation per oocyte donation cycle is €1000.
- A maximum of six newborns is allowed per donor.
- Oocyte donation is discouraged in recipients aged over 50 (Table 14.4).

Smoking

Although it is well known that smoking is associated with decreased fertility, the effect of cigarette smoking on pregnancy rates after oocyte donation is unclear. We evaluated the outcome of 462 oocyte-donation cycles according to the smoking status of donor and recipients. Smoking incidence was 45.1% among the donors and 21.4% in the recipients. Donors' outcomes (gonadotropin consumption, number of mature oocytes and fertilization rate) as well as recipients' were, in our experience, not affected by smoking status. Even though we did not find a negative impact on the pregnancy rates of the population studied, we strongly recommend donors and recipients to stop smoking.

Donors' previous fertility

In a retrospective analysis of 605 donors in our oocyte-donation program we found that in 294 cycles oocytes from donors of proven fertility gave rise to 158 pregnancies (53.7%). In the remaining 311 from nulligravid donors, 172 pregnancies were obtained (55.3%). For us, a donor's proven fertility is not a predictive factor for a better outcome in the recipient.

Ovarian stimulation protocols for oocyte donors

Oocyte donors are sometimes under treatment with oral contraceptives, which makes it easier to synchronize the processing of donors and recipients. However, as they later undergo the usual pituitary suppression this means that the response to ovarian stimulation is lower due to the dual suppression (oral contraceptives and GnRH agonists), though there is the advantage of the lower risk of ovarian hyperstimulation syndrome [5].

The incorporation of GnRH antagonists into the stimulation protocols of the oocyte donors makes the treatment more comfortable for them but the recipients' pregnancy rates are significantly reduced. In our experience, although there are no differences in the number of oocytes available in each group or in the number of embryos that are transferred to the recipients, we have observed that the mean quality of the embryos that come from oocytes of donors stimulated under GnRH agonists is significantly higher, which might explain the higher pregnancy rate obtained in these recipients [6]. Later, with the inclusion of more cases in this study, we found that the differences in the pregnancy rates disappeared and the low rates of ovarian hyperstimulation under GnRH antagonist were maintained.

Triggering ovulation was classically carried out with the administration of 10 000 IU of urinary hCG or 250 µg of recombinant hCG. However, treating the donors with GnRH antagonists has the advantage that the ovulatory discharge can be effected with a bolus of GnRH agonist. This strategy reduces very considerably the risk of donor ovarian hyperstimulation.

The evidence currently available confirms the need to obtain an adequate ovarian response from the donors, which must be accompanied by the lowest possible risk of hyperstimulation. With this aim, it is recommendable to use donor oocyte protocols that combine recombinant or urinary gonadotropins with GnRH antagonists, in which ovulation is triggered with a bolus of GnRH agonist.

Endometrial preparation of the recipients

Oocyte recipients with ovarian function were inhibited with a depot GnRH agonist (Decapeptyl 3.75, Ipsen Laboratory, Spain) administered in the midluteal phase of the previous cycle. More recently and in order to make synchronization between donor and recipient easier, we have been using a short suppression of the recipient with daily doses of GnRH antagonist (Cetrorelix 0.25, Merck Serono Laboratory) starting after 7 days of estrogen preparation. Results obtained so far are very promising (Table 14.5). Endometrium was primed with 6 mg of estradiol valerate per day for a minimum of 14 days (Progynova 1 mg, Schering Laboratories, Spain) and additional vaginal administration of micronized progesterone 600 mg per day starting on the day of the oocyte recovery of the donor and for 14 days (Utrogestan 200 mg, Seid Laboratories, Spain).

Other protocols using transdermal estrogen, intramuscular progesterone, and/or a bolus of a GnRH agonist administration can also be applied but the standard regime with oral estrogens and vaginal progesterone is very efficient and easy to follow.

Table 14.5 GnRH antagonists for oocyte recipients

	Recipients (n)	Embryos replaced ($\bar{X} \pm DS$)	Pregnancies (n)	Pregn/ replacement (%)
Agonist	63	2.0 ± 0.2	29	46.0
Antagonist	76	1.9 ± 0.2	41	53.09

No significant difference.

Table 14.6 Oocyte donation results by number of optimal embryos transferred

	Number of optimal embryos transferred			P
	0	1	2	
Pregnancy rate (%)	43.5 (64/147)	46.9 (91/194)	60.6 (366/604)	< 0.05
Multiple pregnancy rate (%)	23.4 (15/64)	35.2 (32/91)	39.1 (143/366)	0.054
Implantation rate (%)	27	32	42	< 0.001

Risk of multiple pregnancy

In our experience, by transferring a maximum of two embryos whenever possible in a population of 945 recipients we had a multiple pregnancy rate of 36%. Considering this percentage to be excessive we wanted to find out which factors were associated with a higher risk of multiple pregnancy. After a multivariate analysis of our material we found that the ages of the donor and recipient were not decisive, but that the number of high-quality embryos that were transferred was a decisive factor (Table 14.6).

Reducing the excessive multiple pregnancy rate requires policies of selective transfer of a single embryo selected from the pool of available embryos (eSET). This strategy is particularly important in patients over 45 with a high potential risk of obstetric complications. To reach this objective, it will be necessary to raise awareness among doctors and patients about the advantages of eSET and about the obstetric, perinatal and psychosocial risks of multiple pregnancies [7]. We must also explain to them that cumulative pregnancy rates combining eSET and subsequent frozen embryo transfers are really efficient in achieving optimal pregnancy rates and a reduction of multiple pregnancy rates [8,9].

Patients with Turner syndrome

Patients with ovarian failure due to Turner syndrome attend our hospitals asking to be included in the oocyte-donation programs. It is very important to remember that in women with Turner syndrome the risk of aortic dissection or rupture during pregnancy may be 2% and the risk of death during pregnancy is increased as much as 100-fold. Cardiology consultation and careful screening for cardiac abnormalities is a prerequisite for any planned attempt at pregnancy via oocyte donation. An echocardiogram revealing any significant abnormality represents an absolute contraindication to attempting pregnancy in a patient with a Turner syndrome.

If a pregnancy is established in a Turner syndrome recipient, special control of a possible hypertension and serial echocardiographic controls are mandatory. Patients in stable condition having an aortic diameter less than 4 cm may have a vaginal delivery under epidural anesthesia. Women showing progressive aortic root dilatation should have an elective cesarean section under epidural anesthesia [10].

Ethical aspects of oocyte donation

We have shown that oocyte-donation programs are highly effective, although their application in day-to-day clinical practice can sometimes involve a number of ethically compromising situations.

First, we are concerned about the protection of the donors, who must be protected as they are sometimes very young, ill-informed and unaware of the potential risks of the technique, something that is of particular importance in donors who have not previously had children. It is important for them to be given as much information as possible and to be closely monitored, and mild stimulation protocols must be applied that involve a low risk of hyperstimulation. Nor must we overlook the requirement to keep records of donors, both for the traceability of possible complications in the offspring and for long-term risks in the donors themselves [11].

We believe that anonymity is important and beneficial but we have respect for opinions that allow and support non-anonymous donations in what has come to be called "intrafamilial medically assisted reproduction". There is no doubt that this could be an option to consider in special situations provided that there is no compromise to the expectations of donors and recipients before starting an oocyte-donation process [12].

It is also important for recipients to be accompanied from the psychological point of view as they may present difficulties in taking decisions, concern about the donor's background, and inadequate handling of confidentiality with anxiety that can reach considerable levels.

Finally, we would like to refer to what is now known as "cross-border reproductive care", i.e. cases of patients who have to leave their own countries and travel abroad to receive the treatment that is not available to them in their own countries. The reasons why patients should travel abroad for infertility treatment are legal and financial, and are a consequence of post-modern society, with a multitude of moral and religious views, which in the field of reproduction have given rise to a mosaic of different laws in a regional context such as Europe, and of poor public provision for infertility care which promotes private-based reproductive medicine.

This insufficient public funding must be improved with better access and distributive justice. If this is done, it will reduce this ill-named "reproductive tourism", which acts as a safety valve that decreases the pressure for internal law reform.

Oocyte-donation programs are an example of technical simplicity, high healthcare effectiveness, and social complexity. We must not overlook all of the parties involved in the process. Donors and recipients deserve our attention and our greatest respect.

References

1. Lutjen P, Trounson A, Leeton J, *et al.* The establishment and maintenance of pregnancy using in vitro fertilization and embryo donation in a patient with primary ovarian failure. *Nature* 1984; **307**(5947): 174–5.

2. Kramer W, Schneider J, Schultz N. US oocyte donors: a retrospective study of

medical and psychosocial issues. *Hum Reprod* 2009; **24**(12): 3144–9.

3. Coroleu B, Martinez F, Veiga A, Calderón G, Barri PN. Programa de donación de ovocitos en el Instituto Dexeus. *Progr Obstet Ginecol* 1988; 31–9.

4. Barri PN, Coroleu B, Martinez F, *et al.* Indications for oocyte donation. *Hum Reprod* 1992; **7**(Suppl 1) : 85–8.

5. Martinez F, Boada M, Coroleu B, *et al.* A prospective trial comparing oocyte donor ovarian response and recipient pregnancy rates between suppression with gonadotrophin-releasing hormone agonist (GnRHa) alone and dual suppression with a contraceptive vaginal ring and GnRH. *Hum Reprod* 2006; **21**(8): 2121–5.

6. Martinez F, Clua E, Parera N, *et al.* Prospective randomized, comparative study of leuprorelin + human menopausal gonadotropins versus ganirelix+ recombinant FSH in oocyte donors and pregnancy rates among the corresponding recipients. *Gynecol Endocrinol* 2008; **24**(1): 1–6.

7. Tur R, Coroleu B, Torelló MJ, *et al.* Prevention of multiple pregnancy following IVF in Spain. *RBMOnline* 2006; **13**(6): 856–63.

8. Practice Committee of the Society for Assisted Reproductive Technology and the Practice Committee of the American Society of Reproductive Medicine. Guidelines on number of embryos transferred. *Fertil Steril* 2008; **90**(Suppl 3): 163–4.

9. Vilska S, Unkila-Kallio I, Punamäki RL, *et al.* Mental health of mothers and fathers of twins conceived via assisted reproduction treatment: a 1-year prospective study. *Hum Reprod* 2009; **24**: 367–77.

10. College National des Gynecologues et Obstetriciens Français. *Syndrome de Turner et grossesse. Recommandations pour la pratique clinique RPC.* Agence de la Biomedicine, 2009; 1–19.

11. Purewal S, van den Akker OB. A study of the effect of message framing on oocyte donation. *Hum Reprod* 2009; **24**(12): 3136–43.

12. Kramer W, Schneider J, Schultz N. US oocyte donors: a retrospective study of medical and psychosocial issues. *Hum Reprod* 2009; **24**(12): 3144–9.

Embryo donation: practice and ethical dilemmas

F. Shenfield

Most treatments in assisted reproduction raise ethical issues, but embryo donation raises more than others, in view of the emotional (personal) and symbolic (societal) values attached to this entity, which represents our future. This chapter will cover both the practice of embryo donation, the ethical and legal aspects, whether for reproductive purpose or for research.

Since the inception of the complex, although now routine, technique of IVF, the human embryo may be observed outside the body, and this has captured the world's imagination, in a different way than the older technique of sperm donation. The donation of embryos is more complex than sperm or egg donation, as it involves the consent of the two people who provided the gametes. Furthermore, one also has to take into account the consent of the recipient woman and her partner if present. Thus, from the outset, up to four people may be involved in the reproductive project, which complicates ethical and legal matters. However, when embryo donation is for the purpose of research, the gamete providers are the prime agents for consent, although the interests of society at large are also at stake.

Thus, embryos may be given for the reproductive project of another couple, or a single woman where the law allows it (as in the UK), or may be given/donated for research. Human embryo research has also led to many debates since its inception and the newer issues around stem cell research, a subject of major current interest, have been rekindled by the therapeutic hopes from stem cell research. More specifically embryonic stem cells, with or without somatic cell nuclear transfer technology (SCNT), have been much in the news and public mind, although induced pluripotent stem cells may actually offer more practical therapeutic applications in the near future.

We will first outline the general principles and ethical questions surrounding gamete/embryo donation.

Embryo (and gamete) donation in general

Two main controversial issues for gamete(s) or embryo donation are anonymity and payment. Traditionally gamete donors were anonymous, but recently this has been questioned, with the right of the offspring to have access to his/her origins being recognized as important to their sense of identity. The other issue is older still, but often rekindled, especially when donation becomes more scarce: should donors be paid, or (highly) compensated for their donation, and what is fair compensation?

The Subfertility Handbook: A Clinician's Guide, Second Edition ed. Gab Kovacs. Published by Cambridge University Press. © Cambridge University Press 2011.

Indeed it seems obvious, at least from a semantic point of view, that a gift should be free. Furthermore, the fact is that if society intends to pay gamete donors, the term "donation" itself should be changed to "sale" of gametes and embryos. However, in most countries where gamete donation is used as a means of solving infertility problems, those who recruit the donors have difficulties in matching the supply to the demand, especially oocytes and embryos. Thus, it has been argued that pragmatism should prevail in a scarce-supply environment and that some type of financial inducement should certainly not be forbidden. In the UK, this, of course, must be within the frame of English law, which states that "no money or other kind of benefit shall be given or received in respect of any supply of gametes or embryos unless authorized by directions" [1]. The notion of gifting is also enshrined, among others, in the law in France, but Spain differs slightly, where compensation is given as a maximum lump sum to egg donors [2].

With the conviction that the human body and its parts and products should remain outside commerce, one can attempt a rational argument in the realm of ethics, for altruistic donation. The special quality of respect due to the person was most cogently articulated over 200 years ago by Immanuel Kant. It stems from the observance of the second formulation of the categorical imperative, "to treat all humanity always at the same time as an end and never merely as a means". The opposite utilitarian attitude has proposed that in a scarce-supply environment, one might choose to pay donors. But negative consequences identified by Titmus [3] about the payment for blood donation can be applied to gamete donation: this may deter genuine altruistic donors, there may be an increased risk of transmitting disease by donors motivated by gain only and willing to falsify information, and especially there is the risk of potential exploitation of the weakest socioeconomic groups of society. This very argument of potential coercion is used by opponents of egg sharing, a pragmatic approach used in the UK to increase oocyte donation, where a woman who is being stimulated donates some of her oocytes to a third party, who then share the costs. The HFE Act 1990 allowed benefits for female donors (those allowed being treatment services and sterilization), and the debate can be thus summed up: is this a form of coercion to donate, a form of payment, or is it an acceptable "exchange"?

Interestingly however, the US literature has no qualms mentioning payment for embryos [4], something which would be totally unacceptable in Europe. Indeed an initiative of the Abraham Center of Life of San Antonio in Texas, enrolling brilliant sperm donors and beautiful oocyte donors to create embryos for donation, led a French colleague to ask when "embryos would be submitted to auctions" [5].

Although evidence for one path or the other is lacking [6], a recent change in UK law passed in 2005 specifies that all new gamete donors must undertake to give their name when the offspring reaches majority. Sweden passed this law in 1985 and whether this will deter new donors (especially egg sharers who would find out 18 years later that their recipient was successful if they were not), time only will tell. However, national figures collated by the HFEA already show a decrease in the number of donors in 2005. As far as embryo donation for reproduction is concerned, recent information obtained under the Freedom of Information Act also shows a sharp decline since 2005 in embryos given to others for (reproductive) treatment (Table 15.1). This is not surprising when considering the required undertaking, since 2005, of being named if required by the offspring when he/she reaches legal majority. If most embryo donors are likely to be actual or future parents, it must be rather awe-inspiring to think of meeting one day full genetic siblings to one's own legal and gestated child(ren).

Table 15.1 Numbers of embryos donated

Year	Number of embryos donated – for research	Number of embryos donated – for treatment
2002	4518	197
2003	3737	140
2004	3627	205
2005	4493	243
2006	3346	91
2007	4209	84

New studies concerning children who have been told of their origins will offer evidence on the lack of secrecy of the procedure of gamete donation, but we may have to wait a long time before being able to observe the effects of known embryo donation on children. For instance in the UK no offspring from donated embryos will have reached majority before 2023. The important question is the meaning of "knowing one's origins", a matter of importance to each and everyone of us, but one which has many different meanings, historical, psychological, and anthropological, while arguably the meaning of genetic origins is historically newer to humans than that of kinship.

Powerful voices of anger and distress of some children of sperm donation have been heard [7], arguing that they have been deprived of specific knowledge, the identity of the genetic sperm provider (avoiding the legal and emotional term father), information without which they do not find their sense of identity complete. We know, however, that in most cases, the interests of children and parents seem to coincide as several studies have already shown that children conceived by "assisted reproduction" fare very well in the measured personal and social criteria, when compared to children conceived "naturally" or adopted [8,9]. Another argument used is this of "the right of the child" to know of his/her "origins" and the potentially divisive role of secrets in families. When one enters the area of rights and finds a conflict of interests between those claiming rights, it is difficult to ascertain what might take precedence, as for instance, between the "right to privacy" of the parents and donors or the "right to know" of the prospective child. Arguably, what may matter most to the child to be is the concern of the future/intended parents (the recipient couple), as their attitude will directly influence the well-being and welfare of the child. The current evidence that the outcome is generally as good as for naturally conceived offspring is reassuring, but we must not forget our (ethical) responsibility to these children as a profession, and indeed our (legal) duty of care whether general or specific as it is in UK law. It is indeed our duty to look prospectively and reflect on different approaches. For the time being, it would seem that democratic openness to different approaches in families and the respect of their privacy favors a double-stranded approach with all the consequences for the children for whom we are jointly responsible. This has, however, been rejected by many regulators on the grounds that it would entail unequal treatment for the donation offspring.

Finally, recent studies on gamete donors' offspring seeking their partial genetic roots shows their interest in their half-siblings [10,11]. The case of embryo donation is further complicated of course by the fact that such offspring might seek information or a meeting with their full genetic siblings. To make the matter even more complex, the HFE Act 2008 allows such sharing of information with donation siblings but not with the donor's offspring, wishing to protect the donor's family from his/her generous decision. What the children/offspring will make of this is everyone's guess, and only research will be able to enlighten us, in many years to come. But this model, copied on the openness of the adoption model, has recently been commented upon by the ASRM ethics committee, which stated that "embryo donation is not adoption". Indeed the major difference is that one cannot claim that a donation offspring was "abandoned", as in the case of adoption.

Embryo donation to another couple

What makes patients give their embryos to others has been the subject of much research. A recent Canadian study of 49 couples with embryos in storage for over 3 years showed that factors for prediction of donation were linked to "comfort with sharing information with a recipient couple" and probability increased if the choice of "conditional donation" [12], with a choice of donation according to their own preference, was included. This theme of conditional donation recurs in an Australian study, which concluded that "motivation to donate" depended on knowing more about the recipients [13]: amongst "clients ... surveyed, of which 99 women (35%) and 66 men (23%) responded, only 4% indicated it was likely they would donate to other couples; 48% thought donors should be able to specify characteristics of recipients; and 41% indicated they would be more likely to donate if donation was conditional". The authors concluded that "a sense of ownership and responsibility for the well-being of the offspring underpinned reluctance to donate, (and that) ... perceived control over the caretaking environment was seen as an advantage of conditional donation". Another study from Brazil stated that "decisions to donate embryos to another couple or discard them were colored by strong values about human life" [14]. Finally "concerns were also raised about the need for donors to relinquish control", but another important aspect which concerns all regulatory authorities and clinics internationally was the "accumulation of unclaimed embryos" and the difficulties in maintaining contact with the couple from whom they originated.

In Victoria, Australian legislation governing fertility treatment provides that surplus human embryos must not be stored for longer than 5 years. In searching how to facilitate decisions about surplus embryos, a survey was performed to reflect how couples could be helped to decide between one of three options: discard, donate to research, or donate to another infertile couple. The authors surveyed 42 people who agreed to participate in either a structured interview or a group discussion [13]. All participants had completed IVF treatment and had surplus embryos in storage. The aim of the interviews was to discuss participants' decision-making regarding their surplus embryos. Most participants described the decision-making process as difficult and emotional. They concluded "that participants could be assisted by more information about each of their current options, and opportunities to talk to others in similar situations", and that "many responded positively to the idea of having more options, including choice about which research projects to donate to (directed research), and about the recipients of their donated embryos (directed donation)". This is a sad indictment of the amount of information they had been given, prior to treatment or cryopreservation, or remembered. Indeed this information (and its understanding) is, in general as well as in particular, the major key to their proper consent. If verbal information is not enough, written information is a necesarry adjunct.

Interestingly, whilst the previous studies were performed with couples thinking of donating embryos, a US study found that "selling" was sometimes acceptable [8]: the authors found "statistically significantly lower support for selling embryos among patients who were Hispanic (relative to Caucasians) or had never been pregnant, whereas significantly greater support was observed among Hindu and secular women, patients being treated for male factor infertility, and those who in the past had or were currently undergoing intrauterine insemination". They also found that "age, education, marital status, and parity were not statistically significantly associated with the opinions about selling extra embryos to other couples".

This is, however, the only study where "selling" was mentioned. By contrast, another US survey [15] sought to correlate other values than monetary to the likelihood of donation, and found they mostly related to a view of the embryos as possible future child(ren). Drapkin Lyerly and colleagues [15] found in a multi-institutional survey that 54% of respondents with cryopreserved embryos were very likely to use them for reproduction, 21% were very likely to donate for research, 7% or fewer were very likely to choose any other option, and that respondents who ascribed high importance to concerns about the health or well-being of the embryo, fetus, or future child were more likely to thaw and discard embryos or freeze them indefinitely. They concluded that "fertility patients frequently prefer disposition options that are not available to them or find the available options unacceptable". They advise "restructuring and standardizing the informed consent process and ensuring availability of all disposition options may benefit patients, facilitate disposition decisions, and address problems of long term storage". Again we find that the key to proper consent is good information, a common feature of many published papers, which indeed leads one to wonder about the quality of patients' information and support prior to formal consent in writing. It is also possible that couples underestimate the intensity of the feelings they may have towards this entity created with their gametes, which they have not been able to see prior to IVF. Belgian colleagues [16] interviewed 7 couples and 11 female patients, also in order to find out how they conceptualize their embryos. Six major themes emerged from the narratives of the participants when they spoke about their embryos: (i) a medical-technical perspective; (ii) feelings; (iii) genetic link to oneself and/or one's partner; (iv) symbolic meaning of the relationship between the infertile partners; (v) moral status; and (vi) instrumental value. The investigators found that, when patients considered donation to another couple for reproductive purposes, the presence of the themes "genetic link" and "symbol of the relationship" was linked with a clear reluctance to donate, and that (later), "in the second step of the decision-making process, the option of donation for research and discarding were considered".

Thus, it transpires from all these studies that giving one's embryos for research is less emotionally difficult than giving them for reproductive purpose, a fact which fits the psychological image of "potential child" attached to the embryos conceived after fertility treatment. We have to remember that these patients often had a long path prior to and during IVF, and have invested much emotion in the process.

In practice, for the UK, Table 15.1 also shows the number of embryos given to research projects approved by the HFEA, over a period of 6 years. This number is much larger than the number given to another couple for reproductive purpose, by a factor of 10 to 20. The message seems to be very clear: it is easier to give an "entity" to research, which might have become a baby after many hurdles, than to give the same entity to a couple in need, for whom it may become a child, after a live birth.

Donating embryos for research

In some cases, embryos may be donated for very specific research. Indeed when the couple is undergoing IVF with PGD in order to have a healthy child, the decision to donate super-numerary embryos for research in the field of their specific pathology might arguably be easier than for couples who do not carry the burden of passing on serious disease to their offspring. Thus several researchers found donation of such embryos for research posed little problem as it was likely to help people in the same boat, by furthering research in the very disease they had fallen prey to. Indeed a registry of stem cells issued from such embryos has been created [17].

Otherwise embryos may be donated for fundamental research, or for stem cell research, from embryos created with or without somatic cell nuclear transfer (SCNT). What has been called "therapeutic cloning" by the press and lay public, with the advent of Dolly the cloned sheep created by SCNT, has not been helpful in the debates on the status and nature of the human embryo. The repulsion caused almost universally by reproductive cloning has not been universally matched by the same feelings or arguments on the use of stem cells from human embryos. Indeed, Britain was the first state to allow research for "therapeutic" cloning. Embryo research had been licensed under strict conditions since the HFE Act 1990, permitting only research linked to reproduction. After a report by the Chief Medical Officer and a vote in both chambers of Parliament, new categories were added to Statute 31 January 2001, and confirmed in the new ART legislation of 2008, allowing this time "research for serious disease."

Furthermore, one must also remember the importance of semantics and terminology when describing the embryo. Aware of the potential exploitation of semantic games when discussing embryo research in general, the ESHRE taskforce defined the preimplantation embryo in its first ethics consideration on behalf of the society. The ESHRE taskforce for Ethics and Law [18] stressed that this term was descriptive, meaning the embryo out of the body before it is given a chance of becoming a fetus and then a legal person by embryo transfer to a uterus. But such a descriptive term does not imply a lesser quality; it is nevertheless a human embryo, with special consideration needed.

Meanwhile, specific issues arise from the possible application of stem cell animal research to the human embryo. With this in mind, the ESHRE taskforce on law and ethics considered the matter of stem cell technology [19]. It stated that many fundamental ethical questions in this field are far from new. Indeed, consent must be obtained for research, reflecting the principle of autonomy. But the taskforce stressed also that "in view of the special nature of stem cells and their longevity, it should be specifically mentioned that the embryos will be used for research into the establishment of cell lines which can be kept indefinitely, may eventually be used for therapeutic purposes, and will never be replaced into a uterus. It should also be made clear whether the cells may be used for commercial and/or clinical purposes. This is therefore specific rather than general consent", to be discussed with the gamete providers.

Finally, as "there are also specific ethical considerations according to source of cells, and especially regarding the creation of embryos specifically for research: (we added that) embryos specifically created for the purpose is appropriate only if the information cannot be obtained by research on supernumerary zygotes". Indeed, this question of the creation of embryos for research is especially vexed. While article 18 of the European Convention on Human Rights and Biomedicine [20] specifically forbids this, in the UK the HFEA is charged with overseeing embryo research within the limits by a licensing system: the creation of embryos de novo for research is not unlawful, but its "necessity" must be demonstrated, ensuring that embryos are not created for futile reasons. Obviously, creating embryos for research is only needed for a specific aim, and again the specific consent of the gamete providers will be required, but the feelings will necessarily be different than those of a couple giving their "spare" embryos to research.

There is also a good deal of research into the mindset and attitudes of couples asked to consider the gift of embryos for research, and what might influence their decision. First, (implication) counseling is obviously important in helping the couples to make a decision: sampling IVF patients about their intention to donate their spare embryos for stem cell research, a Scottish survey of 508 couples found that 69% expressed an interest in research on their initial consent form, and that further consent was strengthened by counseling by a dedicated nurse [21]. Whilst a US survey found that "few sought formal counseling" [22], the apparent difference may be due to the fact that counseling was indeed offered to all in the UK study. Furthermore, the couples' values are also relevant, as in for donation for reproduction, but foremost is naturally the fact that there may be "supernumerary" embryos to give. A review [23] from the USA in 2008 found that "research purpose, treatment stage, embryo quality, religious beliefs and altruism seemed important factors for donation"; (indeed) "being at the beginning of treatment, not knowing" the aim of the research, or having good-quality embryos "were more related to a decision not to donate, confirming again the emotional importance of the embryos seen as potential future children". But whatever the motivation, it is obvious that "psychological support (must) be offered" [24]. The embryo's "moral status" is indeed a salient factor in the decision-making of the embryo donors [25], but "consider(ing)" its social status as well is more puzzling. To be a member of society one has to be alive and participating, at whatever level, from infancy to old age, whether one is more or less cognizant of one's environment. What kind of "social" status indeed may an embryo have when there is no legislation which recognizes the embryo in vitro as a person, as Ms Evans, in spite of her diagnosis of ovarian cancer, found from the European Court of Human Rights [26], who refused her the transfer of her frozen embryos conceived with her ex-husband after he denied his consent? The court firmly denied the embryo the "right to life", and a fortiori a status of legal "person".

As far as national law is concerned, there are wide differences between countries regarding the rules for embryo donation for reproductive purpose, symbolized by the difference between the UK and France, where potential parents of a donated embryo must be seen by a judge in order to assess their "suitability", prior to the cycle's initiation and after clinical consultation. This feels more like an adoption process, alhough there is agreement that embryo donation is very different from adoption [27].

The clinical aspects of embryo donation

The technique of embryo donation is very simple [28]: it is a frozen embryo transfer (FET), where the embryo originated from another couple and not the woman who is having the implantation. This can be performed in either a hormone replacement therapy (HRT) cycle, or in a natural cycle. As most couples "adopt" donated embryos because the female is not producing oocytes (and therefore regular spontaneous ovulation is unlikely), HRT cycles are used most often.

This requires the use of estrogen to induce endometrial proliferation, ultrasound confirmation that this has occurred, and then the administration of a progestogen to induce secretory change for the appropriate number of days that the embryo was frozen on. Transfer is then performed, and the HRT is continued till towards the end of the first trimester when the placenta takes over steroid hormone production.

In natural cycle transfers, ovulation is detected by luteinizing hormone (LH) assays, and the embryo(s) is (are) transferred on the appropriate post-ovulation day.

The donation of frozen embryos by couples who have completed their families and still have embryos in cryostorage is a very efficient use of valuable resources. It is yet another way of parenting in the twenty-first century.

Conclusion

We can conclude that, emotionally, donating embryos is a difficult decision, which certainly challenges the notion of "genetic relatedness" [29], especially when it is for another couple's reproductive plans. Indeed, the practice of embryo donation has implications at national and international levels, as do many others in our specialty. With regard to the concerns about "abandoned embryos", or gamete providers changing their mind together or singly, various legal solutions can be recommended [30]. However, the individual dimension is often the most poignant, and this is what practitioners and counselors certainly face in their daily practice. Nevertheless, international comparisons with the study of different sociocultural approaches help us to challenge dogma. Indeed, one must mention that in some countries it is allowed to create embryos for research, if "necessary", a word with a very specific legal meaning, that in practice the research project would not be feasible with available super-numerary embryos.

Might one also create embryos for donation to others for reproductive purposes, what will the difference be for the offspring emotionally, especially if the recipient desires to only have embryos with the assurance that none others are created for the same purpose for another family? Although one psychoanalyst is firmly against this process, stating that it merely avoids incestuous fantasies concerning the future offspring, this refusal in France may have more to do with the legislator trying to find a "use" for the roughly 200 000 abandoned embryos (in 2005), a number increasing yearly by about 20 000.

A final legal caveat resides in the rare possibility of mistakes in transfer of the embryos to the uterus, which happened in the USA in September 2009 [31] where a mother of three was pregnant with the embryo of another infertile couple. In this case of "unwilling donation" and "wrong recipient", she agreed to surrender the child at delivery to his/her genetic parents. Whether or not adoption is needed in such a case would depend on the national legislation, and especially whether surrogacy is allowed or not, as this generous lady is in fact a gesta-tional surrogate for the gamete providers who did not receive their embryos.

These complex cases do show that we have not yet seen the end of the debate about embryo donation, but also confirm that prior information and implication counseling are the only tools which may help the donors and recipients to understand and rationalize their emotions. Education of the public at large must also be a tool to enable all to make enlightened plans about this very specific reproductive project and donation for embryo research. The decision may well be time- and especially experience-dependent, as couples who become parents are more likely to see the spare embryo as "cells" rather than a future child, and give such spare entities for research [23], a step which appears always easier than giving to another couple. The priority is always to have a baby, for the donors as much as for the receivers. Finally, time will only tell whether it will be even more difficult to find embryo donors, either for reproduction or for research, when single embryo transfer or soft stimulation programs become more common practice.

References

1. HFE Act 2008. Available at: www.dh.gov. uk/en/ . . . /Legislation/Actsandbills/ DH_080211.

2. IFFS Surveillance. Available at: www.iffs-reproduction.org/documents/ Surveillance_07.pdf.

3. Titmus R. *The Gift Relationship: From Human Blood to Social Policy*. London: Allen and Unwin, 1971.

4. Jain T, Stacey A, Missmer S. Support for selling embryos among infertility patients. *Fertil Steril*, 2009; **90**(3): 564–8.

5. Sureau C. A quand les embryons aux encheres? *Rev Pract Gynecol Obstet* 2006; **107**: 7.

6. Shenfield F, Steele SJ. What are the effects of anonymity and secrecy on the welfare of the child in gamete donation? *Hum Reprod* 1997; **12**: 392–5.

7. Gollancz D. Donor insemination: a question of rights. *Hum Fertil* 2001; **4**: 164–7.

8. Golombock S, Breaways A, Cook R, *et al.* The European study of assisted reproduction families: family functioning and child development. *Hum Reprod* 1996; **11**: 2324–31.

9. Pennings G. The double track policy for donor anonymity. *Hum Reprod* 1997; **12**: 2839–44.

10. Freeman T, Jadva V, Kramer W, Golombok S. Gamete donation: parents' experiences of searching for their child's donor siblings and donor. *Hum Reprod* 2009; **24**: 505–16.

11. Scheib JE, Ruby A. Contact among families who share the same sperm donor. *Fertil Steril* 2008; **90**: 33–7.

12. McMahon C, Saunders DM. Attitudes of couples with stored frozen embryos toward conditional embryo donation. *Fertil Steril* 2009; **91**: 140–7.

13. Fuscalo G, Russell S, Gillam L. How to facilitate decisions about surplus embryos:

patients' views. *Hum Reprod* 2007; **22**: 3129–38.

14. Massaro Melamed RM, De Sousa Bonetti TC, De Almeida Ferreira Braga DP, *et al.* Deciding the fate of supernumerary frozen embryos: parents' choices. *Human Fert* 2009; **12**: 185–90.

15. Drapkin Lyerly A, Steinhauser K, Voils C, *et al.* Fertility patients' views about frozen embryo disposition: results of a multi-institutional US survey. *Fertil Steril* 2010; **2**: 499–509.

16. Provoost V, Pennings G, De Sutter P, *et al.* Patients' conceptualization of cryopreserved embryos used in their fertility treatment. *Hum Reprod* 2010; **25**: 705–13.

17. Sermon KD, Simon C, Braude P, *et al.* Creation of a registry for human embryonic stem cells carrying an inherited defect: joint collaboration between ESHRE and hESCreg. *Hum Reprod* 2009; **24**: 1556–60.

18. ESHRE Ethics and Law taskforce I. The embryo. *Hum Reprod* 2001; **16**: 1046–8.

19. ESHRE Ethics and Law taskforce IV. Stem cells. *Hum Reprod* 2002; **17**: 1409–10.

20. European Convention of Human Rights and Bioethics 1997. Available at: www.xolopo.de/ . . . /oviedo_convention_a_european_legal_ framework_15982.html.

21. Brett S, Livie M, Thomas G, McConnell A, Rajkhowa M. Report on the donation of supernumerary embryos from fresh IVF and ICSI treatment cycles for human stem cell research. *Human Fertil* 2009; **12**: 34–9.

22. Newton CR, McDermid A, Tekpetey F, Tummon IS. Embryo donation: attitudes towards donation procedures and factors predicting willingness to donate. *Hum Reprod* 2003; **18**: 878–84.

23. Hug K. Motivation to donate or not donate surplus embryos for stem-cell research: literature review. *Fertil Steril* 2008; **89**: 263–77.

24. Zweifel J, Christianson M, Jaeger A, Olive D, Lindheim SR. Needs assessment for those donating to stem cell research. *Fertil Steril* 2007; **88**: 560–4.

25. Haimes E, Taylor K. Fresh embryo donation for human embryonic stem cell (hESC) research: the experiences and values of IVF couples asked to be embryo donors. *Hum Reprod* 2009; **24**: 2142–50.

26. Evans v. U K, European Court of Human Rights 2007. Available at: www.echr.coe.int/Library/annexes/Bulletin%202008–3.

27. MacCallum F. Embryo donation parents' attitudes towards donors: comparison with adoption. *Hum Reprod* 2009: **24**: 517–23.

28. Kovacs G, Breheny S, Dear M. An audit of embryo donation at an Australian university in vitro fertilization clinic: donation and outcomes. *Med J Aust* 2003; **178**: 127–9.

29. Fuscaldo G, Savulescu J. Spare embryos: 3000 reasons to rethink the significance of genetic relatedness. *Reprod Biomed Online* 2005; **10**(2): 164–8.

30. ESHRE Ethics and Law taskforce II. The cryopreservation of human embryos. *Hum Reprod* 2001; **18**(5): 1049–50.

31. Taylor A. Embryo mix up mother will give child to biological parents. *Bionews* 2010; **527**. Available at: www.bionews.org.uk.

Chapter 16

Endometriosis and its treatment

G. David Adamson and Wendy B. Shelly

Introduction

Endometriosis is estimated to affect 6–10% of reproductive-age women. The prevalence of endometriosis is higher in the infertile population, in which it is estimated to be about 20%[1]. Though endometriosis may not be the sole cause of infertility in such patients, it is now widely believed that endometriosis reduces overall fecundity [2].

The specific role that endometriosis plays in infertility is controversial and remains an area of active study. The anatomic distortion created by scarring and adhesions from endometriosis offers a clear mechanism for reduced pregnancy rates. Adhesions disrupt necessary anatomic relationships and disrupt oocyte pick-up. Scarring can cause tubal blockage with consequent failure of sperm–oocyte interaction. However, in the absence of anatomic distortion, the cause of subfertility in endometriosis is uncertain. Various other mechanisms have also been postulated, including hormonal disruption, local inflammation and altered immune response [3]. As new scientific data emerge regarding the mechanisms of endometriosis-associated infertility, we may better tailor our management strategies in this challenging population.

Diagnosis

Pelvic pain is the most common presenting symptom of endometriosis, occurring in 80% of patients [4]. Dyspareunia and dysmenorrhea are both common, though endometriosis-associated pain can be seen throughout the menstrual cycle. Pain can vary in character and location and may even be associated with bowel activity and micturition. Endometriosis can also be pain-free and identified only when undergoing evaluation for infertility or other abdominal pathology. There appears to be no consistent relationship between pain presentation and the extent or type of endometriosis lesion. Broadly, though, clinicians usually associate endometriomas with unilateral pain, bladder lesions with bladder symptoms, bowel lesions with dyschezia or other bowel symptoms, and posterior cul-de-sac/rectovaginal septum lesions with dyspareunia.

This variability in presentation contributes to the difficulty in diagnosing endometriosis and probably accounts for the significant delay in diagnosis experienced by many patients, which averages 8–9 years. Diagnosis, first and foremost, requires a thorough history and physical examination, including rectal exam. Performance of pelvic and rectal examination at the time of menses increases the probability of detecting lesions. Ultrasonography and MRI are of variable accuracy in diagnosing deeply infiltrating endometriosis, with sensitivity

The Subfertility Handbook: A Clinician's Guide, Second Edition ed. Gab Kovacs. Published by Cambridge University Press. © Cambridge University Press 2011.

ranging between 33 and 83%, based on location of lesions [5]. Diagnostic laparoscopy or laparotomy is the only definitive way to diagnose pelvic endometriosis [6]. Laparoscopy is thought to be superior to laparotomy in the hands of an experienced surgeon due to superior visualization. Pathology, though not necessary, can be a useful adjunct in diagnosis.

Various staging systems have been proposed once endometriosis has been diagnosed. One popular staging system has been that of the American Fertility Society (now the American Society for Reproductive Medicine) in 1979 and modified in 1985 [7,8]. The prevailing complaint regarding this and other staging systems in use is their inability to predict clinical outcomes such as pregnancy rate. In an effort to address this valid concern, a new validated staging system has been designed using prospective clinical data on 801 patients and comprehensive statistical analysis. The Endometriosis Fertility Index (EFI) incorporates historical, surgical, and functional data to assign a score to each patient (Figure 16.1). This score can then be used to estimate pregnancy rate [9]. With widespread use and further validation, the EFI will hopefully provide clinicians with a tool that can facilitate treatment plans in patients with infertility as a result of endometriosis.

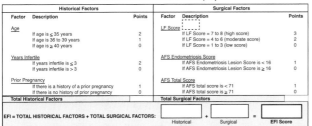

ENDOMETRIOSIS FERTILITY INDEX (EFI) SURGERY FORM

Figure 16.1 Endometriosis Fertility Index (EFI) surgery form. Image courtesy of G. David Adamson and *Fertility and Sterility* (Elsevier). See color plates.

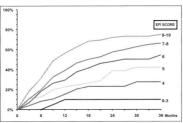

Treatment

Treatment options for patients with endometriosis are dictated by both current and long-term reproductive goals, pain symptoms and the extent of disease. In patients not actively interested in conception, medical management with progestins, gonadotropin-releasing hormone agonists and aromatase inhibitors as well as surgical resection/ablation and neurectomy offer variable control of symptoms. However, in those patients whose reproductive goals are to restore or improve fertility, medical treatment in particular has not been shown to improve pregnancy rates [10]. Interventions in fertility patients instead focus on destruction of pelvic implants and restoration of anatomy, enhancement of fertility with the aid of ovarian stimulation drugs and assisted reproductive technologies (ART) or some combination of these. It is the specific treatments available to patients with endometriosis-associated infertility on which we focus in the remainder of this chapter.

Ovarian suppression

Ovarian suppression was long held as the standard in treatment of endometriosis-associated infertility. Methods of suppression included progestins, danazol, and gonadotropin-releasing hormone agonists. One obvious shortcoming of suppressive therapy was the prolongation of infertility associated with the period of treatment, typically 6 months. Ultimately, multiple randomized controlled trials comparing the various suppression regimens and/or placebo have demonstrated no differences in treatment outcomes [10,11]. Meta-analyses have been performed by Hughes *et al.* [10] and Adamson and Pasta [12]. The pregnancy rate was not different between ovarian suppression and no treatment (relative risk (RR) 0.98, confidence interval (CI) 0.81–1.15), with no difference noted amongst the various suppression medications. Given the evidence and associated prolongation of infertility due to duration of treatment, there does not appear to be a role for ovarian suppression in the treatment of endometriosis-associated infertility.

Surgery

Surgery provides important diagnostic information regarding the extent of disease in cases of endometriosis. It is also a valuable treatment tool for endometriosis-associated infertility. Surgical intervention addresses two mechanisms proposed for infertility caused by endometriosis: the presence of endometriosis lesions and the anatomic distortion caused by adhesions and scarring. Surgical treatment of endometriosis is typically accomplished via laparotomy or laparoscopy. Though ultimately dictated by the expertise of the surgeon, laparoscopy is widely held as the surgical approach of choice in the management of endometriosis. Adamson and Pasta [12] showed that in cases of moderate to severe disease, laparoscopy was superior to laparotomy with a relative risk (RR) of pregnancy of 1.87 ($P = 0.031$). Laparoscopy offers improved visualization, which is key in evaluating the extent of disease. Laparoscopy has also been shown to reduce adhesion formation and reduce tissue trauma [13]. From the perspective of the patient, laparoscopy offers quicker recovery with little or no hospitalization time and improved cosmesis over laparotomy. Laparoscopic techniques available for the destruction of endometriosis lesions include sharp excision, laser excision or ablation, and electrosurgical excision or ablation. Though each method confers its own set of advantages and disadvantages, the method of choice is best dictated by surgeon comfort and skill level.

Surgery may also address other mechanisms by which endometriosis causes infertility by eliminating the endometriosis lesions. Research investigating the immunobiology of endometriosis has determined that the peritoneal fluid from women with endometriosis contains compounds that alter cumulus–fimbria interaction with the potential to negatively affect gamete and fallopian tube function [14]. Others have suggested that the presence of endometriosis instigates chronic inflammation and the build-up of cytotoxic leukocytes, leading to altered gamete function and poor embryo development [15–18]. Thus, surgical management may actually address multiple components of the reproductive process, leading to the increased pregnancy rates seen in patients after surgical intervention.

Observation in minimal or mild endometriosis

Despite the clinician's inclination to treat when disease has been diagnosed, there is evidence to suggest that observation alone is a reasonable option in cases of minimal or mild endometriosis. While surgery can address pain or anatomical distortion, it is of limited value in cases of minimal to mild disease. The ENDOCAN randomized controlled trial from Canada showed a higher pregnancy rate at 9 months with surgery (37.5%) vs. no treatment (22.5%), with a number needed to treat to achieve pregnancy of 7.7 [19]. A second trial from Italy did not show any difference in similarly randomized groups, with pregnancy rates of 19.6% with treatment vs. 22.2% with no treatment [20]. De novo adhesion formation after surgery is also of concern, especially in a population with minimal disease. Taking these factors into consideration, surgical intervention in this population may be of limited benefit. Thus, in at least some patients with minimal to mild disease and no other symptoms aside from the inability to conceive, observation is a viable option. The anatomical distortion typically associated with more severe endometriosis would preclude this alternative in patients with moderate to severe disease.

In considering observation in any treatment plan, thorough evaluation to determine extent of disease is obviously paramount (see Figure 16.2).

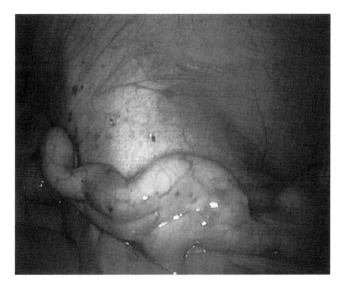

Figure 16.2 Mild endometriosis with multiple "powder-burn" lesions on pelvic sidewall. Photograph courtesy of Fertility Physicians of Northern California. See color plates.

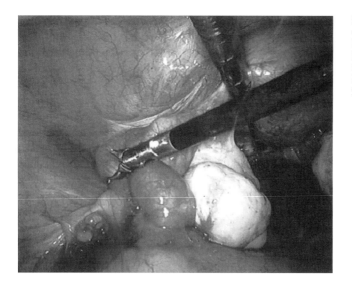

Figure 16.3 Severe endometriosis with adhesions between ovary, fallopian tube, bowel, and pelvic sidewall. Photograph courtesy of Fertility Physicians of Northern California. See color plates.

Surgery in moderate to severe endometriosis

Moderate to severe endometriosis is most often associated with significant anatomic distortion and a low spontaneous pregnancy rate if left untreated. It is widely believed that surgical intervention improves pregnancy rates by restoring anatomic relationships and reducing the impact of endometriosis lesions as addressed above. Despite this, there is a paucity of randomized data in the literature to prove this assumption. Nonetheless, given the general consensus among physicians, in the face of few data, surgical treatment is recommended in cases of moderate to severe endometriosis (see Figure 16.3). Repeat surgery has not been demonstrated to be effective by any large randomized trials. Patients who do not achieve pregnancy within a reasonable time period after appropriate surgical treatment are best served by in vitro fertilization [6].

Endometriomas

Ovarian endometriomas can be managed with either laparoscopy or laparotomy, with the cyst being removed by stripping, ablation, drainage, or excision. Complete resection of the cyst wall allows for minimal thermal exposure from electrosurgery to healthy ovarian tissue and the benefit of a pathological diagnosis. It does not appear that the number or size of the endometriomas has an impact on pregnancy outcomes. The greatest concern regarding endometrioma removal in cases of infertility is the potential loss of viable ovarian tissue and subsequent decreased ovarian reserve. Studies have shown disparate findings regarding the retention of ovarian function after operation [21–23]. The presence of an ovarian endometrioma at the time of IVF did not negatively affect pregnancy rates on meta-analysis [24]. A prospective, randomized trial of ovarian cystectomy prior to IVF versus IVF alone found poorer ovarian response in the cystectomy group, but no difference in implantation (16.5% vs. 18.5%) or pregnancy rates (34 vs. 38%) [25]. Given the outcomes of these analyses, the benefit of cystectomy for endometriomas, especially for those less than 4 cm in diameter, in the setting of IVF is questionable.

Ovarian suppression with surgery

Historically, ovarian suppression has often been used in advance of operative intervention for endometriosis. Theoretical advantages include reduced bulk of disease at time of surgery, reduced vascularity, reduced size of endometrioma and potential improvement in treatment success. Negatives for preoperative suppression therapy include potential change in the appearance of endometriosis at the time of surgery leading to incorrect assessment of extent of disease, delay in treatment as well as side effects and cost. There are no data in the literature to conclusively show benefit of preoperative treatment. Postoperative suppression treatment has been shown to be of no benefit. A Cochrane review in 2004 showed an odds ratio (OR) of 0.83 for ovarian suppression vs. no treatment [26].

Surgical treatment for endometriosis-associated infertility is thus beneficial in most circumstances. In addition to the obvious benefits of pain management and restoration of anatomy, surgery also offers accurate diagnosis and provides for well-informed management discussions with patients. Surgical intervention also allows for the possible diagnosis of other abdominal pathology which may have an impact on fertility, such as myomas. Finally, additional diagnostic procedures such as hysteroscopy can be performed concurrently, affording the opportunity to address fertility-compromising issues such as intrauterine polyps, fibroids, septae, and adhesions.

Assisted reproductive technologies

Life-table analysis performed by Adamson *et al.* found monthly fecundity rates postoperatively were 4.4% in the first year, 2.9% in the second year and 0.6% in the third year [27]. With fecundity fairly consistent for up to 9 to 15 months, it is reasonable to allow patients the opportunity to conceive for this duration prior to additional intervention. Beyond 15 months, alternative therapies should be proposed. Re-operation, as discussed above, is of limited utility if the first procedure was deemed adequate. In this setting, the most appropriate treatment is assisted reproductive technologies.

Another clinical question concerns the effect of endometriosis on IVF outcomes. Numerous deleterious effects have been proposed, including lower pregnancy rates, poorer response to stimulation, reduced number of oocytes retrieved, reduced fertilization rates, reduced implantation rates, and even poorer oocyte and embryo quality. Unfortunately, randomized controlled trials have yet to address these issues and non-randomized data are equivocal. A retrospective study found no effect of stage of endometriosis in general on pregnancy rates with IVF [28]. A meta-analysis of 22 papers assessing similar data showed a pregnancy rate OR of 0.56 (CI 0.44–0.70) in IVF cycles where endometriosis was diagnosed compared to tubal factor controls [29]. Collected data from the Society for Assisted Reproductive Technology have thus far shown no difference in pregnancy rates with IVF [30]. With this disparity in data, most clinicians do not feel that endometriosis alone has a significant impact on pregnancy rates when assisted reproductive technologies are used unless reduced ovarian reserve is present because of ovarian disease and/or prior ovarian surgery.

Complementary and alternative medicine sources

The surge in public interest in complementary and alternative medicine sources has led clinicians to consider such treatments in the management of endometriosis-associated infertility. A recent Cochrane review evaluated available scientific data regarding the efficacy of Chinese herbal medicine in the treatment of endometriosis, including the role it may play in enhancing fertility. One study contained in the review showed no difference in pregnancy rates when Chinese herbal medicine was compared to gestrinone [31]. Other practitioners have proposed acupuncture as an alternative therapy in the treatment of endometriosis-associated infertility, but no trials are yet available in the literature. Further study of complementary and alternative medicine will hopefully yield new treatment options for patients in the future.

Conclusion

Endometriosis can be a debilitating condition with respect to pain and disruption of the activities of daily living. This is further worsened when the endometriosis contributes to or causes infertility in the reproductive-age woman. An accurate diagnosis and discussion of long-term goals is paramount when choosing the most appropriate therapy. Diagnosis with thorough history-taking and physical exam can be confirmed with either laparoscopy or laparotomy. Use of staging systems such as the new Endometriosis Fertility Index can estimate outcomes with respect to fertility and offer clinicians and patients guidance when designing a treatment strategy.

Pregnancy rates are dictated by patient characteristics, extent of disease, and type of intervention. Aggregated pregnancy rates following treatment of endometriosis-associated infertility are shown in Table 16.1. In cases of minimal or mild endometriosis, observation alone offers a pregnancy rate of 2–10% per month. Life-table analysis reveals a pregnancy rate at 2 years after laparoscopic intervention at 60% for minimal or mild disease, 50% for moderate disease and 40% for severe disease [27]. Treatment options must take into account extent of disease and are tailored to specific patient goals for reproduction. They can include observation, medical management, surgery, and assisted reproductive technologies. Scientific investigation of complementary and alternative medicine may offer additional treatment options in the future. Overall, with appropriate diagnosis and the use of various treatments, the overall prognosis for pregnancy in women with endometriosis is very favorable.

Table 16.1 Pregnancy rates following treatment of endometriosis-associated infertility

Treatment	Stage / monthly fecundity (%)		
	Minimal/mild	Moderate	Severe
Expectant	3	3	0
Ovarian suppression[a]	3	4	1
Surgical	5	5	3
IVF per cycle (age< 35/35–40/ > 40)	40/30/15	40/30/15	35/25/10

[a] After discontinuation of ovarian suppression medication.

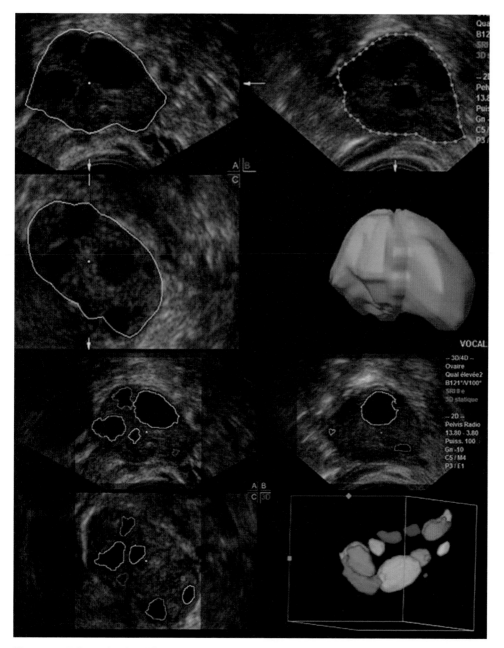

Figure 6.1 Software developed for automatic detection of follicles.

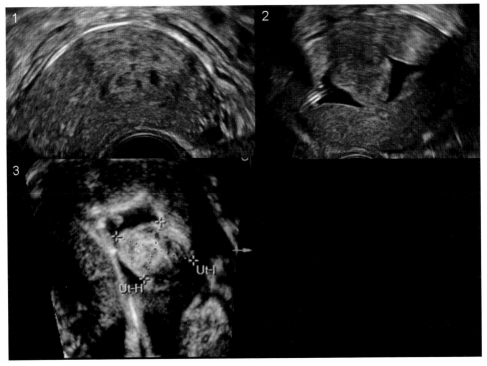

Figure 6.4 Submucosal myoma in 3D hysterosonography: (1) without preparation: localization of the myoma difficult to specify; (2) after filling: good display of intramural and intra-cavitary components (2D image); (3) reconstruction in the coronal plane (3D).

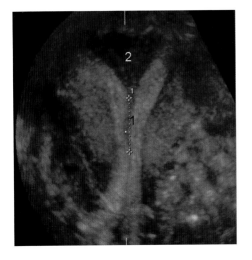

Figure 6.8 Septate uterus in 3D, with partition having a fibrous portion (1) and a muscular portion (2). Coronal reconstruction.

ENDOMETRIOSIS FERTILITY INDEX (EFI) SURGERY FORM

LEAST FUNCTION (LF) SCORE AT <u>CONCLUSION</u> OF SURGERY

Score	Description		Left		Right	
4 =	Normal	Fallopian Tube	☐	+	☐	
3 =	Mild Dysfunction					
2 =	Moderate Dysfunction	Fimbria	☐	+	☐	
1 =	Severe Dysfunction					
0 =	Absent or Nonfunctional	Ovary	☐	+	☐	

To calculate the LF score, add together the lowest score for the left side and the lowest score for the right side. If an ovary is absent on one side, the LF score is obtained by doubling the lowest score on the side with the ovary.

	Left		Right		LF Score
Lowest Score	☐	+	☐	=	☐

ENDOMETRIOSIS FERTILITY INDEX (EFI)

Historical Factors			Surgical Factors		
Factor	Description	Points	Factor	Description	Points
Age			**LF Score**		
	If age is ≤ 35 years	2		If LF Score = 7 to 8 (high score)	3
	If age is 36 to 39 years	1		If LF Score = 4 to 6 (moderate score)	2
	If age is ≥ 40 years	0		If LF Score = 1 to 3 (low score)	0
Years Infertile			**AFS Endometriosis Score**		
	If years infertile is ≤ 3	2		If AFS Endometriosis Lesion Score is < 16	1
	If years infertile is > 3	0		If AFS Endometriosis Lesion Score is ≥ 16	0
Prior Pregnancy			**AFS Total Score**		
	If there is a history of a prior pregnancy	1		If AFS total score is < 71	1
	If there is no history of prior pregnancy	0		If AFS total score is ≥ 71	0
Total Historical Factors			**Total Surgical Factors**		

EFI = TOTAL HISTORICAL FACTORS + TOTAL SURGICAL FACTORS: ☐ Historical + ☐ Surgical = ☐ EFI Score

ESTIMATED PERCENT PREGNANT BY EFI SCORE

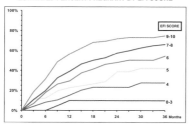

EFI SCORE
9–10
7–8
6
5
4
0–3

Figure 16.1 Endometriosis Fertility Index (EFI) surgery form. Image courtesy of G. David Adamson and *Fertility and Sterility* (Elsevier).

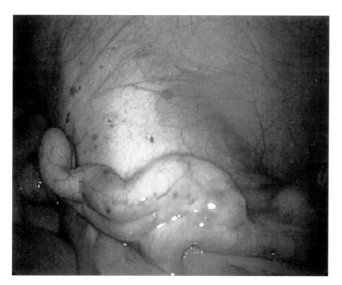

Figure 16.2 Mild endometriosis with multiple "powder-burn" lesions on pelvic sidewall. Photograph courtesy of Fertility Physicians of Northern California.

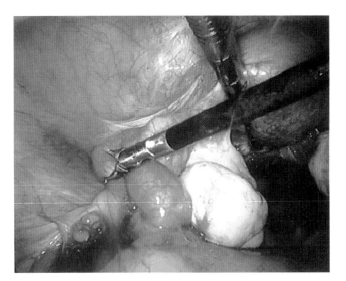

Figure 16.3 Severe endometriosis with adhesions between ovary, fallopian tube, bowel, and pelvic sidewall. Photograph courtesy of Fertility Physicians of Northern California.

References

1. Eskenazi B, Warner ML. Epidemiology of endometriosis. *Obstet Gynecol Clin North Am* 1997; **24**: 235–58.

2. Hammond MG, Jordan S, Sloan CS. Factors affecting pregnancy rates in a donor insemination program using frozen semen. *Am J Obstet Gynecol* 1986; **155**: 480–5.

3. Harada T, Iwabe T, Terakawa N. Role of cytokines in endometriosis. *Fertil Steril* 2001; **76**: 1–10.

4. Adamson GD. Diagnosis and clinical presentation of endometriosis. *Am J Obstet Gynecol* 1990; **162**: 568–9.

5. Grasso RF, Di Giacomo V, Sedati P, *et al.* Diagnosis of deep infiltrating endometriosis: accuracy of magnetic resonance imaging and transvaginal 3D ultrasonography. *Abdom Imaging* 2009 [Epub ahead of print].

6. The Practice Committee of the American Society for Reproductive Medicine. Endometriosis and infertility. *Fertil Steril* 2006; **86**(Suppl 4): S156–60.

7. American Fertility Society. Classification of endometriosis. *Fertil Steril* 1979; **32**: 633–4.

8. American Fertility Society. Revised American Fertility Society classification of endometriosis: 1985. *Fertil Steril* 1985; **43**: 351–2.

9. Adamson GD, Pasta DJ. Endometriosis fertility index: the new, validated endometriosis staging system. *Fertil Steril* 2009; in press.

10. Hughes EG, Fedorkow DM, Collins JA. A quantitative overview of controlled trials in endometriosis-associated infertility. *Fertil Steril* 1993; **59**: 963–70.

11. Olive DL, Pritts EA. The treatment of endometriosis: a review of the evidence. *Ann NY Acad Sci* 2002; **955**: 360–72.

12. Adamson GD, Pasta DJ. Surgical treatment of endometriosis-associated infertility: meta-analysis compared with survival analysis. *Am J Obstet Gynecol* 1994; **171**: 1488–504.

13. Operative Laparoscopy Study Group. Postoperative adhesion development following operative laparoscopy: evaluation at early second-look procedures. *Fertil Steril* 1991; **55**: 700–4.

14. Suginami H, Yano K. An ovum capture inhibitor (OCI) in endometriosis peritoneal fluid: an OCI-related membrane responsible for fimbrial failure of ovum capture. *Fertil Steril* 1988; **50**: 648–53.

15. Halme J, Becker S, Hammond MG, Raj MH, Raj S. Increased activation of pelvic macrophages in infertile women with mild endometriosis. *Am J Obstet Gynecol* 1983; **145**: 333–7.

16. Olive DL, Weinberg JB, Haney AF. Peritoneal macrophages and infertility: the association between cell number and pelvic pathology. *Fertil Steril* 1985; **44**: 772–7.

17. Oral E, Arici A, Olive DL, Huszar G. Peritoneal fluid from women with moderate or severe endometriosis inhibits sperm motility: the role of seminal fluid components. *Fertil Steril* 1996; **66**: 787–92.

18. Morcos RN, Gibbons WE, Findley WE. Effect of peritoneal fluid on in vitro cleavage of 2-cell mouse embryos: possible role in infertility associated with endometriosis. *Fertil Steril* 1985; **44**: 678–83.

19. Marcoux S, Maheux R, Berube S. Laparoscopic surgery in infertile women with minimal or mild endometriosis. *N Engl J Med* 1997; **337**: 217–22.

20. Gruppo Italiano per lo Studio dell' Endometriosi. Ablation of lesions or no treatment in minimal-mild endometriosis in infertile women: a randomized trial. *Hum Reprod* 1999; **14**: 1332–4.

21. Marconi G, Vilela M, Quintana R, Sueldo C. Laparoscopic ovarian cystectomy of endometriomas does not affect the ovarian response to gonadotropin stimulation. *Fertil Steril* 2002; **78**: 876–8.

22. Loh FH, Tan AT, Kumar J, Ng SC. Ovarian response after laparoscopic ovarian cystectomy for endometriotic cysts in 132 monitored cycles. *Fertil Steril* 1999; **72**: 316–21.

23. Canis M, Pouly JL, Tamburro S, *et al.* Ovarian response during IVF-embryo

transfer cycles after laparoscopic ovarian cystectomy for endometriotic cysts of > 3 cm in diameter. *Hum Reprod* 2001; **16**: 2583–6.

24. Gupta S, Agarwal A, Agarwal R, Loret de Mola JR. Impact of ovarian endometriomas on assisted reproduction outcomes. *Reprod Biomed Online* 2006; **13**: 349–60.

25. Demirol A, Guven S, Baykal C, Gurgan T. Effect of endometrioma cystectomy on IVF outcome: a prospective randomized study. *Reprod Biomed Online* 2006; **12**: 639–43.

26. Yap C, Furness S, Farquhar C. Pre and post operative medical therapy for endometriosis surgery. *Cochrane Database Syst Rev* 2004; **3**: CD003678.

27. Adamson GD, Hurd SJ, Pasta DJ, Rodriguez BD. Laparoscopic endometriosis treatment: is it better? *Fertil Steril* 1993; **59**: 35–44.

28. Olivennes F, Feldberg D, Liu HC, *et al*. Endometriosis: a stage by stage analysis – the role of in vitro fertilization. *Fertil Steril* 1995; **64**: 392–8.

29. Barnhart K, Dunsmoor-Su R, Coutifaris C. Effect of endometriosis on in vitro fertilization. *Fertil Steril* 2002; **77**: 1148–55.

30. Society for Assisted Reproductive Technology, American Society for Reproductive Medicine. Assisted reproductive technology in the United States: 2000 results generated from the American Society for Reproductive Medicine/Society for Assisted Reproductive Technology Registry. *Fertil Steril* 2004; **81**: 1207–20.

31. Flower A, Liu JP, Chen S, Lewith G, Little P. Chinese herbal medicine for endometriosis. *Cochrane Database Syst Rev* 2009; **3**: CD006568.

The role of surgery in female subfertility

B. Hédon, H. Déchaud and C. Dechanet

Introduction

Surgery was, not so long ago, the only means to alleviate female subfertility in many situations, when the pelvic organs developed abnormally or were altered by an acquired, often infectious, disease. Techniques have been developed, using the classical open route through the abdominal wall, with, in some situations, the use of magnification in order to increase the accuracy of surgical repair [1]. More recently, endoscopic techniques have replaced the majority of the open techniques, producing a less invasive and potentially less destructive surgery [2].

Today, the place of surgery is questioned by the wide use of assisted procreation techniques. Their efficacy is demonstrated in many situations when not so long ago surgery would have been the only possible option. Infertility specialists tend to be more specialized in assisted procreation than in reproductive surgery, and naturally favor the procedures with which they feel at ease. Even the patients consider surgical procedures as being more invasive and potentially more risky than an attempt at assisted procreation.

Nevertheless, surgical procedures are part of the global management an infertility center should be able to offer to its patients. There are cases when surgery is a better choice for the patient and should be offered as first-line therapy. There are cases when surgery should come as back-up therapy when assisted procreation has failed. There are also cases when surgery is necessary before assisted procreation in order to optimize the chances of obtaining a pregnancy.

Moreover, reproductive surgery is not only a reconstructive surgery aimed at a better functioning of the reproductive organs, but it is also more and more a preventive procedure, aimed at the protection and the conservation of the reproductive potential when it is put at risk because of a malignant disease and potentially sterilizing therapies.

For all these reasons, reproductive surgery must be part of the training program of infertility specialists. Whether the same physicians must be both surgeons and assisted procreation specialists is debatable. But reproductive surgeons and assisted procreation specialists must be part of the same team and be able to discuss each case in order to offer the best possible treatment scheme for the patient. It is using this approach that the best potential cumulative pregnancy rate can be offered [3].

Note: Surgery of ectopic pregnancies and surgery of endometriosis, both diseases that can require surgery for their treatment, with potential reproductive consequences, are not covered in this chapter and should be found in the corresponding chapters.

The Subfertility Handbook: A Clinician's Guide, Second Edition ed. Gab Kovacs. Published by Cambridge University Press. © Cambridge University Press 2011.

Reconstructive surgery of pelvic organs

Tubes

Treating tubal damage requires not only an appropriate surgical technique, but also a profound knowledge of tubal physiology and pathophysiology. Fallopian tubes cannot be considered as mere plumbing pipes for which patency is the alpha and the omega of diagnosis. Reproductive surgeons know that the tubes are active functional organs. Patency is of course required, but also a good potential function, with a mucosa safeguarding a proper percentage of ciliated and mucosal cells, and a tubal wall with a good muscular layer. Some parts of the tubes require special attention: the fimbria plays a specific role for the capturing of the oocyte. Moreover, a minimal tubal length is necessary, in particular for the ampulla.

Distal disease

Hydrosalpinx is the most common pathological finding. It results from the complete obstruction of the tubal distal ostium because of the coalescence of the fimbriae between themselves. Infertility results from the lack of patency, but also from the transport deficiency of the fimbria, as well as from the cellular destruction of the ciliated cells that should be at a high density in this part of the tube.

The surgical procedure to alleviate this condition is called "neosalpingostomy" because it results in the creation of a neo-ostium surrounded by a neo-fimbria. A crucial key is the re-establishment of a proper tubo-ovarian relationship with the tubo-ovarian fimbria bridging the two organs and conducting the egg towards the tubal lumen.

When disease has not reached the stage of a complete distal tubal obstruction with accumulation of mucus and tubal distension, the condition is described as being a "phymosis". The distal tubal plasty in order to recreate a fimbria is called a "fimbrioplasty".

These procedures are nowadays commonly performed via laparoscopy [4]. The expected results depend on the quality of the surgery performed, but the main limitation comes from the intensity of the initial disease and the subsequent sequelae [5]. Various scores have been described in order to classify the selection of patients who can take advantage of surgery, and refer the others directly for IVF [6].

Proximal disease

Two different conditions have been described as "proximal disease": There are cases with pure tubal obstruction, without involvement and destruction of the tubal wall. These cases are described as "intraluminal plug", or simple coalescence of the mucosa in this narrow part of the tube. Re-establishing patency can be done by selective catheterization of the uterine tubal ostium followed by injection of liquid under pressure in the tubal lumen. This simple procedure can be done either under radiological control (and in this case it is usually performed by the radiologist at the time of hysterosalpingography) or under hysteroscopic control. In this latter case, it is performed by the reproductive gynecologist and the procedure is often linked with a laparoscopic evaluation of the pelvis and a dye test, which allows one to check the re-establishment of patency.

The results of these cures of pure proximal tubal obstruction are often good. Not only does the absence of tubal damage maximize the chances of obtaining normal functioning tubes once their patency has been restored, but also it is possible that the proximal obstruction has played the opportune role of protecting the distal part of the tube from being involved by the spread of the infectious and inflammatory disease.

The other condition is called "salpingitis isthmica nodosa". It is characterized by a parietal destruction of the proximal part of the tube, where the muscular layer is more developed. The tubal wall is invaded by diverticulae surrounded by an intense fibrosis. These diverticulae are open in the tubal lumen and often lined by endometrial cells. This histological condition has brought some confusion with endometriosis, but, in this case, it is clearly of infectious origin.

Surgically, it is possible to dissect the fibrotic node from the surrounding uterine muscular layers and to reanastomose the tube after suppression of the diseased part. This can be done with a microsurgical technique only, via a laparotomy [7]. Results depend on the severity of the disease and the quality of the tubal reanastomosis.

Key points:

- Tubal pathological conditions are usually bilateral, even though not always strictly symmetrical
- Bifocal lesions (proximal and distal on the same tube) are the equivalent of multifocal lesions, contraindicating reconstructive surgery
- In the case of asymmetry of disease, the better tube makes the prognosis.

Tubo-tubal anastomosis for reversal of sterilization

In theory, this should be the ideal situation in order to recover a normal tubal function after the re-establishment of patency [8]. The results of reversal of sterilisation by tubo-tubal anastomosis depend on:

- the remaining length of the tube, and in particular of the ampulla; a minimal length of 2 cm of ampulla is required
- the localization of the tubal interruption: an isthmo-isthmic reanastomosis is preferable to an isthmo-ampullary anastomosis (luminal discrepancy between both parts) and to an ampullo-ampullary anastomosis
- the type of severing of the tube done at the time of sterilization: an electric cauterization creates more damage than a surgical ligation or a tubal ring or a tubal clip
- the time since the sterilization: not only does the more time elapsed since sterilization mean that the patient is older, but also tubal damage and deciliation can develop in the ligated tube.

No study has been performed in order to compare the results of assisted procreation and surgery in this specific case of sterilization reversal. Both techniques depend very much on age of the patient. Because of the effectiveness of surgery and also because of potential ovarian stimulation difficulties encountered in older patients, surgery should be preferred in most situations.

Ovaries

Ovarian drilling

Ovarian drilling is done via laparoscopy in clomiphene-resistant PCO patients.

The procedure consists of puncturing the ovarian capsule with electric cautery or laser, in order to make four to ten holes through the cortex down to the medulla of each ovary. It is a common finding that ovarian drilling is usually followed in anovulatory PCO patients by several cycles with a normal ovulation.

A meta-analysis of nine prospective controlled trials comparing the efficacy of ovarian drilling and of gonadotropins for the treatment of infertility concludes there is a similar chance of obtaining a live birth, but with a significantly decreased risk of developing a hyperstimulation syndrome or obtaining a multiple gestation after an ovarian drilling [9].

Nevertheless, ovarian drilling is a second-intention therapy, in clomiphene-resistant PCO patients only, and should be a unique procedure, a repeat drilling carrying the potential risk of creating an ovarian deficiency.

Cystectomy

Ovarian cysts are not associated with infertility, except in the case of endometriosis. Nevertheless, surgery of benign ovarian cysts is considered as being a standard gynecological procedure, but carries the potential risk of creating an ovarian insufficiency with infertility. For this reason, a proper technique must be applied. Usually performed under the laparoscope, an ovarian cystectomy should preserve as much normal ovarian tissue as possible. Repeat or multiple cystectomies are specially at risk of subsequent ovarian deficiency and should always be avoided [10].

Uterus

Uterine septum

The presence of an abnormal uterine septum is associated with an increased risk of missed abortion and premature birth. For these obstetrical reasons, section of the septum is often proposed in infertile patients, with the main reason that in the case of a pregnancy, a good deal of risk can be avoided.

In fact, experience in patients treated by assisted procreation techniques shows that embryos implant with a higher frequency when both uterine cavities, separated by the abnormal septum, have been reunified.

Section of a uterine septum is nowadays a hysteroscopic technique, after considering the thickness of the uterine fundus [11]. In this regard it is necessary to differentiate between a double uterus, where the division includes both the cavity and the uterine wall, in which section of the septum cannot be performed, and a so-called septate uterus where the uterine corpus is unique. This diagnosis can be made with a proper ultrasonographic evaluation of the uterus, as well as by magnetic resonance imaging and/or laparoscopy.

Myoma

Uterine myomas are frequently found in infertile patients, but their implication in the infertility process is often unclear. For this reason the surgical treatment of myomas in infertile patients cannot be standardized. Sub-mucous myomas are associated with a significant reduction in live birth rates (70 %), while intramural fibroids decrease this rate by 30%. Sub-serous myomas are not associated with a decrease in birth rates.

Sub-mucous myomas should be treated by hysteroscopic resection. Limits of this technique are: volume of the myoma (< 10 cm), development of the myoma in the interstitium (more than half of the volume should be protruding in the cavity in order to benefit from hysteroscopic resection) and volume of the uterine cavity (if the cavity is enlarged, the uterus is globally fibrotic, and results of hysteroscopic resection are altered).

Hysteroscopic resection has gained in safety since the use of isoosmotic saline solutions, bipolar electrodes and controlled intrauterine pressure of the liquid injected for distension and lavage [12]. Hysteroscopic resection of fibroids is commonly followed one or two months later, after the menses, by a hysteroscopic review in order to detect a starting synechia on the wound of the resection. This viscous adhesion could, with time, develop into a fibrotic adhesion, more difficult to treat. When detected early, it is easily cured by the distension of the cavity with the distension liquid and the hysteroscope.

In some cases, the volume of the sub-mucous myoma necessitates several procedures in order to complete resection and re-establish a near-normal uterine cavity.

Interstitial myomas are treated by conservative myomectomy. This can be done via the laparoscope, depending on the volume, the situation of the myoma and the number of myomas present. Only experienced laparoscopic surgeons should undertake such a procedure as it can be very hemorrhagic and dissecting the myoma from the surrounding uterine tissue is sometimes quite difficult.

In a majority of cases, interstitial myomas are best treated via a laparotomy. Special care must be undertaken in order to avoid postoperative adhesions. Careful tissue handling and hemostasis, as well as meticulous repair of the uterine surface, are the best prevention. The use of anti-adhesion barriers can, in selected cases, add some preventive efficacy.

The main concern with interstitial fibroid myomectomy is the indication [13]. Its efficacy in order to improve the fertility of the patient is debatable. In patients older than 35 years with more than 2 years of infertility, its benefit is not significant [14].

Polyps, synechiae

Their detection is part of the infertility work-up, because they interfere with embryo implantation and development. Intrauterine anomalies are a cause of infertility and their correction is needed both in order to try and alleviate infertility in the couple and allow a spontaneous pregnancy to occur, and also before any assisted procreation. Results of hysteroscopic treatment of intrauterine anomalies are very encouraging.

Peritoneum

Peritoneal disease associated with infertility is represented by adhesions [15]. They are caused by the inflammatory process associated with infection in cases of pelvic inflammatory disease. They can also occur after surgery, in particular when a significant amount of tissue handling has been necessary, or when tissues are severed and hemostasis is incomplete. Adhesions are also part of the endometriotic syndrome and in this case are often intimate, fibrotic, and difficult to alleviate without risk for the organs involved. This type of adhesion tends to recur, whatever surgical precaution is taken. They fix a limit to pelvic reconstructive surgery, whose principles should always be:

- pelvic reconstructive surgery for treatment of infertility is indicated only if sufficient pelvic repair can be obtained in order to improve the chances for the woman to get pregnant
- pelvic reconstructive surgery should not put at risk the other organs situated in the pelvis
- pelvic reconstructive surgery is useless if repeat disease is highly probable.

Surgical preparation of assisted procreation

Salpingectomy

There are now several prospective randomized studies giving consistent indications that a diseased tube can impair embryo implantation when transferred into the uterine cavity after in vitro fertilization.

In patients with hydrosalpinges, a meta-analysis of five randomized controlled trials shows that there is a benefit in favor of salpingectomy before IVF in comparison with no surgery. Not only is the pregnancy rate increased, but also the rate of live births [16].

There are discussions about whether all hydrosalpinges are deleterious, or only the bigger ones as detected by ultrasound, and whether it is more the inflammatory status of the tube that needs to be treated rather than the hydrosalpinx itself. If salpingectomy has proven to be efficient in improving the implantation rate of embryos, the same evidence does not exist yet in favor of proximal tubal occlusion (interrupting the flow of tubal mucous towards the uterine cavity) or in favor of salpingostomy (allowing tubal drainage towards the abdominal cavity).

The consensus is that salpingectomy should be performed only in patients with severe tubal disease, unable to take advantage of pelvic reconstructive surgery, and whose chances rely solely on assisted procreation [17].

In the case of unilateral hydrosalpinx, ablation of the diseased tube has been shown to improve both the chances of obtaining a spontaneous pregnancy (via the remaining tube) and the chances of obtaining an embryo implantation after IVF.

Uterine septum

Resection of a significant uterine septum before IVF is associated with an improved pregnancy rate after embryo transfer. Some surgeons tend to wait after one or two implantation failures, but, because the hysteroscopic procedure is well standardized and bears a minimal risk, section of the septum is usually done before any embryo transfer.

Other procedures

Adhesiolysis or previous surgical treatment of endometriosis is not associated with a subsequent improved pregnancy rate after IVF. They are not recommended when IVF is indicated, unless there is a reason such as pain or other pathological condition requiring a specific treatment.

Surgical procedures for prevention of infertility

Protection of ovaries

The surgical procedures aimed at placing the ovaries in a protected area are more and more obsolete. They are of course useless in the case of chemotherapy. It is only in specific cases of radiotherapy, and in particular when local radiotherapy is applied for the treatment of cervical cancer, that displacing the ovaries has some rationale.

Results are disappointing and often inconsistent and unpredictable. For these reasons, displacing techniques are currently no longer performed and are replaced by preventive ovariectomy in order to cryopreserve the ovocytic potential of the ovary.

Cryopreservation of ovaries

Consensus is that cryopreservation of ovarian tissue should be proposed whenever a sterilizing treatment becomes necessary in a young girl or woman who has not completed her family.

Techniques are not fully evolved yet, and numerous discussions take place between those who advocate cryopreservation of the whole ovary and those who prefer to take parts of the ovaries or even superficial bands containing the primordial follicles [18].

Similarly, when usage of the tissues becomes necessary, there is no specific technique that demonstrates its superiority. The ovary can be replaced in vivo in order to allow in vivo maturation of the follicles and IVF is performed. Others rely on in vitro maturation before IVF.

There is a chance that ovocyte vitrification can gain in efficacy and replace cryopreservation of ovarian tissue whenever a follicular stimulation can be performed before applying the sterilizing treatment [19].

Conclusion

Fertility enhancement surgical techniques are numerous and require both surgical skills and a thorough knowledge of human reproduction physiology and pathology. They are best practiced by infertility centers which can offer a global service to infertile couples. If a center is specialized in assisted procreation techniques, the temptation is high to treat every patient with these techniques and to forget the proper place of surgery. On the other hand, an isolated surgeon, whatever his skills, will never be able to offer the best pregnancy rates possible if he considers surgery as the only choice to offer to the patient. Cases must be individually considered and discussed between infertility specialists with surgical and endoscopic potential as well as with direct access to assisted procreation whenever required.

References

1. Hedon B, Wineman M, Winston RML. Loupes or microscope for tubal anastomosis? An experimental study. *Fertil Steril* 1980; **34**: 264.

2. Tulandi T. Reconstructive tubal surgery by laparoscopy. *Obstet Gynecol Surv* 1987; **42**: 193–8.

3. Audibert F, Hedon B, Arnal F, *et al.* Therapeutic strategies in tubal infertility with distal pathology. *Hum Reprod* 1991; **6**: 1439–42.

4. Ahmad G, Watson AJ, Metwally M. Laparoscopy or laparotomy for distal tubal surgery? A meta-analysis. *Hum Fertil* 2007; **10**: 43–7.

5. Audebert AJ, Pouly JL, Von Theobald P. Laparoscopic fimbrioplasty: an evaluation of 35 cases. *Hum Reprod* 1998; **13**: 1496–9.

6. Mage G, Pouly JL, de Joliniere JB, *et al.* A preoperative classification to predict the intrauterine and ectopic pregnancy rates after distal tubal microsurgery. *Fertil Steril* 1986; **46**: 807–10.

7. Dubuisson JB, Chapron C, Ansquer Y, Vacher-Lavenu MC. Proximal tubal occlusion: is there an alternative to microsurgery? *Hum Reprod* 1997; **12**: 692–8.

8. Gomel V. Tubal reanastomosis by microsurgery. *Fertil Steril* 1977; **28**: 59–65.

9. Farquhar C, Lilford RJ, Marjoribanks J, Vandekerckhove P. Laparoscopic 'drilling' by diathermy or laser for ovulation induction in anovulatory polycystic ovary syndrome. *Cochrane Database Syst Rev*

2007; **3**: CD001122. doi: 10.1002/14651858. CD001122.pub3.

10. Canis M, Pouly JL, Tamburro S, *et al.* Ovarian response during IVF-embryo transfer cycles after laparoscopic ovarian cystectomy for endometriotic cysts of > 3 cm in diameter. *Hum Reprod* 2001; **16**: 2583–6.

11. Zabak K, Benifla JL, Uzan S. Septate uterus and reproduction disorders: current results of hysteroscopic septoplasty. *Gynecol Obstet Fertil* 2001; **29**: 829–40.

12. Griffiths A, D'Angelo A, Amso N. Surgical treatment of fibroids for subfertility. *Cochrane Database Syst Rev* 2006; **3**: CD003857. doi: 10.1002/14651858. CD003857.pub2.

13. Pritts EA, Parker WH, Olive DL. Fibroids and infertility: an updated systematic review of the evidence. *Fertil Steril* 2009; **91**: 1215–23.

14. Vercellini P, Maddalena S, De Giorgi O, *et al.* Determinants of reproductive outcome after abdominal myomectomy for infertility. *Fertil Steril* 1999; **72**: 109–14.

15. Bruhat MA, Mage G, Manhes H, *et al.* Laparoscopy procedures to promote fertility ovariolysis and salpingolysis. Results of 93 selected cases. *Acta Eur Fertil* **14**: 113–15.

16. Strandell A, Waldenstrom U, Nilsson L, Hamberger L. Hydrosalpinx reduces in-vitro fertilization/embryo transfer pregnancy rates. *Hum Reprod* 1994; **9**: 861–3.

17. Dechaud H, Daures JP, Arnal F, Humeau C, Hedon B. Does previous salpingectomy improve implantation and pregnancy rates in patients with severe tubal factor infertility who are undergoing in vitro fertilization ? A pilot prospective randomized study. *Fertil Steril* 1998; **69**: 1020–5.

18. Donnez J, Dolmans M, Demylle D, *et al.* Livebirth after orthotopic transplantation of cryopreserved ovarian tissue. *Lancet* 2004; **364**(9443): 1405–10.

19. Porcu E, Venturoli S, Damiano G, *et al.* Healthy twins delivered after oocyte cryopreservation and bilateral ovariectomy for ovarian cancer. *Reprod Biomed Online* 2008; **17**: 265–7.

Chapter 18

Laboratory techniques in IVF

George A. Thouas and David K. Gardner

Introduction

Since their adaptation from animal and veterinary sciences in the 1970s, clinical embryology laboratories around the world have functioned as purpose-built biotechnology facilities dedicated to preimplantation embryo production by in vitro fertilization (IVF), using assisted reproduction technologies (ARTs). Typically, patients are treated by obstetrics and gynecology specialists using the procedures of oocyte retrieval and embryo replacement, with intervention in the interim from embryologists engaged in gamete and embryo micro-manipulation, culture, and storage. While these laboratories house specialized technologies for use in multi-step procedures, they remain heavily dependent on careful, dedicated, and responsible manual operation by highly trained personnel.

ART procedures are similar between laboratories and countries. Importantly, the legislative regulation of clinical ART practices is relatively strict, and under continuous revision, owing to the unique level of responsibility imparted to any person licensed to handle human gametes and embryos for reproductive purposes. There is a necessity for rigorous standardization of procedures, reporting, and implementation of safety measures, both internally and externally. Amongst these requirements is the ongoing need for quality control of the IVF laboratory, to ensure a consistent level of embryo quality, which, together with an acceptable standard of treatment outcomes, forms a quality management system. This chapter will provide an overview of current and future practices in IVF laboratories, with discussion of key biological and logistical considerations that optimize embryo quality and subsequent pregnancy outcomes.

Management of IVF laboratory practices

It is important to consider that IVF laboratories are multifactorial systems, with many individual factors contributing cumulatively to influence embryo quality, which is ultimately reflected in clinical pregnancy outcomes. These factors include the embryologists, laboratory environment in which they work, and the procedures that they perform. No single laboratory variable should be considered less significant than the next, from a clinical management perspective. Indeed, in order to optimize the IVF treatment cycle, it is imperative to consider all procedures in a holistic fashion, given their impact on each other (Figure 18.1).

In common with any biotechnology facility for the handling and culture of live tissue in vitro, appropriate levels of containment and biosafety are also necessarily maintained.

The Subfertility Handbook: A Clinician's Guide, Second Edition ed. Gab Kovacs. Published by Cambridge University Press. © Cambridge University Press 2011.

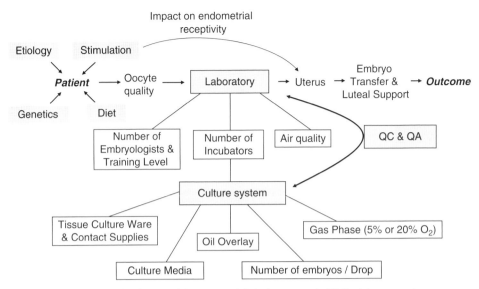

Figure 18.1 Interrelationships between laboratory and clinical outcomes in IVF. The laboratory culture system, operated by the embryologist, is composed of multiple steps that constitute embryo production. Compromise in any of these steps can potentially impact on embryo quality. These steps mediate the transition from oocyte to transferable embryo, and are subject to internal quality control. Modified from reference 26.

Attention will be paid in this section to description of the basic aspects of IVF laboratory conditions, operation, safety procedures, and quality control.

Managing the laboratory environment

Design and environmental control factors are of particular importance to ART laboratories, in addition to the standard legal requirements for medical laboratories. A range of unique architectural and structural considerations influence the establishment of IVF laboratories, including the choice and chemical composition of building materials and number of wall and ceiling penetrations [1]. These latter two factors can have a direct bearing on the internal leaching of airborne organics, as well as introduction of external airborne contaminants. Hence control of air handling in an established laboratory represents an example of an environmental control parameter; preventative measures such as HEPA filtration for sub-micron airborne particulates, and activated carbon filtration for airborne organics have also been recommended. This and other aspects of quality assurance/control (QA/QC) have been extensively discussed in the wider context of total quality management [2].

Containment represents another basic security and safety consideration, effective at several levels. Restriction of access to qualified personnel represents a higher level of containment, with a further subdivision of laboratory space forming part of or adjoining an operating room complex. This common practice of restricting access to clinical and nursing staff, operating room staff, patients, and embryologists limits the transmission of airborne pathogens, carried by aerosols generated from living tissue, biological fluids, and the solutions used to contain them. The cohabitation of laboratories within surgical suites also facilitates the direct hand-over of follicle aspirates and biopsy material directly to the embryologist, while allowing for maintenance of aseptic conditions during the embryo production process. To this end, biohazard containment hoods are widely employed as a secondary containment system, providing a working environment that: (a) protects embryologists from airborne pathogens originating in the sample; (b) prevents spread of pathogens to the samples from embryologists and other personnel; and (c) prevents cross-contamination between samples, or to other laboratory areas. Such precautions are imperative in isolated cases where patients are carriers or sufferers of known virulent pathogens such as hepatitis B/C and HIV.

Laboratory personnel

Maintenance of containment, safety, hygiene, and environmental monitoring are integral to the routine operating procedures of a clinical IVF laboratory, at the level of the embryologist. Routine safety precautions such as protective barrier equipment and disinfection are intended to prevent pathogen transmission. A practical example is the correct containment of medical waste such as sorted follicle aspirates, tissue biopsies, and spent consumables. Other safety measures protect against non-biological hazards (manual handling, chemical, temperature, etc.) associated with microscopy, cryopreservation, reagent handling, and sanitation. Examples of the more dangerous hazards include the potential for asphyxia from exposure to liquid nitrogen, and repetitive strain injury during micromanipulation. Often, IVF protocols contain combinations of hazards, including biological and manual handling hazards associated with sharps and glass pipettes.

In spite of responsible occupational safety standards for maintained well-being of the embryologist, their occupational performance can still impact on the output of the IVF laboratory, with regard to the number of personnel, level of expertise, and compliance with established protocols. Inconsistencies in embryo production, due to continual minor perturbations such as incubator over-use, prolonged or continual exposure of the embryos to non-physiological conditions and manual handling artifacts can all have detrimental cumulative affects on outcomes. Investment in appropriate training and ongoing monitoring of procedures is therefore essential, with the recommendation that all laboratory staff undergo a biannual review of all procedures.

Managing embryo quality

Control of variables within the laboratory environment, including the operation of specific technology and how specific protocols are performed (e.g. incubation times, oxygen or carbon dioxide levels within incubators, microinjection efficiency), all combine to influence embryo quality. While there is a host of known variables that adversely affect the developmental and implantation potential of the embryo, when such factors are controlled collectively measurable improvements in these outcomes can be obtained [3].

Specific laboratory QC tests, including the mouse embryo assay (MEA) and the sperm motility assay, have been developed over several decades, originating from methods in experimental embryology to assess the embryo-toxicity of laboratory components used for clinical IVF [4]. Unless tested using such assays, it is best to consider all contact supplies as potentially toxic. Ultimately the best quality indicator measure remains the consistency of laboratory output parameters, including fertilization rate, embryo score, and implantation rate [5].

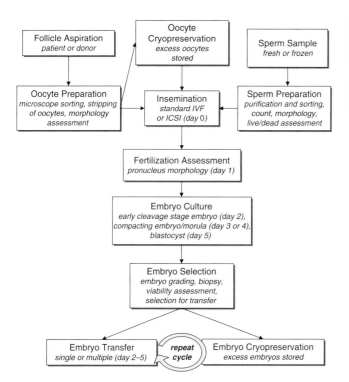

Figure 18.2 Work-flow of a typical IVF laboratory. Diagrammatic representation of the procedures involved in IVF, starting with gamete manipulation and insemination, followed by embryo manipulation, culture, transfer, and storage.

Choice of laboratory protocols and work-flow

Following gonadotropin stimulation for the recruitment of several follicles to facilitate the collection of multiple mature oocytes, follicular contents are aspirated surgically using transvaginal ultrasound-guided needle biopsy. On the same day, spermatozoa are purified from ejaculates produced by the male partner or donor. The IVF procedure begins at the time of surgery on day 0, when the embryologist performs the basic procedures outlined in Figure 18.2.

This work-flow forms the backbone of a typical IVF laboratory. Laboratory personnel are assigned to specific tasks in this process, depending on the workload, patient requirements, and operating room schedule. Each task requires a specific range of equipment and supplies available in the IVF laboratory, either transiently or continuously (Table 18.1).

While the procedures and equipment are widely available and implemented in a relatively standard fashion across laboratories, there are minor variations in preference. Examples include differences in the source and type of culture media and consumables, specific culture conditions, embryologist differences in routine handling steps during oocyte treatments, choice of embryo handling instruments (e.g. pipetting techniques), and a host of others. Standardization of the consistency of lab protocols may suffice to prevent sudden declines in embryo quality and implantation rate, which can occur randomly, and are difficult to diagnose. Prevention is therefore the main method of procedural control, dependent on continued vigilance of embryology practices, and the implementation of and commitment to a quality management system [2].

Table 18.1 Equipment requirements for IVF protocols

List of equipment required for a typical IVF laboratory, listed with corresponding methods and indications according to which is used. Note that multiple equipment and consumables are often used for one protocol, which represents increased manual handling and risk to laboratory outcomes.

Laboratory equipment	IVF procedure								
	Oocyte preparation	Sperm preparation	Insemination	Fertilization check	Embryo culture	Embryo biopsy	Embryo selection	Embryo transfer	Cryo-preservation
Biohazard laminar flow hood	•	•	•			•			•
Upright stereomicroscope			•						
Micropipettor	•	•	•	•	•	•	•	•	•
Inverted stereo-microscope				•		•	•	•	
Compound microscope						•			
Centrifuge		•	•						
Micromanipulators and microtools						•			
Cytometer		•					•		
Nutrient media	•	•	•		•	•		•	•
Benchtop balance	•	•			•				
Refrigerator	•	•	•	•	•	•			•
Freezer	•	•	•	•	•	•			•
Disposable plasticware (Petri dishes, tubes, syringes, pipettes, etc.)	•	•	•		•	•	•	•	•
Benchtop tools (e.g. warming plates, tube holders)	•	•	•	•	•	•	•	•	•

Table 18.1 (cont.)

Laboratory equipment	IVF procedure								
	Oocyte preparation	Sperm preparation	Insemination	Fertilization check	Embryo culture	Embryo biopsy	Embryo selection	Embryo transfer	Cryopreservation
Liquid-handling tools	•	•	•	•	•	•		•	•
Cell culture incubators with gas supply	•		•	•	•	•			
Slow freezing machine									•
Liquid nitrogen (supply and storage tanks)		•							•
Cryopreservation tools (storage containers, vitrification equipment)		•							•
Viability detection device							•		
Imaging equipment						•	•		
Zona-drilling laser						•			

In summary, the IVF laboratory represents a dedicated biomedical facility operating in conjunction with clinical procedures for the treatment of infertile and subfertile couples. The level of ethical and technical responsibility in operating these laboratories imparts unique regulatory considerations, owing to the specialized technique of manual oocyte insemination, embryo production and replacement. It should be emphasized that the conditions and competence that reside within a modern embryology laboratory have a significant impact on the outcome of an IVF cycle. The following section will discuss current practices in clinical IVF laboratories in relation to embryo quality as a key laboratory outcome.

Oocyte and embryo manipulation

Standard insemination

The method of standard IVF involves insemination of mature oocytes with a known concentration of spermatozoa purified from an ejaculate, using a variety of separation methods. The two preferred techniques are density gradient centrifugation ($\approx$20 min) and swim-up ($\approx$30–60 min), which are often performed in tandem. The gradient method is recommended since it can markedly reduce the percentage of chromatin-damaged sperm in the extract [6]. Standard IVF protocols have changed little since their original clinical applications, as far as the basic steps of co-incubation of sperm and oocytes for a known period in a dedicated medium, followed by manual removal of excess zona-bound sperm and re-incubation of the inseminated oocyte in fresh culture medium. Variations in this technique typically include optimization of the sperm exposure time (short: 1–4 hours, or long: 16–20 hours) and sperm concentration per oocyte (low: 10–25 000/ml, or up to 100 000/ml), depending on sperm quality, with a general preference for short exposures at low concentrations. Normal fertilization is then indicated after 18–24 hours by the presence of a single male and female pronucleus within the central ooplasm, visualized at $\times$100–200 magnification, on an inverted phase-contrast microscope fitted with an appropriate stage warmer.

Fertilization rate, the number of normally fertilized oocytes as a proportion of mature oocytes inseminated, is a key indicator of stimulation and IVF efficiency. Diagnosing the reason for a failed fertilization in a cycle is difficult, with a host of potential biological factors at the cellular and genetic level that could be responsible. These can be associated with anomalies of sperm (e.g. failure of decondensation) or oocyte (e.g. failed activation, incomplete cortical reaction). Morphological quality of the inseminating sperm is far easier to assess than oocyte problems. There are also a range of abnormal post-fertilization events that have been described, including variable pronucleus number (polyspermy), presence of micronuclei, and spontaneous activation of an oocyte. Many of these effects can be ascribed to male factor subfertility, in relation to the total number of viable sperm, their normality and motility.

Intracytoplasmic sperm injection (ICSI)

For severe male factor infertility, including severe oligozoospermia and asthenospermia, where deficits in quantity and normality prevent the use of a purified extract, ICSI is the method of choice. While standard IVF is still widely practiced, a majority of fresh cycles involve insemination using ICSI. The method itself evolved from earlier techniques such as partial zona dissection to expose sperm passively to the oolemma, or microinjection sperm directly into the subzonal space. Due to complications such as polyspermic fertilization, such approaches proved less feasible than ICSI, whereby direct injection of one sperm into the ooplasm is performed, thus bypassing the zona and oolemma altogether [7].

During ICSI, a single sperm is immobilized and aspirated into a narrower glass injection pipette, which is then pushed through the zona pellucida and underlying oolemma into the ooplasm. Immediately prior to sperm expulsion, the oolemma is typically ruptured under a negative pressure to assist penetration of the sperm into the ooplasm. Care must be taken to avoid artifacts resulting from incorrect sperm immobilization, incorrect orientation of the injection site relative to oocyte axes, incomplete penetration of the oolemma, and incomplete displacement of the ooplasm following sperm entry. While ICSI has proven a clinically safe technique and is routinely performed, it remains a form of physical manipulation of the oocyte, and therefore represents a potential source of perturbation to the oocyte.

In addition to sperm quality and normality as the main concerns for the success of ICSI, oocyte normality also plays an important role. The oocyte represents a fragile stage of development, when maternally inherited mechanisms are held in stasis until they are activated by the sperm, triggering preimplantation development. An increased incidence of cytopathology in oocytes from aging and subfertile women, including chromosomal aneuploidy, may contribute to increase the likelihood of arrested development at key stages of oocyte maturation and activation, pronucleus formation, and embryo cleavage divisions. There is additional speculation that oocytes may incur epigenetic errors, depending on how they were inseminated. Dumoulin and colleagues have observed gender-specific differences in embryos derived by ICSI, but not in those produced by standard insemination [8]. Despite these concerns, ongoing long-term follow-up of ICSI cases continues to show that both standard IVF and ICSI insemination are comparable in terms of live birth rate and child development [9].

Embryo biopsy

The same technology and protocols used for ICSI have also been modified for use in the biopsy of oocytes and embryos for genetic analysis. Clinical laboratories have applied methods including single blastomere removal from cleavage-stage embryos [10] and trophectoderm removal from blastocysts [11]. Biopsied blastomeres can then be analyzed using a range of molecular genetic techniques, including chromosome-specific in situ hybridization for aneuploidy detection, polymerase chain reaction (PCR) for mutatation detection in specific chromosomes, and other genome-wide screening techniques. The most recent advances have included high-resolution whole genome arrays, such as single nucleotide polymorphism arrays [12]. Embryo biopsy in conjunction with preimplantation genetic diagnosis (PGD) has therefore become a more broad diagnostic screening system, with the potential for obtaining global information about the genetics of embryos from subfertile populations.

At present, a majority of PGD programs employ biopsy of day 3 embryos. While removal of a significant proportion of the embryo does not completely impede ongoing development, biopsied day 3 embryos are relatively less viable than non-manipulated controls [13]. Other concerns with cleavage stages include testing artifacts such as allelic drop-out and mosaicism that may contribute to potential false negatives, which have made the sampling of a second blastomere a common practice. A landmark randomized controlled trial published in 2007 showed for the first time that in females between 35 and 41 years of age, PGD testing of cleavage-stage embryos actually resulted in a significant decrease in ongoing pregnancy rate after transfer, compared to embryos without biopsy [14]. Circumventing this negative effect might be possible by delaying the biopsy procedure to the blastocyst stage, when a smaller proportion of cells is removed relative to the embryo, and those embryos surviving extended culture are less likely to carry genetic abnormalities, relative to those arresting earlier [15].

Embryo production methods

Clinical IVF is unique with respect to the directness of translation of laboratory techniques from experimental embryology using mammalian models. Even today, embryo production by IVF and associated manipulation procedures in human or veterinary medicine and in reproductive biology are essentially the same. Laboratory procedures have been optimized to the point that most of the developmental blocks observed in previous decades have been eliminated, and embryos can be cultured for extended periods if desired.

In vitro oocyte maturation

The capability of embryo production has widened, from the retrieval and fertilization of mature oocytes and culture to day 2 in the 1980s and 1990s, to earlier oocyte retrievals and extended embryo cultures. As an alternative to the isolation of mature pre-ovulatory oocytes, use of immature oocytes followed by in vitro maturation (IVM) has provided a viable alternative for certain groups of subfertile women, as reviewed previously [16], with recent advances that have dramatically improved laboratory outcomes, including the concept of induced maturation [17]. Further details of IVM procedures and advances are described in Chapter 12.

Cleavage-stage embryo culture

Traditionally, a single bicarbonate-buffered medium has been used for IVF and embryo culture, within a humidified culture incubator with automated control of carbon dioxide, and temperature level [18]. A chemically buffered (e.g. HEPES or MOPS) equivalent of the same medium is used for handling the gametes and embryos outside this physiological environment, unless embryology workstations are fitted with gassing facilities. While test-tubes were commonly used for oocyte insemination and embryo culture in the early years of assisted human conception, typically such procedures now occur in Petri dishes (35 or 60 mm) containing reduced volumes of media (50–100 μl) under an overlay of paraffin oil, preferably in a reduced oxygen concentration (5–7%).

Significant improvements have been made in the area of culture medium formulation, based on successes in the survival and development of embryos from mammalian species [19]. Part of this approach has been the formulation of chemically defined media, involving the removal of embryo-toxic components, reduction of necessary factors that have dosage-dependent toxicity, and inclusion of factors with known beneficial effects. Milestones in this evolution have been the abolition of maternal serum as the protein macromolecule, in preference for purified serum albumins and glycosaminoglycans, as well as additional essential nutrients such as vitamins.

A pivotal change to improving the developmental potential and viability of cleavage-stage embryos has been the inclusion of amino acids [20], which has led to a phasing out of simple media in preference for chemically defined, nutritionally optimized complex media. This

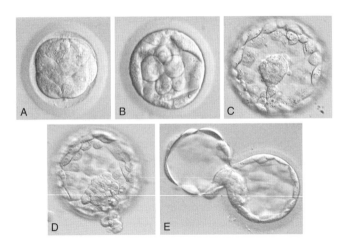

Figure 18.3 Morphology of post-compaction human embryos. Bright-field photomicrographs of in vitro produced embryos at different stages of blastocyst development. (A) and (B) early blastocyst stage, when blastocoel formation has begun – inner cell mass blastomeres (B) can be seen surrounded by flattened trophectoderm epithelium; (C) expanded blastocyst stage, when the blastocoele cavity has increased in size to occupy a majority of the embryo, with a tightly packed inner cell mass and trophectoderm layer with many cells; (D) and (E) partially hatched blastocyst stage, when the trophectoderm eventually breaches and escapes the zona pellucida.

step improved embryo development, thereby facilitating a widespread preference for replacing later-stage day 3 and 4 embryos, rather than day 2 embryos, with reductions in fragmentation and better cryosurvival [21]. While artifacts such as fragmentation still occur on day 3, and a spread of embryo morphologies is evident, there is also a clearer indication of which embryos are the more developmentally competent, based on their relative kinetics. Overall, extending culture by an additional 24 hours to day 3 has not had any overt detrimental effects, with modest improvements in implantation and pregnancy outcomes.

Blastocyst culture

The global imperative for single embryo transfer (SET) as a benchmark to prevent multiple pregnancies has been a driver behind the trend toward extended embryo culture and selection of the most viable embryo in a cohort [22]. Considering that natural implantation ensues around the blastocyst stage, development to blastocyst is a useful indicator of the implantation potential of the embryo. Consequently, pregnancy rates following blastocyst transfer are markedly better than following cleavage-stage embryo transfer, even in combination with SET [23], with up to approximately half of normally fertilized oocytes typically surviving to this stage.

Blastocyst development involves a dramatic change in embryo morphology and growth, between days 3 and 5 of development, the so-called post-compaction stages. Adjacent blastomeres merge to form a compacted clump (morula) marked by tight junction formation and membrane fusion, followed by a rapid onset of cell division. During this proliferative phase, most blastomeres differentiate to form an outer trophectoderm (TE) epithelial layer that contains the blastocoel, a fluid-filled spherical microenvironment that supports a small population of undifferentiated inner cell mass (ICM) cells, the embryo progenitor cells (Figure 18.3).

Accompanied with this increased blastocyst cell proliferation is an increased metabolic demand, predominantly reliant on glucose as the key carbohydrate, a shift from pyruvate during early cleavage [24]. This developmental shift has guided the optimization of medium formulations, including sequential media, which are stage-specific versions of the same medium used in tandem from day 1 to 5. Irrespective of the medium type (sequential or monophasic), all media need to be renewed after 48 hours to avoid toxicity to the embryo, as well as to avoid depletion of carbohydrates and other substrates. Clinical application of blastocyst culture using sequential media have resulted in markedly improved embryo development and pregnancy rates, especially when incorporated holistically with optimized laboratory and culture conditions, blastocyst grading criteria, and an effective quality management scheme [3,25].

Blastocyst culture and transfer has provided an important alternative to cleavage-stage embryo transfer. Advantages of the technique have included the potential to more efficiently synchronize the stage of embryo development with uterine receptivity, the clearer distinction between morphologically advanced embryos, declines in the incidence of genetically abnormal embryos, and improvements in post-biopsy survival. From a total of 17 independent randomized controlled trials, as summarized previously [26], eight comparisons of cleavage-stage versus blastocyst-stage transfers report significantly improved pregnancy rates, whereas eight report comparable outcomes and one reports a significant decrease. In support of the evidence for improved outcomes after blastocyst transfer, a recent Cochrane review of 50 randomized controlled trials found that in those fitting the report criteria, a significant improvement is observed in implantation, pregnancy, and live birth rates after blastocyst transfer [27].

Pre-transfer embryo treatment

While the transfer procedure itself remains more in the clinical domain than that of IVF laboratory protocols, post-transfer outcomes rely heavily on the quality of IVF embryos. This includes not only the success of the embryo production process, but also the preservation of embryo quality immediately prior to transfer, when they may be subjected to a range of transient environmental perturbations (e.g. cold exposure during catheterization, physical insults during injection, osmotic fluctuations from uterine secretions), thereby influencing the implantation and pregnancy rate. It is worth noting that some IVF laboratory interventions have therefore extended past embryo production, to the pre-treatment of embryos immediately prior to transfer.

An example is the use of hyaluronan, a proteoglycan secreted by the female reproductive tract, as a supplement to the transfer medium. Improvements in implantation and fetal formation in the mouse [28] have previously been reported using this supplement. A clinical trial of the same supplement in an enriched transfer medium has since shown it to increase clinical pregnancy and implantation rates after blastocyst transfer [29]. In all, consideration of embryo treatments to preserve embryo quality prior to transfer may better ensure their implantation potential, especially for SET.

Assessment of embryo development and viability

Embryo morphology

Visual assessment of preimplantation embryo morphology remains the most widely used method of determining embryo development in vitro. This is typically performed

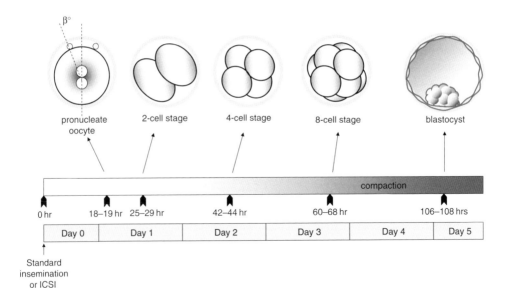

Figure 18.4 Timeline of in vitro preimplantation embryo production. Expected times of known morphological stages of embryo development, in hours post-insemination and in days of culture. Normally fertilized pronucleate oocytes typically have two centrally located symmetrical vesicles; angle beta should be less than 50°; 2-cell stage embryos should have no fragments, 4-cell embryos should have no less than 20% fragmentation; on day 3, embryos will have anywhere from 6 to 8 cells, with no less than 20% fragmentation; following compaction of blastomeres and morula formation, the resultant blastocyst should have a cohesive trophectoderm layer with many cells, surrounding a tightly packed inner cell mass with many cells.

by laboratory personnel using bright-field phase-contrast microscopy, with high magnification capability (up to × 400). Immediately evident using this approach are two parameters of embryo quality and development. First is the kinetic development of the embryo, as indicated by the stage-specific hallmarks including cell number, size, and presence of structural features (e.g. compacting blastomeres, a blastocoele cavity, hatched TE). To eliminate the subjectivity involved in these manual observations, a range of methods of embryo grading have been devised according to a numerical classification, as reviewed previously [5]. These form the basis of quantitative criteria used for selection of embryos for transfer and cryopreservation, a way of benchmarking embryo quality across clinics (Figure 18.4).

A second parameter is the normality of the embryo, indicated by the degree of fragmentation, arrested development or other cellular defects (e.g. vacuoles, micronuclei), which are often seen in infertile and subfertile patient cohorts. Several micro-imaging methods have been used for the detection of fine cytostructural abnormalities in oocytes and embryos, including transmission electron microscopy and quantitative epifluorescence microscopy. These methods have, however, been restricted to spare oocytes or embryos, owing to their invasiveness due to preservation of cytoarchitecture. Clinically amenable methods for assessing normality must therefore not be detrimental to the developmental competence of the embryo. With this in mind, the technique of non-invasive polarized-light microscopy has therefore proven useful for the non-invasive determination of meiotic spindle normality and geometry in mature oocytes [30].

Kinetic assessment of embryo development is usually based on measurement of the timing of morphological stages as they occur in the developing embryo. Several recent advances have been made in continuous monitoring techniques, with more accuracy and less environmental disturbances than the standard daily or bi-daily manual assessments. Time-lapse videography has been used to this end, providing minute-by-minute detail of morphological changes from day 1 through to day 5 of development. In a recent study by Pribenszky and colleagues [31], a compact digital imaging microscope system designed for accommodating culture dishes was used to continuously monitor individual embryos while being maintained under incubation conditions, without need for incubator door opening. Similar methods for continuous monitoring have correlated pregnancy outcome to the timing of morphological changes in developing embryos [32], in support of previous manual observations, such as the predictive value of elapsed first cleavage times [33]. Collectively, these studies lend support to an integrated strategy of embryo selection proposed by Sakkas and Gardner, which takes into account early and late morphological events within their established time-frames, spanning the entire period from pronuclear oocyte to blastocyst, rather than a single point measure in a single window of development [5].

Embryo physiology and functional endpoints

The dynamic morphological changes in embryo development are driven by metabolism. Metabolic activity has been found to correlate closely with developmental competence of many mammalian species. While comparatively less evidence exists on human embryos, they still exhibit similar profiles including the characteristic shift from pyruvate to glucose metabolism after compaction [24]. Also, nutritional improvements in human embryo culture medium based on this information have been highly successful in improving embryo quality in many clinics.

Like morphological parameters, physiological parameters can correlate with both expected "normal" ranges of embryo development, while also indicating clinically relevant abnormalities. Added benefits include that metabolic information can be effectively quantitated using automated approaches [34], with changes occurring at the metabolic level providing a more sensitive indicator of the physiological health of the embryo than at the morphological level. Also, metabolic processes are highly sensitive to environmental stresses, which can induce a range of mutagenic and apoptogenic molecular damage. A corollary to this is that embryos have an inherent capacity for adaptation and recovery from transient or cumulative shocks, imparted by factors such as redundancy in metabolic pathways and antioxidant mechanisms that prevent nonspecific molecular damage.

So from a laboratory viewpoint, it is important to identify and quantify the parameters that constitute normal embryo physiology, as well as minimize the insults incurred as a result of ART procedures. Regarding the former, a range of assays have been developed that are gradually becoming more adaptable to clinical IVF, as biotechnology becomes more readily translated from applications in the life-sciences (described in the following section). Regarding the latter, many environmental factors in the laboratory have been identified as toxic or harmful to embryo development in animal models, including atmospheric oxygen, paraffin oil overlays, ambient light, transient thermal shocks, cryopreservation injury, chemical toxicity, and manual handling artifacts [35]. Controlling these variables has formed part of risk management in the establishment of successful blastocyst transfer programs, and improvements in these laboratory modifications are reflected in improved embryo physiology [3].

Diagnostic assays for viability detection

Quantitative methods for assessment of embryo physiology, particularly metabolism, are predictive of embryo viability, again the product of extensive work in mammalian experimental embryology. These methods have been dominated by the biochemical detection of nutrient exchange in culture medium using microfluorometry [34]. Accurate measurement of the consumption of specific substrates (glucose, pyruvate, lactate, oxygen, amino acids) and metabolites (lactate, ammonium, carbon dioxide) can be performed, establishing a profile of metabolic normality of the developing embryo, while highlighting environmental disturbances. This approach is technologically demanding, mainly because measurements are typically performed on samples of media from single embryos.

Screening techniques for the detection of multiple metabolites have also been applied to the analysis of embryos and culture media samples. HPLC has been able to provide profiles of consumption and production of all 20 amino acids, following non-invasive analysis of culture media [36]. More recently, systematic technologies for quantitative screening of the embryo metabolome (all low-molecular-weight by-products of metabolism) have been applied to the analysis of embryo culture media, [37]. Like other "Omics" technologies, metabolomics analysis involves systematic chemical separation, automated spectroscopy and bioinformatics sorting of data to produce "molecular profiles" that correlate with embryo physiology. Using such an approach, it is now possible to obtain a biological algorithm of a single embryo, which is indicative of pregnancy outcomes [38]. These techniques are conveniently non-invasive, owing to their method of sampling the embryo culture medium itself. Other complementary Omics techniques are capable of invasive analysis of individual embryos or biopsied cells. Functional genomics (e.g. gene microarrays) and proteomics (e.g. MALDI-TOF and SELDI-TOF mass spectroscopy) platforms have also been used to screen global genetic and protein complements of human embryos and their secretory proteins [39].

These emerging biotechologies hold great promise for advancing the capability and safety of clinical IVF procedures. In combination with other innovative techniques such as lab-on-a-chip approaches [40], these analytical screening platforms represent a highly sensitive and accurate means of selecting for embryo quality and viability based on quantitating their biochemistry and physiology. This is potentially very important for subfertile couples, where differences between the quality of sibling embryos are more subtle and difficult to detect, and only marginally below expected clinical values. There is also the inherent value of these assays as diagnostic tools to better understand the etiology of the couple, on a case-specific basis, based on the diversity of molecular information contained within the samples.

Oocyte and embryo cryopreservation

Embryos not selected for transfer are preserved in liquid nitrogen storage ("cryopreserved" or "cryostored") as a standard practice. This procedure is employed by a majority of clinical IVF laboratories, although laboratory-specific differences exist in the type of chemical treatments used during the procedure. Chemical treatment of embryos involves two main processes: (a) displacement of water from the cytoplasmic compartments of the embryo with cryoprotectant agents and (b) osmotic adjustment of the embryo to relatively high concentrations of permeable and non-permeable cryoprotectants. These steps result in a lowering of the temperature of the embryo, protection against intracellular and extracellular ice crystal formation and subsequent micro-fracturing within the embryo (cryoinjury), as well as maintaining membrane fluidity and preventing osmotic shock due to increased viscosity of the incubation medium and permeants.

Traditional cryopreservation has involved the process of slow-freezing, whereby the environmental temperature around the embryo container is decreased at a gradual rate of 3–8°C/minute, using a controlled-rate freezing device [41]. This method has remained relatively unchanged since the 1980s, and has proven highly effective in achieving pregnancies in patients returning after a previous failed cycle. The technique is therefore clinically safe, despite negative effects such as cryoprotectant toxicity and compromised post-thaw survival of the embryo that lead to artifacts such as blastomere lysis and retarded development.

Since 2000, the process of rapid cooling (vitrification) has provided a viable alternative to slow freezing. Vitrification involves the induction of a far more rapid drop in temperature surrounding the embryo container, which typically contains lower volume of freezing medium (less than 5 μl) compared to those used for slow-freezing (200–500 μl). The end result is a supercooling of the oocyte or embryo, preserving it in a glass-like suspended liquid state, rather than a crystalline solid [42]. In terms of patient outcomes, vitrification is currently proving to be relatively more efficient for the post-cryopreservation survival, fertilization, and embryo viability of oocytes in comparison with slow-freezing [43].

While long-term follow-up of vitrification is ongoing, high rates of post-warming survival of oocytes and embryos suggest that this method could ultimately supercede slow-freezing as the standard method of cryopreservation in IVF. The higher survival rate for oocytes using vitrification is of particular interest to clinics not permitted by law to store excess embryos; for patients who have undergone IVM/IVF; for clinical groups outside fertility treatment such as cancer patients, who wish to preserve their gametes; and as a potential fertility preservation facility for women who wish to circumvent the advancing age effects of delayed parenthood.

Summary and perspective

- A clinical IVF laboratory is a controlled biotechnology facility, operated by specialized embryology staff, who assist clinicians in the treatment of subfertile patients, using ARTs
- Clinicians have a duty of care to the patient in choosing the appropriate laboratory protocol on a case-specific basis
- IVF essentially involves the manipulation of sperm and oocytes, fertilization of the oocytes to generate preimplantation embryos, assessment and selection of these embryos for intrauterine transfer, and excess gamete or embryo cryopreservation
- IVF laboratories represent a multifactorial system. Compromises in individual aspects can have a cumulative detriment to patient outcomes, by adversely affecting embryo quality. Hence a holistic and integrated process of quality control should be adopted, to maintain the consistency of patient outcomes
- Emerging technologies are continuing to improve the capability and safety of all facets of existing ARTs, particularly in the areas of extended embryo culture, improved embryo viability, innovations in embryo assessment and selection, and innovations in cryopreservation techniques

References

1. Cohen J, Gilligan A, Garrisi J. Setting up an ART laboratory. In Gardner DK, Weissman A, Howles CM, Shoham Z, eds. *Textbook of Assisted Reproductive Technologies: Laboratory and Clinical Perspectives*, 3rd edn. London: Informa Healthcare, 2009; 1–8.

2. Mortimer D, Mortimer ST. *Quality and Risk Management in the IVF Laboratory*. Cambridge: Cambridge University Press, 2005; 24–44.

3. Schoolcraft WB, Gardner DK. Blastocyst culture and transfer increases the efficiency of oocyte donation. *Fertil Steril* 2000; **74**(3): 482–6.

4. Gardner DK, Reed L, Linck D, Sheehan C, Lane M. Quality control in human in vitro fertilization. *Semin Reprod Med* 2005; **23**(4): 319–24.

5. Sakkas D, Gardner DK. Evaluation of embryo quality: new strategies to facilitate single embryo transfer. In Gardner DK, Weissman A, Howles CM, Shoham Z, eds. *Textbook of Assisted Reproductive Technologies: Laboratory and Clinical Perspectives*, 3rd edn. London: Informa Healthcare, 2009; 241–54.

6. Sakkas D, Manicardi GC, Tomlinson M, *et al.* The use of two density gradient centrifugation techniques and the swim-up method to separate spermatozoa with chromatin and nuclear DNA anomalies. *Hum Reprod* 2000; **15**(5): 1112–16.

7. Palermo P, Joris H, Devroey P, Van Steirteghem AC. Pregnancies after intracytoplasmic injection of a single spermatazoon into an oocyte. *Lancet* 1992; **340**: 17–18.

8. Dumoulin JC, Derhaag JG, Bras M, *et al.* Growth rate of human preimplantation embryos is sex dependent after ICSI but not after IVF. *Hum Reprod* 2005; **20**(2): 484–91.

9. Palermo GD, Neri QV, Takeuchi T, Rosenwaks Z. ICSI: where we have been and where we are going. *Semin Reprod Med* 2009; **27**(2): 191–201.

10. Hardy K, Handyside AH. Biopsy of cleavage stage human embryos and diagnosis of single gene defects by DNA amplification. *Arch Pathol Lab Med* 1992; **116**(4): 388–92.

11. Muggleton-Harris AL, Glazier AM, Pickering SJ. Biopsy of the human blastocyst and polymerase chain reaction (PCR) amplification of the beta-globin gene and a dinucleotide repeat motif from 2–6 trophectoderm cells. *Hum Reprod* 1993; **8**(12): 2197–205.

12. Treff NR, Su J, Tao X, Levy B, Scott RT Jr. Accurate single cell 24 chromosome aneuploidy screening using whole genome amplification and single nucleotide polymorphism microarrays. *Fertil Steril* 2010 Feb 24 [Epub ahead of print].

13. Tarin JJ, Conaghan J, Winston RM, Handyside AH. Human embryo biopsy on the 2nd day after insemination for preimplantation diagnosis: removal of a quarter of embryo retards cleavage. *Fertil Steril* 1992; **58**(5): 970–6.

14. Mastenbroek S, Twisk M, van Echten-Arends J, *et al.* In vitro fertilization with preimplantation genetic screening. *N Engl J Med* 2007; **357**(1): 9–17.

15. Fragouli E, Lenzi M, Ross R, *et al.* Comprehensive molecular cytogenetic analysis of the human blastocyst stage. *Hum Reprod* 2008; **23**(11): 2596–608.

16. Papanikolaou EG, Platteau P, Albano C, *et al.* Immature oocyte in-vitro maturation: clinical aspects. *Reprod Biomed Online* 2005; **10**(5): 587–92.

17. Gilchrist RB, Lane M, Thompson JG. Oocyte-secreted factors: regulators of cumulus cell function and oocyte quality. *Hum Reprod Update*. 2008; **14**(2): 159–77.

18. Quinn P, Warnes GM, Kerin JF, Kirby C. Culture factors affecting the success rate of in vitro fertilization and embryo transfer. *Ann N Y Acad Sci* 1985; **442**: 195–204.

19. Gardner DK, Lane M. Amino acids and ammonium regulate mouse embryo development in culture. *Biol Reprod* 1993; **48**(2): 377–85.

20. Devreker F, Hardy K, Van den Bergh M, *et al.* Amino acids promote human blastocyst development in vitro. *Hum Reprod* 2001; **16**(4): 749–56.

21. Balaban B, Urman B. Embryo culture as a diagnostic tool. *Reprod Biomed Online* 2003; 7(6): 671–82.

22. Van Royen E, Mangelschots K, De Neubourg D, *et al.* Characterization of a top quality embryo, a step towards single-embryo transfer. *Hum Reprod* 1999; **14**(9): 2345–9.

23. Gardner DK, Surrey E, Minjarez D, *et al.* Single blastocyst transfer: a prospective randomized trial. *Fertil Steril* 2004; **81**(3): 551–5.

24. Gott AL, Hardy K, Winston RM, Leese HJ. Non-invasive measurement of pyruvate and glucose uptake and lactate production by single human preimplantation embryos. *Hum Reprod* 1990; 5(1): 104–8.

25. Gardner DK, Schoolcraft WB, Wagley L, *et al.* A prospective randomized trial of blastocyst culture and transfer in in-vitro fertilization. *Hum Reprod* 1998; **13**(12): 3434–40.

26. Gardner DK, Lane M. Culture systems for the human embryo. In Gardner DK, Weissman A, Howles CM, Shoham Z, eds. *Textbook of Assisted Reproductive Technologies: Laboratory and Clinical Perspectives*, 3rd edn. London: Informa Healthcare, 2009; 219–40.

27. Blake DA, Farquhar CM, Johnson N, Proctor M. Cleavage stage versus blastocyst stage embryo transfer in assisted conception. *Cochrane Database Syst Rev* 2007; 4: CD002118.

28. Gardner DK, Rodriegez-Martinez H, Lane M. Fetal development after transfer is increased by replacing protein with the glycosaminoglycan hyaluronan for mouse embryo culture and transfer. *Hum Reprod* 1999; **14**(10): 2575–80.

29. Urman B, Yakin K, Ata B, Isiklar A, Balaban B. Effect of hyaluronan-enriched transfer medium on implantation and pregnancy rates after day 3 and day 5 embryo transfers: a prospective randomized study. *Fertil Steril* 2008; **90**(3): 604–12.

30. Wang WH, Meng L, Hackett RJ, Odenbourg R, Keefe DL. The spindle observation and its relationship with fertilization after intracytoplasmic sperm injection in living human oocytes. *Fertil Steril* 2001; **75**(2): 348–53.

31. Pribenszky C, Losonczi E, Molnar M, *et al.* Prediction of in-vitro developmental competence of early cleavage-stage mouse embryos with compact time-lapse equipment. *Reprod Biomed Online* 2010; **20**(3): 371–9.

32. Lemmen JG, Agerholm I, Ziebe S. Kinetic markers of human embryo quality using time-lapse recordings of IVF/ICSI-fertilized oocytes. *Reprod Biomed Online* 2008; **17**(3): 385–91.

33. Lundin K, Bergh C, Hardarson T. Early embryo cleavage is a strong indicator of embryo quality in human IVF. *Hum Reprod* 2001; **16**(12): 2652–7.

34. Gardner DK, Leese HJ. Assessment of embryo metabolism and viability. In Trounson A, Gardner DK, eds. *Handbook of In Vitro Fertilization*. Boca Raton, FL: CRC Press, 1999; 347–72.

35. Gardner DK, Lane M. Embryo culture systems. In Trounson A, Gardner DK, eds. *Handbook of In Vitro Fertilization*. Boca Raton, FL: CRC Press, 2000; 205–64.

36. Brison DR, Houghton FD, Falconer D, *et al.* Identification of viable embryos in IVF by non-invasive measurement of amino acid turnover. *Hum Reprod* 2004; **19**(10): 2319–24.

37. Houghton FD, Hawkhead JA, Humpherson PG, *et al.* Non-invasive amino acid turnover predicts human embryo developmental capacity. *Hum Reprod* 2002; **17**(4): 999–1005.

38. Seli E, Sakkas D, Scott R, *et al.* Noninvasive metabolomic profiling of embryo culture media using Raman and near-infrared spectroscopy correlates with reproductive potential of embryos in women undergoing in vitro fertilization. *Fertil Steril* 2007; **88**(5): 1350–7.

39. Katz-Jaffe MG, McReynolds S, Gardner DK, Schoolcraft WB. The role of proteomics in defining the human embryonic secretome. *Mol Hum Reprod* 2009; **15**(5): 271–7.

40. Urbanski JP, Johnson MT, Craig DD, *et al.* Noninvasive metabolic profiling using microfluidics for analysis of single preimplantation embryos. *Anal Chem* 2008; **80**(17): 6500–7.

41. Leibo SP. Cryopreservation of mammaliam oocytes. In Tulandi T, Gosden RG, eds. *Preservation of Fertility.* London: Taylor and Francis, 2004; 141–55.

42. Vajta G, Nagy ZP, Cobo A, Conceicao J, Yovich J. Vitrification in assisted reproduction: myths, mistakes, disbeliefs and confusion. *Reprod Biomed Online* 2009; **19** Suppl 3: 1–7.

43. Kuwayama M, Vajta G, Ieda S, Kato O. Vitrification of human embryos using CryoTip™ method. *Reprod BioMed Online* 2005; **11**: 608–14.

Chapter 9

Infertility counseling

Linda Hammer Burns

Human reproduction is universally recognized as a psychosocial and biological imperative. Subfertile individuals, throughout antiquity and across all cultures, have been stigmatized and ostracized, willing to pursue remedies for childlessness through available medical practices, spiritual/cultural rituals, and/or social realignment (e.g. adoption, divorce) [1]. This pursuit of "a baby at any price" – regardless of physical, social, medical, or emotional cost to intended parents, offspring, or reproductive helpers is a powerful consumer force influencing reproductive care. While historically medical remedies for infertility were primitive and ineffective, psychological care was irrelevant or left to spiritual advisors. In the twenty-first century, the advent of assisted reproductive technologies (ARTs), maternal/fetal medicine, human genome therapy, and gamete manipulation, as well as infertility counseling have offered hope and success to an array of subfertile patients worldwide. Still, these miraculous successes have not come without concomitant ethical dilemmas, medical risks for parents, offspring and reproductive helpers, legal dilemmas, social upheaval, and psychosocial distress [2].

The twenty-first century has also seen a shift in the role of mental health care in reproductive medicine. In the middle of the twentieth century, it was the responsibility of psychiatrists to cure neurosis (primarily in women) who were thought to be subfertile as a result of ambivalent feelings about motherhood, sexuality, pregnancy, or her relationship with her own mother [3]. Psychiatrists and psychologists were expected to cure these neuroses in order to restore fertility. But as the diagnosis of subfertility of unknown etiology declined, the role of infertility counseling evolved from curing neurosis to a more complex caregiving role [3]. Infertility counselors today offer patients and caregivers assistance along their reproductive journey, helping patients maintain cultural and moral compasses, marital and familial stability, and, most importantly, individual emotional well-being. As such, they enhance not only the well-being of subfertile individuals but the emotional well-being of the children created via assisted and complex reproduction [4].

The aim of this chapter is to provide:

- an overview of the psychological experience of infertility (before, during, and after care) and the importance of infertility counseling in maintaining healthy patients physically and mentally throughout their reproductive journey
- an overview of the definition of infertility counseling; minimum standards of education, training, credentialing, and professional development; and laws and professional guidelines worldwide that define the practice of infertility counseling

The Subfertility Handbook: A Clinician's Guide, Second Edition ed. Gab Kovacs. Published by Cambridge University Press. © Cambridge University Press 2011.

- an outline of methods for providing infertility counseling (independent practitioner, consultant to a reproductive treatment clinic, and as a member of the treatment clinic/ team) and the pros and cons of the approaches for patients and medical caregivers
- a summary of the literature on clinical issues and therapeutic interventions that best benefit patient well-being and medical treatment outcomes
- an overview of the complex psychosocial issues of third-party reproduction and the important role of the infertility counseling in these family-building methods.

The psychology of infertility

Involuntary childlessness, or the inability to procreate as desired, can disturb one's fundamental assumptions about a predictable and stable world [3]. Today, reliable birth control allows women to "control" their reproductive lives – parenthood is not only an assumption, it is a deliberate decision. When conception and birth do not go according to plan, shock and disbelief emerge as couples realize that, despite their best efforts (e.g. prayers, herbal remedies, ARTs) the outcome they want and deserve has eluded them. Subfertility is a very deceptively inclusive term referring to involuntary childlessness, secondary infertility, repeated miscarriage, ectopic pregnancy, chemical pregnancy, or molar pregnancy or pregnancy loss in a gestational carrier/surrogate, difficulty conceiving after successful reproduction in a previous relationship, and failure of third-party reproduction. The inclusivity of subfertility also reflects the complexity of reproductive medical treatments including in vitro fertilization (IVF), preimplantation genetic diagnosis (PGD), intracytoplasmic sperm injection (ICSI), embryo cryopreservation and transplant, as well as those on the horizon (e.g. ovarian tissue transplant, uterine transplantation, and cloning). Infertility counseling is a dynamic, ever-changing and evolving field that reflects the dynamic nature of reproductive medicine itself.

Some degree of emotional distress in response to infertility and/or its treatment is anticipated and predictable. Typical emotional responses to infertility include anger, guilt, shock, lowered self-esteem, sexual dysfunction, marital distress, and social isolation (Table 19.1). Worldwide, reproductive failure involves significant losses for both men and women, although they have emotionally different responses to subfertility, with women experiencing and expressing more distress than their male partners. The exception is male factor infertility diagnosis, in which men experience and express more emotional distress [5].

While the vast majority of individuals are able to manage the experience of infertility effectively, some individuals experience exacerbations of preexisting psychiatric disorders or clinically significant emotional problems (Table 19.2). This may also be the case for some reproductive collaborators such as gestational carriers or oocyte donors participating in reproductive medical treatments. Researchers investigating the prevalence of psychiatric morbidity (preexisting and/or newly emergent) in individuals attending a fertility clinic found that 69% of women and 21% of men had a psychiatric diagnosis. Adjustment and anxiety disorders were the most common, with depression twice as prevalent in infertile women with a history of depression [6].

Subfertility and its treatment can adversely impact not only emotional well-being but physical well-being – particularly when an individual has a concomitant medical condition. Some subfertile couples enter reproductive treatment well aware of a medical condition adversely impacting their reproductive ability. As a result, they may have more realistic expectations of treatment success and greater comfort with medical system and treatment protocols – although this may not be true for their partners. Other subfertile patients learn

Table 19.1 Observed psychological effects of infertility [4]

A. Emotional effects

  1. Grieving/depression

  2. Anger/frustration

  3. Guilt

  4. Shock/denial

  5. Anxiety

B. Loss of control

  1. Loss of control over activities, body, emotions

  2. Inability to predict and plan future

  3. Loss of health

  4. Loss of security (about a predictable future)

C. Effects on self-esteem, identity, beliefs

  1. Loss of self-esteem and self-confidence, feelings of inadequacy

  2. Identity problems or shifts, loss of status or prestige

  3. Changes in world views

D. Social effects

  1. Effects on marital interactions and satisfaction (positive and negative)

  2. Effects on sexual functioning

  3. Different social network interactions, changes in relationships with network members, loneliness, embarrassment

E. Loss of a (potential) relationship

  1. Loss of fantasy or hope of fulfilling an important fantasy

  2. Loss of something or someone of great symbolic value

  3. Loss of future and past in one person

Adapted from: Stanton AL, Dunkel-Schetter L. Psychological reactions to infertility. In Stanton AL, Dunkel-Schetter L (Eds.). *Infertility: Perspectives from Stress and Coping Research.* New York: Plenum Press, 1991; 31; and Mahlstedt PP. The psychological component of infertility. *Fertil Steril* 1985; 43: 335–56.

about a medical condition impacting reproduction during the infertility work-up. Both partners must adjust to a new medical diagnosis as well as subfertility treatment, which can trigger significant psychosocial distress requiring reconfiguration of life plans, treatment goals, and/or family-building options [7].

Subfertility is a multigenerational developmental life crisis in which the infertile couple is unable to assume the roles and responsibilities of adulthood which parenthood bestows and also prevents their parents from moving into the next stage of their lives: grandparenthood. The family system is impacted by the subfertile couple's childlessness particularly if the

Table 19.2 Psychiatric responses to infertility [4]

Depression/dysthymia	Anorgasmia
	Post-traumatic stress disorder
Anxiety disorders	Factitious disorders
Obsessive/compulsive disorder	Noncompliance with treatment
Panic attacks	Bereavement (complicated or delayed)
Sleep problems	Occupational problems
Eating disorders	Identity problems
Body dysphoria	Religious or spiritual problems
Personality disorders	Acculturation problems
Anger management/violence	Phase of life problems
Impulsivity	Legal problems
Pathological or excessive grief	Abuse/addiction problems
Marital and/or sexual problems	Alcohol
Somatization disorder	Gambling
Sexual problems	Prescription medication
History of rape, trauma	Tobacco
Low libido	Recreational drugs
Infrequent or no sexual intercourse	Sex

family system is unable to appropriately grieve and/or adapt to other forms of family-building (e.g. donor gametes, adoption) [3]. The subfertile couple's inability to achieve parenthood may shake their confidence in their ability to manage the challenges of medical treatment and/or the emotional maelstrom.

Infertility counseling

Psychiatry emerged as a new field of medicine late in the nineteenth century. As noted earlier, by the middle of the twentith century psychiatry's role in treating the subfertile was medical: cure the neurotic disease thereby restoring reproductive ability. Infertility counseling is a synthesis of two medical specialties: reproductive medicine and psychiatry. Infertility counseling is a term used to represent the wide array of mental health professionals working in reproductive medicine: psychologists, social workers, psychiatrists, psychiatric nurses, marriage and family therapists, and counselors. Although some countries have a defined sub-specialty status (e.g. in the USA: National Association of Perinatal Social Workers), these are guidelines and not a recognized specialty [8]. To date, no mental health profession recognizes infertility counseling as a distinct specialty, or provides specific training or credentialing in the field. One exception is that obstetricians/gynecologists in Germany, Austria, and

Switzerland may pursue additional training and credentialing in psychosomatic women's health although this is not specific to infertility [9].

"Counseling" is a protected and legislated mental health field in some states, provinces, or countries, but is not universally recognized as a mental health profession primarily because "counseling" is used both professionally and colloquially. For example, genetic counseling is a recognized and regulated professional field requiring graduate-level education, while counseling can also mean advisor to a student or guidance from a clergy member, neither of whom have mental health training. Most professionals understand the difference between counseling and psychotherapy, but most patients do not. Still, the term infertility counseling became the adopted term because it included all mental health professionals, avoided the debate of whether subfertile individuals should be required to receive mental health "treatment" when the majority had no mental health "diagnosis", and avoided conflict about the kind of counseling which was/is understanding based on the professional education and training of the mental health professional [8]. In defining the specialty of infertility counseling, academic and clinical training, scope of practice, codes of ethics and professional values vary across delineated mental health specialties, significantly influencing how the mental health professional practices and provides infertility counseling. While some traditional, client-centered psychotherapeutic approaches promote a non-directive approach, others provide educational guidance, advice, evaluation, and mental health assessment [8]. Although infertility counseling may not be the ideal terminology for the field, it is the one that has evolved and is generally used as part of the reproductive medicine lexicon.

The evolution of the field of infertility counseling began in the early 1980s influenced by efforts on three significantly different fronts: (1) government legislation and regulation in some countries and jurisdictions that included specific requirements for the provision of counseling as part of reproductive care (e.g. Australia, UK); (2) professional infertility counseling associations that established national (e.g. USA) or pan-national (e.g. Europe) infertility counseling guidelines, professional education, and contributions to research, practice standards, and policy development; and (3) the development of the International Infertility Counseling Organization to support collaboration among infertility counselors worldwide [8].

Australia and the UK were among the first countries to legally mandate infertility counseling and establish the first autonomous professional infertility counseling associations – although the educational background of the counselor was less well defined. In the UK pre-legislative reports in 1984 and 1985 and the subsequent Human Fertilisation and Embryology Authority (HFEA) recommended in 1990 that counseling be made freely available at all licensed clinics. The HFEA Code of Practice identified three distinct types of counseling: (1) implications counseling, (2) support counseling, and (3) therapeutic counseling. The British Infertility Counselling Association (BICA), established in 1988, is an independent and autonomous infertility counseling organization and the only one with a journal. In 1991 BICA published its first *Infertility Counselling Guidelines*, which identified four elements integral to the provision of infertility counseling:

- the welfare of the resultant child and other children who may be affected
- the needs of the infertile people
- the needs of the prospective donor
- the desire for assurance at a societal level that the infertility services are conducted responsibly.

To date, the only training and credentialing program in infertility counseling is in the UK. It was established by BICA in conjunction with the University of Sheffield, Sheffield, UK, and offers education, training, mentoring, and certification but only for mental health professionals who are trained and practice in the UK (www.bica.org) [8].

The Australian state of Victoria passed legislation in 1984 that required that counseling be freely available to all patients at all times and mandated pre-treatment counseling for all parties prior to in vitro fertilization treatment and third-party reproduction. Subsequently, in 1990 the Australian National Bioethics Consultative attempted to clarify the definition of "counseling" by identifying four types of counseling: (1) information provision, (2) facilitation of decision-making (especially in relation to the use of donor gametes), (3) emotional support, and (4) therapeutic counseling. Emotional support and therapeutic counseling were considered the responsibility of a professionally trained counselor, regardless of professional training. Special training in "donor-linking" counseling was developed for infertility counselors to facilitate communication between gamete donors, donor offspring, and their parents [10]. The Australia/New Zealand Infertility Counseling Association (ANZICA) was established as an independent society in 1989 and became a special interest group of The Fertility Society of Australia in 2005.

In the USA the professional infertility counseling organization was established in 1985 as a special interest group within the American Society of Reproductive Medicine (ASRM). In 1995 it became a professional interest group. Original guidelines outlined minimum standards for infertility counselors (www.asrm.org). Over the years the Mental Health Professional Group (MHPG) has developed and adopted practice guidelines, conducted research, and provided annual postgraduate courses on a wide array of infertility counseling issues (e.g. third-party reproduction, adoption, miscarriage, and ARTs) (www.asrm.org). MHPG members have always been integrated members of ASRM, serving on committees, boards, and related societies. In 1990 MHPG adopted Qualification Guidelines on Mental Health Professions in Reproductive Medicine [3]. In the USA, state requirements for licensure vary, although generally mental health professionals must, at a minimum, have a master's-level graduate degree in a mental health field for licensure. According to the guidelines, a qualified infertility counselor should be able to provide the following services: psychological assessment and screening, psychometric testing (with appropriate training), decision-making/implications counseling, grief counseling, supportive counseling, education/ information counseling, support group counseling, referral/resource counseling, sexual counseling, crisis intervention, couple and family therapy, diagnosis and treatment of mental disorders, psychotherapy, and staff consultation. The guidelines suggest a framework for practice, set a standard for determining an individual's qualifications as an infertility counselor, and help ensure quality and standardized patient care. Continuing education is also recommended, which is made available through MHPG. For many years, Latin Americans and Canadians have participated in MHPG until they developed or reconfigured their own organizations more recently.

The European Society of Human Reproduction and Embryology (ESHRE) is an international multidisciplinary professional society. In 1993 the Psychosocial Special Interest Group (PSIG) was founded with membership open to members of ESHRE (similar to MHPG and ANZICA). PSIG members developed and published in 1999 *Guidelines on Infertility Counseling*, which are currently in the processes of revision (www.eshre.com). The guidelines addressed practice guidelines, special populations (e.g. single women, lesbian couples), third-party reproduction, and specific treatments (e.g. preimplantation genetic diagnosis). PSIG offers educational programs every two years as well as special "campus" courses at different times and sites in Europe. Like MHPG, PSIG members are integrated members of ESHRE, serving on various committees and task forces (www.eshre.org) [8].

Beratungsnetzwerk Kinderwunsch Deutschland (BKid) is an independent professional society for infertility counselors established in 2000 that developed guidelines for accreditation of infertility counselors in 2001. The guidelines are similar to those adopted by MHPG and are based on *Couples Counseling and Therapy for Infertility* published in 2004, based on the work of a group of German researchers in infertility counseling in the late 1990s. BKid offers educational courses in infertility counseling and collaborates with other organizations (www.bkid.de) [8].

Prior to 2003, there were five infertility counseling organizations as described above. At the International Federation of Fertility Societies (IFFS) meeting in Australia in 2001 attendees from around the world discussed establishing an international counseling society similar to IFFS. In 2003 at ESHRE in Madrid representatives of the five existing infertility counseling organizations met to found the International Infertility Counseling Organization (IICO). IICO gained special interest group status from IFFS – although to date IICO is not an integrated member of IFFS. The IICO also presented its first postgraduate course in Montreal in 2004. The aims of IICO are to:

- define quality standards of communicative and counseling interventions within the context of infertility care
- encourage and support international cooperation and education among mental health professionals working in reproductive health and cooperation with other specialized societies in the field of infertility
- establish global professional standards and practice for the provision of psychological care regarding reproductive issues and to develop curricula and training programs for mental health professionals
- organize international meetings and congresses on subjects of infertility counseling at regular intervals in conjunction with (but not exclusive to) the tri-annual meeting of IFFS and meetings of other relevant societies; and
- promote the study of the ethical and psychosocial aspects of reproductive health.

IICO has collaborated with other infertility counseling organizations worldwide in providing educational courses that enhance understanding of global issues and cross-border care. Since IICO began in 2003, more than twenty new infertility counseling organizations have been established (www.iffs-iico.org).

Psychosocial evaluation and therapeutic interventions

Infertility counseling, whether mandatory or voluntary, begins with an interview, the purpose of which is to educate and prepare individuals, couples and third-party reproductive helpers for treatment [11]. In addition, during the interview issues are addressed that may not have been considered, and individuals are assessed for psychopathology to (1) ensure appropriate referral and treatment, (2) determine ability to provide informed consent, and (3) determine ability to manage the demands of the treatment regime. Preparation includes assessment of health behaviors (e.g. usage of tobacco, alcohol, recreational drugs, and herbs) and the provision of education and assistance with improved health efficacy behaviors (e.g. tobacco cessation, weight loss). A template (and not a validated psychometric measure) for the infertility counselor interview is the Comprehensive Psychosocial History of Infertility (CPHI) (Table 19.3). The CPHI provides information gathering in four areas: (1)

Table 19.3 Comprehensive Psychosocial History of Infertility (CPHI)

I. Reproductive history

  A. Infertility

    1. Current infertility: primary or secondary

    2. History of past infertility

  B. Pregnancy

    1. Living children (stepchildren, adopted, donor offspring, placed for adoption)

    2. Therapeutic abortion(s)

    3. Spontaneous abortion(s)

    4. Other perinatal loss: SIDS, death of child

    5. High-risk pregnancy

  C. History of genetic/chromosomal abnormalities

    1. Cancer of the reproductive tract and/or chemotherapy

    2. DES exposure

    3. Congenital abnormalities of the reproductive tract

    4. Family history of genetic disorders

II. Mental status

  A. Psychiatric history

    1. Hospitalization for psychiatric illness

    2. Psychiatric treatment

    3. Treatment with psychotropic medication

    4. Substance abuse

  B. Current mental status

    1. Symptoms of depression

    2. Symptoms of anxiety/panic attacks

    3. Symptoms of obsession

    4. Current use of psychotropic medications

    5. Current problem with substance abuse/addiction

  C. Change in mental status

  D. Exacerbation of prior psychiatric symptoms

III. Sexual history

  A. Frequency and response

  B. Function/dysfunction

  C. Religious or cultural influence on sexual patterns or procreation beliefs

Table 19.3 (cont.)

D. Sexual history

1. Function/dysfunction

2. Sexually transmitted disease

3. Prior sperm donor/surrogate mother/consideration of use of donor gametes

4. Homosexual or ambisexual patterns

5. History of rape or incest

E. Changes in any sexual patterns secondary to infertility or medical treatment.

IV. Relationship status

A. Marital

1. History of marriages/divorces

2. History of marital discord/therapy

3. Extramarital relationships

4. Current satisfaction/dissatisfaction

5. Ambivalence about medical treatment and reproductive technologies

B. Familial

1. History of dysfunctional family of origin

2. Recent deaths or births in family

3. History of numerous familial losses

C. Social

1. Available support system

2. Career disruptions or pressures

3. History of or current legal problems

4. Criminal conduct

Burns LH, Greenfeld DA, for the Mental Health Professional Group. *CPHI: Comprehensive Psychosocial History for Infertility*. Birmingham, AL: American Society for Reproductive Medicine, 1990. www.asrm.org.

reproductive history; (2) mental status; (3) sexual history; and (4) relationship status. Written in 1990, it does not address health efficacy behaviors mentioned earlier (i.e. obesity, smoking cessation, or the use of complementary/alternative medicines). Nevertheless, the CPHI helps identify potential problems, facilitating the infertility counselor's ability to provide supportive psychotherapy, referral to a treatment program, or other appropriate assistance.

Measures of psychopathology have been recommended in professional guidelines for assessing intended parents and third-party helpers, leading to more infertility counselors, regardless of their professional training, obtaining competency in psychological testing and its use in infertility counseling [11–13]. Psychometric testing is a part of the interview/evaluation process (never a substitute for the in-person clinical interview). Test results should be reviewed and interpreted with the patient(s) – either confirming or refuting information gathered during the clinical interview. Reasons for including psychometric testing in the infertility counseling interview/assessment include: additional information from an objective measure; identification of psychologically at-risk individuals; protection of professionals against litigation with data from an objective assessment; and providing a clinical tool that the patient and counselor use collaboratively to identify issues that warrant attention and/or treatment. The measure used most frequently for assessing psychopathology is the Minnesota Multiphasic Personality Inventory-2 (MMPI-2) [14] because it has had the most research in reproductive medicine/counseling, has been translated into the most languages, and has historically been used worldwide for decades as an adjunct to medical treatment [12]. Other measures may be brief assessments of mood (e.g. Beck Depression Inventory) or infertility-specific assessments (e.g. Infertility Questionnaire, FertiQol) [13]. The use of psychological testing is most prevalent in the USA, but has been adopted in other countries – particularly tests that have been translated into other languages, thereby facilitating cross-border care and comparative research. The use of psychometric assessment measures is more about improving the quality of care and less about the denial or postponement of treatment (i.e. gatekeeping). However, if the infertility counselor's role, as part of the treatment team, does involve potentially denying or delaying treatment, then patients must be fully informed and provide consent at the outset [8].

Today the use of psychotropic medications is fairly common, often prescribed by a primary care provider who is unaware of the patient's reproductive treatment/goals and/or is uneducated about possible side effects or drug interactions. Whether the patient is presenting with a newly emergent condition (e.g. depression, anxiety) or a preexisting and/or chronic condition (e.g. bipolar disease, alcoholism), few reproductive physicians have sufficient expertise in psychiatry to take responsibility for mental health care or the management of psychotropic medication [6]. The infertility counselor may provide psychotherapy, education, and/or referral to an appropriate treatment center/psychiatrist to develop a plan for medication management before, during, and after reproductive treatment. This plan may include psychotherapy provided by the patient's therapist or by the infertility counselor in addition to psychiatric medication management. A current or preexisting mental health diagnosis is not, in and of itself, sufficient to deny treatment although the patient's management of the illness or lack thereof may warrant postponement or denial of reproductive treatment. The infertility counselor provides education and support, resources and referrals, assistance with decision-making and problem-solving, setting realistic goals/expectations and/or helping patients when/if treatment is postponed or denied. Reasons for denial of treatment outlined in Table 19.4 represent a compilation of reasons specified in regulations and professional guidelines [15]. It is interesting to note how universal the reasons for denial are globally, whether legislated or in professional guidelines. Regulations/guidelines recommend that reproductive medicine physicians have the right (even responsibility) to refuse treatment when it is their best medical opinion that further treatment would be futile or the prognosis very poor. Physicians are encouraged to fully inform patients to ensure fully informed consent. In addition, physicians should discuss or educate patients about other forms of family-building (e.g. adoption), and encourage infertility counseling. Guidelines/regulations agree that recommendations for treatment denial should be based on a group assessment or review that involves an infertility counselor. Research supporting this approach compared the psychological sequelae for patients who were denied further

Table 19.4 Psychosocial contraindications to infertility treatment [4]

Treatment or pregnancy may significantly worsen an active psychiatric illness
Active substance dependence with concomitant chaotic lifestyle
One partner is coercing the other to proceed with treatment
One or both partners are unable or unwilling to provide consent for the treatment
A legal history related to child endangerment is discovered
Infertility treatment is used to compensate for a sexual dysfunction
Decisions about privacy and disclosure in third-party reproduction cannot be resolved
Use of a family member gamete donor would cause significant familial discord
Custody arrangements for the potential child of a known gamete donor have not been agreed to by all parties
Serious marital discord

treatment by physicians with those for patients who discontinued treatment voluntarily [16]. The researchers found that although at pre-treatment, levels of depression and anxiety did not differ, at post-treatment patients who were denied treatment by the physician reported higher levels of depression and anxiety than those who self-terminated treatment. The researchers concluded that patients who have been denied treatment due to poor prognosis especially needed psychological support as did patients who had self-terminated treatment. Denying treatment for whatever reason is difficult and while patients have difficulty self-terminating, medical caregivers also find it difficult. However, while physicians are being encouraged (or required) to end treatment when appropriate and discuss non-biological family-building, evidence is that patients have severe reactions to such recommendations, and infertility counselors must be prepared to offer not only to facilitate decision-making but also support the treatment team. In addition, infertility counselors must be aware of these dual roles and responsibilities, as well as be prepared to provide counseling in the special circumstances of treatment termination – whether voluntary or mandatory.

Recent research indicates that although infertility counseling may not have significant impact on mental health (e.g. depression, anxiety, and mental distress) it can have a positive impact on increased pregnancy rates [17]. As such, the vast majority of subfertile patients are psychologically resilient and the role of the infertility counselor is to enhance coping skills, provide additional support and education, and encourage positive health efficacy behaviors (e.g. tobacco, alcohol, and drug use cessation, maintaining of ideal body mass index) [18,19]. Infertility counselors may provide assistance with health efficacy behaviors (e.g. stress reduction) or refer to appropriate treatment programs. Helping patients better understand how their own health behaviors can enhance their fertility is not only empowering and a form of active coping; it improves treatment outcomes and reduces the burden on the reproductive treatment team and the overall healthcare system [18]. Infertility counselors are also a valuable resource when the patient has a diagnosed mental illness, and in all third-party reproduction situations for all parties involved before, during, and after.

Infertility counseling and third-party reproduction

Today there are over 50 ways to have a baby without sexual intercourse. Furthermore, one child may have as many as six individuals involved and invested in their conception, birth, and parenting. Increasingly, this involves third-party reproduction: the use of donated sperm, oocytes, embryos and/or gestational carriers or traditional surrogacy (in which the woman's uterus and oocytes are both used in procreation of a child intended to be parented by others). The use of third-party reproduction has grown in popularity worldwide for a variety of reasons primarily related to the individuals pursuing it and not always related to subfertility. Patients may be single women, lesbian couples, homosexual male couples, and single men in addition to traditional heterosexual couples. The reasons for pursuing third-party reproduction are equally varied – chronic illness or congenital anomalies, advanced maternal or paternal age, posthumous reproduction, remarriage, cultural or religious factors, longer life spans, or simply because it is available.

However, there are significant psychosocial issues for all parties in third-party reproduction: intended parents, offspring, gamete or embryo donors, gestational carriers, and/or traditional surrogates. The partners and offspring of the third-party helper are also impacted. Furthermore, there are even more complex issues when the third-party helper is a family member – thereby involving the whole family system. In short, complex reproduction may be medically feasible and even medically easier than it was historically, but it is psychosocially more complex, confounded by patient/consumer-driven expectations facilitated by the media, the Internet, and cross-border care, further underlining the importance of infertility counseling. Guidelines and regulations universally recommend psychological assessment of gamete donors, embryo donors, gestational carriers, and traditional surrogates – usually with their partner or significant other. It is recommended that intended parents undergo the same preparation and education – clinical interview and psychometric testing as third-party reproductive helpers. This is especially important in identified helper situations, in which the infertility counselor meets with all parties for a minimum of one session to ensure all are in agreement about the reproductive plan, prepared to move forward, and there is no evidence of coercion. Although these guidelines/regulations are fairly universal, they are not always adhered to by clinics, for-profit reproductive agencies, or patients/helpers. Consumer demands and treatment-center competition too often result in 'short cuts', with errors of headline-making consequences. Furthermore, there are a variety of ethical issues, including availability of care in underdeveloped countries, cross-border care, the potential for exploitation of donors, gestational carriers, and/or surrogates, payment of third-party helpers, the rights of the child to information about their conception and pregnancy, cultural beliefs about privacy versus secrecy, and inequity of counseling guidelines for egg and embryo donors versus sperm donors [2,20].

Education and preparation in third-party reproduction involves all of the issues of infertility counseling in assisted reproduction as well as the additional issues of the specific form of third-party reproduction and where and how it is being done. The psychosocial issues that should be addressed by the infertility counselor include reasons for participation, readiness to participate, available social support (e.g. partner, family, friends), expectations, questions, and concerns about the process, a personally tailored list of pros and cons of participation, motivation (with special attention to coercion), special physical or emotional circumstances, beliefs about disclosure and contact between donor/surrogate with offspring in future, and feelings about treatment complications and/or failure.

Third-party reproduction is affected by cultural norms, religious beliefs, and personal values related to how infertility is perceived at a personal and social level, dominant religious beliefs, perceptions of genetic versus social relationships in families, the influence of parties providing third-party conception services, and the social and legal recognition of third- party conception. The infertility counselor must address the issue of whether donor-conceived children or children born as a result of a gestational carrier or traditional surrogacy should be informed about their genetic origins and unique conception, and if they should, at what age [4,20].

Countries and regions may regulate (mandate) disclosure, others encourage it, still others allow it under certain circumstances, and others discourage or rigidly oppose disclosure. Whatever the circumstances, it is the infertility counselor's responsibility to address the disclosure issue, inform the participants of current practices as well as the obvious trend toward increasing openness over the past 50 years, and provide information/materials on these trends as well as assistance in how to disclose. It is paramount that the infertility counselor addresses all facets of the situation including that of the offspring created via complex reproduction, the regulations/guidelines where treatment is received as well as where the offspring will be raised if it is a different place. Further, the infertility counselor must examine his/her own personal beliefs, values, and professional ethics so as not to impose them on patients and to prevent transference issues.

The complex relationships and dynamics that are often present in families created by third-party conception highlight the need for the availability of counseling services after the birth of children, especially when donor registries are either government-regulated or voluntary. Infertility counselors worldwide are increasingly becoming trained or offer services in donor–offspring linking counseling, the development of government or profes-sional guidelines, and/or clinic policies on donor anonymity, identified donor, and donor offspring issues. As such, third-party reproduction counseling has become a recognized and valued area of expertise within infertility counseling, addressing the needs of all participants at all stages of the process, including relationships within the resulting families and the well-being of the offspring [4].

References

1. Rosenblatt PC, Peterson P, Portner J, *et al.* A cross-cultural study of responses to childlessness. *Behav Sci Notes* 1973; 8: 221–31.

2. Shenfield F. *Contemporary Ethical Dilemmas in Assisted Reproduction.* New York: Informa Health, 2006.

3. Burns LH, Covington SN, Burns LH. Psychology of infertility. In Covington SN, Burns LH, eds. *Infertility Counseling: A Comprehensive Handbook for Clinicians,* 2nd edn. Cambridge: Cambridge University Press, 2006; 1–19.

4. Greenfeld DA, Klock SC. Assisted reproductive technology and the impact on children. In Covington SN, Burns LH, eds. *Infertility Counseling: A Comprehensive*

Handbook for Clinicians, 2nd edn. Cambridge: Cambridge University Press, 2006; 477–92.

5. Petok W. The psychology of gender specific infertility diagnosis. In Covington SN, Burns LH, eds. *Infertility Counseling: A Comprehensive Handbook for Clinicians,* 2nd edn. Cambridge: Cambridge University Press, 2006; 37–60.

6. Burns, LH. Psychiatric aspects of infertility and infertility treatments. *Psychiatric Clinics of North America*. Philadelphia: North American Psychiatric Clinics, 2007; 689–716.

7. Maier DB, Covington SN, Maier LU. Patients with complicated medical conditions. In Covington SN, Burns LH,

eds. *Infertility Counseling: A Comprehensive Handbook for Clinicians*, 2nd edn. Cambridge: Cambridge University Press, 2006; 237–57.

8. Haase JM, Blyth E. Global perspectives on infertility counseling. In Covington, SN, Burns LH, eds. *Infertility Counseling: A Comprehensive Handbook for Clinicians*, 2nd edn. New York: Cambridge University Press, 2006; 544–57.

9. Strauss B, ed. *Involuntary Childlessness: Psychological Assessment, Counseling, and Psychotherapy*. Seattle: Hogrete & Huber, 2002.

10. Anderson J, Alessi R. Infertility counseling. In Kovacs G, ed. *The Subfertility Handbook: A Clinicians Guide*. Cambridge: Cambridge University Press, 1997; 249–68.

11. Klock SC. Psychosocial evaluation of the infertile patient. In Covington SN, Burns LH, eds. *Infertility Counseling: A Comprehensive Handbook for Clinicians*, 2nd edn. Cambridge: Cambridge University Press, 2006; 83–96.

12. Newton C. Counseling infertile couples. In Covington SN, Burns LH, eds. *Infertility Counseling: A Comprehensive Handbook for Clinicians*, 2nd edn. Cambridge: Cambridge University Press, 2006; 143–55.

13. Boivin J. Evidenced-based approaches to infertility counseling. In Covington SN, Burns LH, eds. *Infertility Counseling: A Comprehensive Handbook for Clinicians*, 2nd edn. Cambridge: Cambridge University Press, 2006; 117–28.

14. Butcher J, Dahlstrom W, Graham J, *et al.* Minnesota Multiphasic Personality Inventory-2 (MMPI-2). *Manual for Administration and Scoring*. Minneapolis: University of Minnesota Press, 1989.

15. Takefman JE. Ending treatment. In Covington SN, Burns LH, eds. *Infertility Counseling: A Comprehensive Handbook for Clinicians*, 2nd edn. Cambridge: Cambridge University Press, 2006; 429–39.

16. Smeenk MJ, Verhaak CM, Stolwijk AM, *et al.* Reasons for dropout in an in vitro fertilization/intracytoplasmic sperm injection program. *Fertil Steril* 2004; **81**: 262–8

17. Hammerli K, Znoj H, Barth J. The efficacy of psychological interventions for infertile patients: a meta-analysis examining mental health and pregnancy rate. *Hum Reprod* 2009; **15**: 279–95.

18. Verhaak C, Burns LH. Behavioral medicine approaches to infertility counseling. In Covington SN, Burns LH, eds. *Infertility Counseling: A Comprehensive Handbook for Clinicians*, 2nd edn. Cambridge: Cambridge University Press, 2006; 169–95.

19. Stanton AL, Dunkel-Schetter C, eds. *Infertility: Perspectives in Stress and Coping Research*. New York: Springer, 1991.

20. Covington SN, Burns LH, eds. *Infertility Counseling: A Comprehensive Handbook for Clinicians*, 2nd edn. Cambridge: Cambridge University Press, 2006; 305–71.

Index

Page numbers in italics represent entries in tables.